2016

The Year Book of VASCULAR SURGERY®

Editor-in-Chief

Marc Passman, MD

Professor of Surgery, Division of Vascular Surgery and Endovascular Therapy, Vice Chair, Department of Surgery, University of Alabama at Birmingham, Birmingham, Alabama

ELSEVIER
MOSBY

ELSEVIER
MOSBY

Vice President, Global Medical Reference: Mary E. Gatsch
Associate Publisher: John Vassallo
Developmental Editor: Meredith Clinton
Production Supervisor, Electronic Year Books: Donna M. Skelton
Electronic Article Manager: Mike Sheets
Illustrations and Permissions Coordinator: Dawn Vohsen

2016 EDITION

Composition by TNQ Books and Journals Pvt Ltd, India

Editorial Office:
Elsevier
Suite 1800
1600 John F. Kennedy Blvd.
Philadelphia, PA 19103-2899

International Standard Serial Number: 0749-4041
International Standard Book Number: 978-0-323-44698-3

Editors

Marc Passman, MD

Professor of Surgery, Division of Vascular Surgery and Endovascular Therapy, Vice Chair, Department of Surgery, University of Alabama at Birmingham, Birmingham, Alabama

Associate Editors

James H. Black III, MD, FACS

The David Goldfarb, MD Associate Professor of Surgery, The Bertram M. Bernheim, MD Associate Professor of Surgery, Chief, Division of Vascular Surgery and Endovascular Therapy, Johns Hopkins Hospital, Baltimore, Maryland

Matthew A. Corriere, MD, MS

Associate Professor, Section on Vascular Surgery, University of Michigan Health Sciences Frankel Cardiovascular Center, Ann Arbor MI

Brian G. Peterson, MD, FACS

Chief of Vascular Surgery, St. Anthony's Medical Center, St. Louis, Missouri

Benjamin W. Starnes, MD

The Alexander W. Clowes MD, Endowed Chair in Vascular Surgery, Professor and Chief, Division of Vascular Surgery; Vice Chair, Department of Surgery, University of Washington, Seattle, Washington

Contributors

Margaret Arnold, MD

Assistant Professor of Surgery, Division of Vascular Surgery, Johns Hopkins Bayview Medical Center, Baltimore, Maryland

Zachary M. Arthurs, MD, FACS

Chief of Vascular Surgery, San Antonio Military Medical Center, San Antonio, Texas

Dawn Coleman, MD

Assistant Professor of Vascular Surgery, Program Director Integrated Vascular Residency Program, University of Michigan, Ann Arbor, Michigan

Yazan Duwayri, MD

Assistant Professor of Surgery, Division of Vascular Surgery and Endovascular Therapy, Department of Surgery, Emory University School of Medicine, Atlanta, Georgia

Robert J. Feezor, MD, FACS

Associate Professor, Program Director of Vascular Fellowship, Division of Vascular Surgery and Endovascular Therapy, Department of Surgery, University of Florida, Gainesville, Florida

Kristine C. Orion, MD

Assistant Professor of Surgery, Section of Vascular Surgery, Yale University School of Medicine, New Haven, Connecticut

Brandon W. Propper, MD, FACS
Assistant Professor of Surgery USUHS, Associate Program Director for General Surgery, San Antonio Military Medical Center, Fort Sam Houston, Texas

Joseph D. Raffetto, MD, FACS, FSVM
Associate Professor of Surgery, Harvard Medical School, Brigham and Women's Hospital; Chief, Vascular Surgery Division, VA Boston Healthcare System, West Roxbury, Massachusetts

Sherene Shalhub, MD, MPH, FACS
Assistant Professor of Surgery, Division of Vascular Surgery, University of Washington, Seattle, Washington

Niten Singh, MD, FACS
Professor of Surgery, Director of Limb Preservation Services, Division of Vascular Surgery, University of Washington, Seattle, Washington

Matthew R. Smeds, MD, FACS
Division of Vascular and Endovasular Surgery, University of Arkansas for Medical Sciences, Little Rock, Arkansas

Michael S. Williams Jr., MD
Assistant Professor of Surgery, Department of Surgery, Division of Vascular Surgery, St. Louis University, St. Louis, Missouri

Table of Contents

Journals Represented

Journals represented in this YEAR BOOK are listed below.

American Heart Journal
American Journal of Cardiology
Annals of Surgery
Annals of Thoracic Surgery
Annals of Vascular Surgery
Canadian Journal of Surgery
Cardiovascular and Interventional Radiological
Circulation
Circulation: Cardiovascular Genetics
Cochrane Database of Systematic Reviews
Diabetes Care
European Journal of Vascular and Endovascular Surgery
Injury
Journal of Cardiothoracic and Vascular Anesthesia
Journal of Rheumatology
Journal of Stroke and Cerebrovascular Diseases
Journal of Surgical Research
Journal of the American College of Cardiology
Journal of the American College of Cardiology Cardiovascular Interventions
Journal of the American College of Surgeons
Journal of the American Heart Association
Journal of the American Medical Association
Journal of Surgical Education
Journal of Thoracic and Cardiovascular Surgery
Journal of Trauma and Acute Care Surgery
Journal of Vascular and Interventional Radiology
Journal of Vascular Surgery
Journal of Vascular Surgery: Venous and Lymphatic Disorders
Neurosurgery
New England Journal of Medicine
Public Library of Science One
Stroke

STANDARD ABBREVIATIONS

The following terms are abbreviated in this edition: acquired immunodeficiency syndrome (AIDS), cardiopulmonary resuscitation (CPR), central nervous system (CNS), cerebrospinal fluid (CSF), computed tomography (CT), deoxyribonucleic acid (DNA), electrocardiography (ECG), health maintenance organization (HMO), human immunodeficiency virus (HIV), intensive care unit (ICU), intramuscular (IM), intravenous (IV), magnetic resonance (MR) imaging (MRI), ribonucleic acid (RNA), and ultrasound (US).

Note

The Year Book of Vascular Surgery® is a literature survey service providing abstracts of articles published in the professional literature. Every effort is made to assure the accuracy of the information presented in these pages. Neither the editors nor the publisher of the Year Book of Vascular Surgery® can be responsible for errors in the original materials. The editors' comments are their own opinions. Mention of specific products within this publication does not constitute endorsement.

To facilitate the use of the Year Book of Vascular Surgery® as a reference tool, all illustrations and tables included in this publication are now identified as they appear in the original article. This change is meant to help the reader recognize that any illustration or table appearing in the Year Book of Vascular Surgery® may be only one of many in the original article. For this reason, figure and table numbers will often appear to be out of sequence within the Year Book of Vascular Surgery®.

1 Basic Consideration

Aortic Disease

Aortic Disease Presentation and Outcome Associated With *ACTA2* Mutations

Regalado ES, Guo D-C, Prakash S, et al (Univ of Texas Health Science Ctr at Houston; et al)

Circ Cardiovasc Genet 8:457-464, 2015

Background.—*ACTA2* mutations are the major cause of familial thoracic aortic aneurysms and dissections. We sought to characterize these aortic diseases in a large case series of individuals with *ACTA2* mutations.

Methods and Results.—Aortic disease, management, and outcome associated with the first aortic event (aortic dissection or aneurysm repair) were abstracted from the medical records of 277 individuals with 41 various *ACTA2* mutations. Aortic events occurred in 48% of these individuals, with the vast majority presenting with thoracic aortic dissections (88%) associated with 25% mortality. Type A dissections were more common than type B dissections (54% versus 21%), but the median age of onset of type B dissections was significantly younger than type A dissections (27 years versus 36 years). Only 12% of aortic events were repair of ascending aortic aneurysms, which variably involved the aortic root, ascending aorta, and aortic arch. Overall, cumulative risk of an aortic event at age 85 years was 0.76 (95% confidence interval, 0.64–0.86). After adjustment for intrafamilial correlation, sex and race, mutations disrupting p.R179 and p.R258 were associated with significantly increased risk for aortic events, whereas p.R185Q and p.R118Q mutations showed significantly lower risk of aortic events compared with other mutations.

Conclusions.—*ACTA2* mutations are associated with high risk of presentation with an acute aortic dissection. The lifetime risk for an aortic event is only 76%, suggesting that additional environmental or genetic factors play a role in expression of aortic disease in individuals with *ACTA2* mutations (Table 3).

▶ *ACTA2* mutation causes aortic dissection, particularly of the thoracic aorta. Because most patients with *ACTA2* mutations have no other physical traits, their presenting symptoms are usually an aortic emergency. Table 3 is a nice

TABLE 3.—Comparison of Aortic Disease Presentation Among Individuals With *FBN1*, *TGFBR2*, and *ACTA2* Mutations

Variable	*FBN1*	*TGFBR2*	*ACTA2*
No. of individuals	243	71	277
Mean age	30±16	29±17	38±20
No. of probands	122	26	81
Percent of probands ascertained because of TAAD	36%	65%	84%
With aortic event*	74 (30%)	25 (35%)	132 (48%)
Thoracic aortic dissection	31 (42%)	13 (52%)	116 (88%)
Type A	23 (31%); 39 ± 9	10 (40%); 38 ± 12	71 (54%); 36 ± 12
Type B	8 (11%); 44 ± 10	3 (12%); 34 ± 6	28 (21%); 29 ± 12
Aneurysm repair	43 (58%); 39 ± 13	12 (48%); 35 ± 16	16 (12%); 33 ± 18
Without aortic event	169 (70%)	46 (65%)	145 (52%)
Ascending aortic aneurysm	135 (80%)	42 (91%)	25 (17%)

TAAD indicates thoracic aortic aneurysm and dissection.
*Frequency of aortic event or diagnosis and mean age ± SD are provided.
Reprinted from Regalado ES, Guo D-C, Prakash S, et al. Aortic Disease Presentation and Outcome Associated With *ACTA2* Mutations. *Circ Cardiovasc Genet.* 2015;8:457-464, with permission from the American Heart Association.

comparison of patients with Marfan syndrome compared with *ACTA2* mutation. It should be noted that the risk of aortic dissection is 2 times higher for *ACTA2* than with *FBN1* mutation. For clinicians treating patients with aortic dissection, this is an important mutation to consider. Too often, dissection alone is attributed to persistent hypertension without a full work-up to include genetic abnormalities. The lifetime risk for *ACTA2* mutation of an aortic event is 76%, making early diagnosis an area for future research. Of those with *ACTA2* mutations, specific mutations predict more aortic complications, and those with positive mutations should have genetic counseling along with vascular surgery evaluation. The authors also believe that outside of genetics environmental factors play a role in triggering aortic events. This mutation is often forgot when considering genetic work-up and should be considered highly in those with thoracic dissection.

B. Propper, MD, FACS

Association Between Fibulin-1 and Aortic Augmentation Index in Male Patients with Peripheral Arterial Disease

Paapstel K, Zilmer M, Eha J, et al (Univ of Tartu, Estonia)
Eur J Vasc Endovasc Surg 51:76-82, 2016

Background.—Fibulin-1 (FBLN-1), a newly identified biomarker for vascular stiffness in type 2 diabetes, may participate in the pathophysiological processes leading to progression of arterial stiffness in atherosclerosis. In the present study, the relationship between FBLN-1 and arterial stiffness was examined in patients with atherosclerosis and in healthy subjects.

Methods.—Thirty-eight patients with peripheral arterial disease (PAD) (age 62.4 ± 9.0 years), 38 patients with coronary artery disease (CAD) (age 64.0 ± 9.5 years), and 30 apparently healthy controls (age 61.1 ± 6.4 years) were studied. Serum FBLN-1, oxidized low density lipoprotein (oxLDL), resistin and plasminogen activator inhibitor-1 (PAI-1) levels were measured using the enzyme linked immunosorbent assay method. The technique of applanation tonometry was used for noninvasive pulse wave analysis and pulse wave velocity assessments.

Results.—The levels of FBLN-1 (PAD = 9.4 [4.9–17.8] vs. CAD = 7.1 [4.8–11.8] vs. controls = 5.6 [4.1–8.4] μg/mL; $p = .005$), carotid-femoral pulse wave velocity (cf-PWV) (9.8 ± 2.2 vs. 9.5 ± 2.2 vs. 8.3 ± 2.2 m/s; $p = .023$) and the heart rate corrected augmentation index (AIx@75) (29.4 ± 7.2 vs. 19.2 ± 7.2 vs. 15.4 ± 7.1%; $p < .001$), differed among the three groups. A correlation between FBLN-1 and AIx@75 was observed only in patients with PAD ($rho = 0.37$, $p = .021$). The relationship retained statistical significance in a multiple regression model after adjustment for potential confounders.

Conclusions.—An independent association was demonstrated between serum FBLN-1 and AIx@75 in the PAD group. Thus, the findings suggest that FBLN-1 may play a role in arterial stiffening in patients with atherosclerosis.

▶ This is the first prospective study showing a relationship between a novel biomarker serum fibulin-1 (FBLN-1) and aortic stiffness in patients with atherosclerosis. FBLN-1 is an extracellular matrix glycoprotein associated with fibronectin, elastin, and basement membranes. Aortic stiffness was obtained by noninvasive means using a commercially available SphygmoCor apparatus. This involves recording 15 sequential high-quality radial waveforms at the left wrist using a high-fidelity micromanometer. The aortic augmentation index is calculated after correction for a heart rate of 75 bpm (AIx@75). Higher values of AIx@75 are thought to indicate increased arterial wave reflection and a reduction in the reservoir function of the aorta. The authors prospectively enrolled 38 with symptomatic peripheral arterial disease (PAD), 38 patients with symptomatic coronary artery disease (CAD), and 30 age-matched clinically healthy controls. All participants were male. Fasting peripheral venous blood samples were collected and serum FBLN-1 levels were detected using enzyme-linked immunoassay. In this small study, FBLN-1 correlated positively with AIx@75 for the PAD patients but not CAD or healthy volunteers. This was found on both univariate and multivariate analysis. The authors conclude that FBLN-1 could serve as a candidate marker for systemic vascular damage, although the exact role of FBLN-1 protein remains to be elucidated.[1-4]

S. Shalhub, MD, MPH, FACS

References

1. Cavalcante JL, Lima JA, Redheuil A, Al-Mallah MH. Aortic stiffness: current understanding and future directions. *J Am Coll Cardiol.* 2011;57:1511-1522.

2. Kals J, Lieberg J, Kampus P, Zagura M, Eha J, Zilmer M. Prognostic impact of arterial stiffness in patients with symptomatic peripheral arterial disease. *Eur J Vasc Endovasc Surg*. 2014;48:308-315.
3. Prenner SB, Chirinos JA. Arterial stiffness in diabetes mellitus. *Atherosclerosis*. 2015;238:370-379.
4. Chue CD, Townend JN, Steeds RP, Ferro CJ. Arterial stiffness in chronic kidney disease: causes and consequences. *Heart*. 2010;96:817-823.

Distinct macrophage phenotype and collagen organization within the intraluminal thrombus of abdominal aortic aneurysm

Rao J, Brown BN, Weinbaum JS, et al (Univ of Pittsburgh, PA; et al)
J Vasc Surg 62:585-593, 2015

Objective.—Little is known about the etiologic factors that lead to the occurrence of intraluminal thrombus (ILT) during abdominal aortic aneurysm (AAA) development. Recent work has suggested that macrophages may play an important role in progression of a number of other vascular diseases, including atherosclerosis; however, whether these cells are present within the ILT of a progressing AAA is unknown. The purpose of this work was to define the presence, phenotype, and spatial distribution of macrophages within the ILT excised from six patients. We hypothesized that the ILT contains a population of activated macrophages with a distinct, nonclassical phenotypic profile.

Methods.—ILT samples were examined using histologic staining and immunofluorescent labeling for multiple markers of activated macrophages (cluster of differentiation [CD]45, CD68, human leukocyte antigen-DR, matrix metalloproteinase 9) and the additional markers a-smooth muscle actin, CD34, CD105, fetal liver kinase-1, and collagen I and III.

Results.—Histologic staining revealed a distinct laminar organization of collagen within the shoulder region of the ILT lumen and a spatially heterogeneous cell composition within the ILT. Most of the cellular constituents of the ILT were in the luminal region and predominantly expressed markers of activated macrophages but also concurrently expressed α-smooth muscle actin, CD105, and synthesized collagen I and III.

Conclusions.—This report presents evidence for the presence of a distinct macrophage population within the luminal region of AAA ILT. These cells express a set of markers indicative of a unique population of activated macrophages. The exact contributions of these previously unrecognized cells to ILT formation and AAA pathobiology remains unknown (Fig 2).

▶ Intraluminal thrombus (ILT) occurs in more than 75% of abdominal aortic aneurysms (AAA) cases. The predominant cells in ILT are platelets, but macrophages have also been observed in lesser quantities. The exact role of macrophages in the formation or maturation of the ILT and overall pathology of AAA is not understood. The authors sought to examine ILT samples using

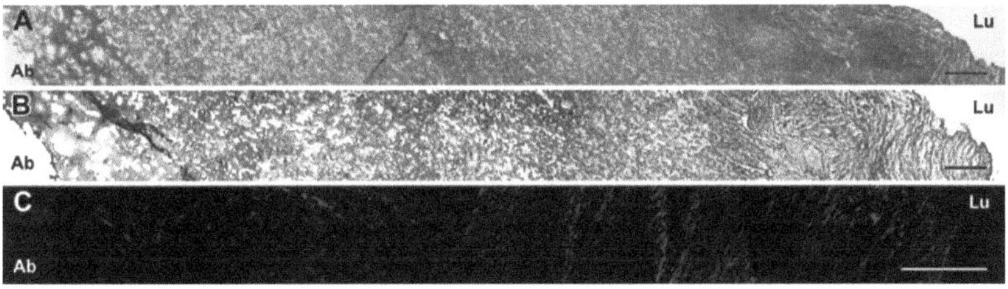

FIGURE 2.—Asymmetric composition of the intraluminal thrombus (ILT) is seen in representative histologic appearance of samples. Samples were stained with (**A**) hematoxylin and eosin, (**B**) Herovici's polychrome, and (**C**) picrosirius red (PSR). Note the distinct appearances of the abluminal (*Ab*), medial, and luminal (*Lu*) regions of the full-thickness ILT sample. **B** and **C**, Herovici's polychrome and PSR staining suggest the presence of collagen within the luminal region of the ILT. *Scale bar* = 250 μm. (Reprinted from Rao J, Brown BN, Weinbaum JS, et al. Distinct macrophage phenotype and collagen organization within the intraluminal thrombus of abdominal aortic aneurysm. *J Vasc Surg*. 2015;62:585-593, with permission from the Society for Vascular Surgery.)

histologic staining and immunofluorescent labeling for markers of activated macrophages to define the phenotype, and distribution of macrophages within the ILT of patients with AAA. Samples of ILT were obtained from 9 men undergoing elective AAA repair for degenerative, fusiform atherosclerotic aneurysms. The histologic appearance of the ILT was that of a layered structure consisting of 3 distinct regions—luminal, medial, and abluminal—as demonstrated in Fig 2. The medial and abluminal regions consisted primarily of fibrin, with a paucity of collagen, whereas the luminal regions contained type I and III collagen. The number of platelets and cells decreased from the luminal to abluminal regions of the ILT. The authors described a "nuclear stratus" within the inner luminal region of the ILT. The cells were found to express common markers of activated macrophages (CD45, CD68, HLA-DR, MMP9) and a-SMA and CD105, in a combination highly suggestive of a fibrocyte-like phenotype. In comparison, cells from the AAA wall expressed only those of indicative of a smooth muscle cell phenotype. The exact role of these cells remains unknown; however, the data from this project would serve as a starting point for further investigations regarding their role, if any, in early AAA progression and ILT formation.[1,2]

S. Shalhub, MD, MPH, FACS

References

1. Folkesson M, Silveira A, Eriksson P, Swedenborg J. Protease activity in the multi-layered intra-luminal thrombus of abdominal aortic aneurysms. *Atherosclerosis*. 2011;218:294-299.
2. Wilson JS, Virag L, Di Achille P, Karsaj I, Humphrey JD. Biochemomechanics of intraluminal thrombus in abdominal aortic aneurysms. *J Biomech Eng*. 2013;135:021011.

Proinflammatory role of stem cells in abdominal aortic aneurysms

Ryer EJ, Garvin RP, Schworer CM, et al (Geisinger Health System, Danville, PA)

J Vasc Surg 62:1303-1311, 2015

Objective.—The pathogenesis of abdominal aortic aneurysm (AAA) formation includes inflammation, vascular smooth muscle cell apoptosis, extracellular matrix degradation, and oxidative stress. That multipotent stem cells have an important role in cardiovascular health and disease has been well established, but the role of stem cells in aortic structural deterioration is poorly defined. We sought to describe the presence of stem cells in human AAA tissue and also investigated the differentiation of stem cells within the aneurysmal aorta.

Methods.—Infrarenal aortic wall specimens were collected from patients (n = 7) undergoing open AAA surgical repair. Nonaneurysmal infrarenal aortic control samples (n = 4) were collected at autopsies. Using immunohistochemistry, we compared the abundance of Stro1-positive ($^+$), c-kit$^+$, and CD34$^+$ cells in aortic tissue. Using double-immunofluorescence staining, we evaluated stem cell differentiation into smooth muscle cells (SM22), fibroblasts (FSP1), and macrophages

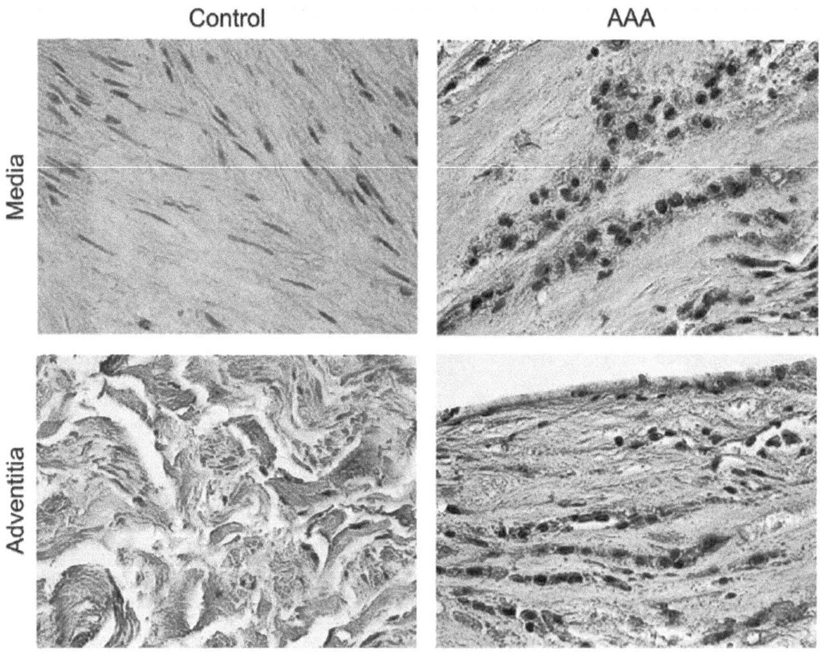

FIGURE 2.—Cells positive for cluster of differentiation (CD) 34 in the media and adventitia layers of a 59-year-old woman with a normally sized aorta (*control*) and 63-year-old woman with a 5.1-cm abdominal aortic aneurysm (*AAA*). Original magnification ×400. (Reprinted from Ryer EJ, Garvin RP, Schworer CM, et al. Proinflammatory role of stem cells in abdominal aortic aneurysms. *J Vasc Surg*. 2015;62:1303-1311, with permission the Society for Vascular Surgery.)

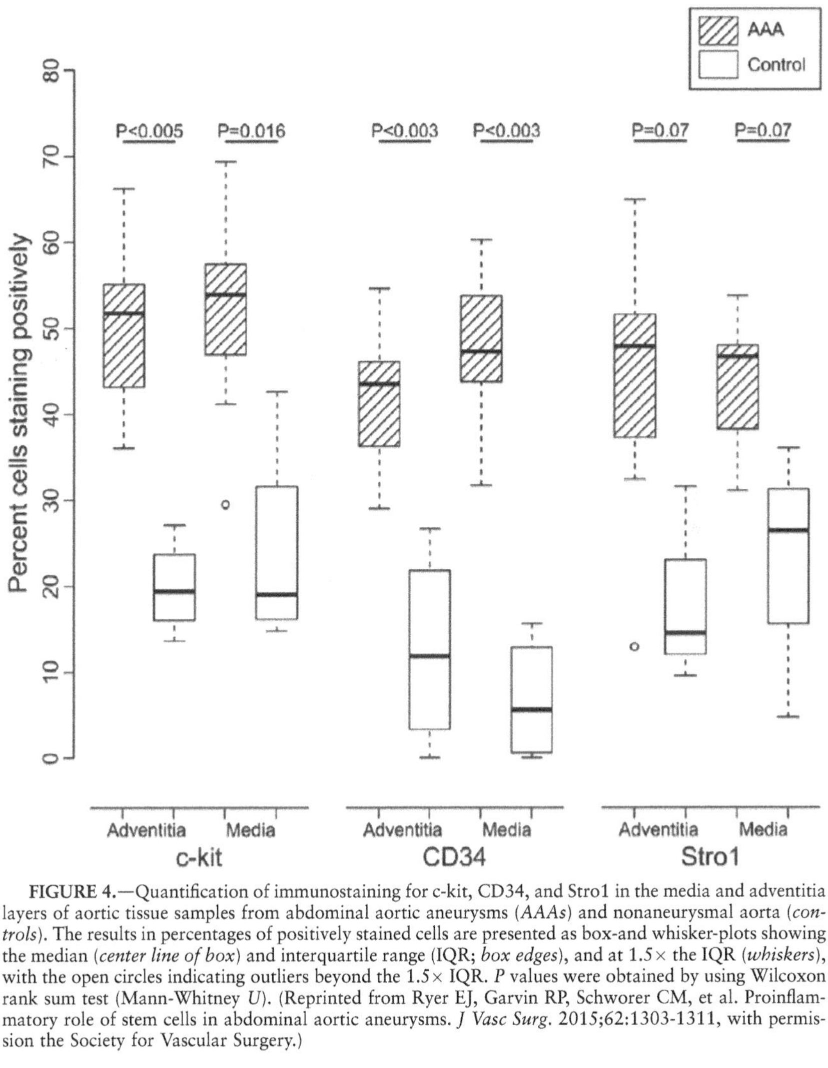

FIGURE 4.—Quantification of immunostaining for c-kit, CD34, and Stro1 in the media and adventitia layers of aortic tissue samples from abdominal aortic aneurysms (*AAAs*) and nonaneurysmal aorta (*controls*). The results in percentages of positively stained cells are presented as box-and whisker-plots showing the median (*center line of box*) and interquartile range (IQR; *box edges*), and at 1.5× the IQR (*whiskers*), with the open circles indicating outliers beyond the 1.5× IQR. *P* values were obtained by using Wilcoxon rank sum test (Mann-Whitney *U*). (Reprinted from Ryer EJ, Garvin RP, Schworer CM, et al. Proinflammatory role of stem cells in abdominal aortic aneurysms. *J Vasc Surg*. 2015;62:1303-1311, with permission the Society for Vascular Surgery.)

(CD68). We then investigated the colocalization of $CD68^+$ cells with the cellular marker of proliferation Ki67.

Results.—The media and adventitia of infrarenal AAA samples both demonstrated a significantly greater number of c-kit^+ and $CD34^+$ cells compared with matched control nonaneurysmal aortic tissues; however, the abundance of $Stro1^+$ cells was not significantly different between the groups. Using double-immunofluorescence staining, we identified that AAA stem cells express the macrophage marker CD68 but not the smooth muscle cell marker SM22 or the fibroblast marker FSP1. $CD68^+$ cells within the aortic wall colocalized with the cellular marker of proliferation Ki67.

Conclusions.—Stem cells are significantly elevated in infrarenal AAA tissue compared with matched control aortic tissue. Our data also demonstrate that AAA stem cells express macrophage surface antigens but not smooth muscle cell or fibroblast markers. Furthermore, $CD68^+$ cells within the aortic wall colocalized with the cellular marker of proliferation Ki67. These finding suggest an inflammatory/immune role of stem cells during AAA pathogenesis and raise the possibility of localized replenishment therapy within the aneurysm wall (Figs 2 and 4).

▶ Stem cell–based regenerative therapy has been effective in repairing myocardium after myocardial infarction, and ongoing clinical trials are evaluating adult stem cell therapy in the treatment of peripheral arterial disease. It is unclear if this treatment strategy would be useful in human abdominal aortic aneurysms (AAA), but animal models suggest that it may be useful. This is the first investigation to examine the prevalence and differentiation of stem cells in human AAA. The investigators compared tissue from infrarenal aortic wall in patients (n = 7) undergoing open AAA repair and nonaneurysmal infrarenal aortic control samples (n = 4) collected at autopsies. The authors demonstrated that stem cells as evidenced by immunostaining of c-kit, CD34, and Stro1 in the media and adventitia layers of the aortic tissue are more abundant in the wall of human infrarenal AAAs compared with controls (Figs 2 and 4). This colocalization of markers suggests that stem cells within the wall of AAAs are differentiating into macrophages but not smooth muscle cells or fibroblasts. The investigators raise the possibility that AAA wall stem cells act as a reservoir for the localized replenishment of aneurysm wall macrophages.[1,2]

S. Shalhub, MD, MPH, FACS

References

1. Shen YH, Hu X, Zou S, Wu D, Coselli JS, LeMaire SA. Stem cells in thoracic aortic aneurysms and dissections: potential contributors to aortic repair. *Ann Thorac Surg*. 2012;93:1524-1533.
2. Wang J, Zhang S, Rabinovich B, et al. Human CD34+ cells in experimental myocardial infarction: long-term survival, sustained functional improvement, and mechanism of action. *Circ Res*. 2010;106:1904-1911.

Carotid and Cerebrovascular Disease

Human Carotid Plaques With High Levels of Interleukin-16 Are Associated With Reduced Risk for Cardiovascular Events

Grönberg C, Bengtsson E, Fredrikson GN, et al (Lund Univ, Sweden)
Stroke 46:2748-2754, 2015

Background and Purpose.—Interleukin-16 (IL-16) functions as a regulator of T-cell growth and acts as an inducer of cell migration. The aim of this study was to determine whether IL-16 measured in human carotid plaques was associated with symptoms (eg, stroke, transient ischemic attack, or amaurosis fugax), markers of plaque stability, and postoperative cardiovascular events.

Methods.—Plaques obtained from patients who had ≥1 cerebrovascular ischemic events within 1 month before endarterectomy (n = 111) were compared with plaques from patients without symptoms (n = 95). Neutral lipids, smooth muscle cell, and macrophage contents were evaluated histologically, and collagen, elastin, and caspase-3 activity were measured biochemically. IL-16, matrix metalloproteinases, and tissue inhibitors of metalloproteinases were measured in plaque homogenates using a multiplex immunoassay. IL-16, CD3, CD4, and FoxP3 mRNA expressions in carotid plaques were analyzed with quantitative real-time polymerase chain reaction.

Results.—Carotid plaques from asymptomatic patients had higher levels of IL-16 mRNA. High plaque IL-16 protein levels (above median) were associated with reduced incidence of postoperative cardiovascular events during a mean follow-up of 21 months (hazard ratio, 0.47; 95% confidence interval, 0.22–0.99; $P = 0.047$). IL-16 levels correlated with the plaque-stabilizing components: elastin, collagen, matrix metalloproteinase-2, tissue inhibitors of metalloproteinase-1, tissue inhibitors of metalloproteinase-2 and FoxP3 mRNA.

Conclusions.—This study shows that high levels of IL-16 are associated with asymptomatic carotid plaques, expression of factors contributing to plaque stability, and decreased risk of new cardiovascular events during a 2-year period after surgery, suggesting that IL-16 might have a protective role in human atherosclerotic disease.

▶ Interleukin-16 (IL-16) is a chemokine expressed by a variety of different cells, including CD8+ T cells, macrophages, and endothelial cells. It has been shown that various T-cell subsets are involved in the inflammatory response in both a positive and negative manner. Here, the authors measured the level of IL-16 messenger RNA (mRNA) and protein in carotid plaques removed at the time of endarterectomy, measured plasma levels of IL-16 in symptomatic and asymptomatic patients, and sought an association between IL-16 and markers of plaque stabilization. They also looked at new cardiovascular events during mean follow-up of 21 months.

Although there was no correlation between plasma levels of IL-16 and levels found in the plaque, IL-16 mRNA expression was found to be significantly higher in the plaques removed from asymptomatic patients compared with symptomatic patients. Additionally, plaque IL-16 mRNA and protein levels were associated with markers of plaque stabilization: collagen, elastin, MMP-2, TIMP-2, and FoxP3 mRNA. During mean follow-up of 21 months, higher IL-16 protein levels in plaques were associated with fewer new cardiovascular events. As the authors mention, there are not many known inflammatory mediators that play an anti-atherosclerotic role and lead to plaque stabilization, thus making IL-16 an attractive target for future studies with potential clinical application.

B. Peterson, MD, FACS

Investigating the Effect of a Single Infusion of Reconstituted High-Density Lipoprotein in Patients with Symptomatic Carotid Plaques

Nasr H, Torsney E, Poston RN, et al (St George's Univ of London, UK; Queen Mary Univ of London, UK; et al)

Ann Vasc Surg 29:1380-1391, 2015

Background.—Elevation of plasma high-density lipoprotein (HDL) cholesterol concentration reduces cardiovascular mortality and morbidity. HDLs have been shown to possess acute anti-inflammatory, antioxidant, and antithrombotic properties. We hypothesize that HDL therapy can acutely alter local and systemic manifestations of plaque instability.

Methods.—Forty patients with early symptomatic carotid disease were randomized to either receive reconstituted HDL (rHDL) 40 mg/kg ($n = 20$) or placebo ($n = 20$). Carotid endarterectomies were performed 24 hr later. Plaques were obtained intraoperatively and used for measurement of thrombomodulatory genes expression. Plasma samples were collected before the infusion, 24 and 48 hr later to measure changes in systemic markers of plaque instability.

Results.—No significant differences were noted in thrombomodulatory genes expression between the 2 groups. Systemic levels of tissue factor, matrix metalloproteinase 9 (MMP-9), and monocyte chemotactic factor-1 (MCP-1) were significantly reduced in the rHDL group. However, the effects on MMP-9 and MCP-1 were abolished in the immediate postoperative period. Although rHDL did not affect plasma interleukin-6 levels 24 hr following the infusion, it prevented the significant postoperative elevation seen in the placebo group.

Conclusions.—A single infusion of rHDL can acutely alter plasma biomarkers associated with plaque instability and cardiovascular morbidity.

► Beneficial effects of elevated levels of high-density lipoprotein (HDL) are well established and create a generalized antiatherogenic process through various mechanisms: anti-inflammatory, antioxidant, and antithrombotic properties; reverse cholesterol transport; and modification of endothelial function. The ERASE trial demonstrated that reconstituted HDL (rHDL) can induce plaque regression in acute coronary syndrome patients.[1] Here, the authors sought to evaluate the acute effects of low-dose infusion of rHDL on carotid plaque characteristics and systemic biomarkers of inflammation in patients with symptomatic carotid artery disease undergoing carotid endarterectomy (CEA).

Forty patients with acute symptoms attributable to carotid artery stenoses > 50% were randomized to receive infusions of low-dose rHDL (n = 20) or placebo (n = 20) 24 hours before undergoing CEA. Systemic biomarkers were collected before infusion and at 24 and 48 hours after CEA. Carotid plaques were also sampled to assess the effect of rHDL on gene expression. Overall, the infusion of rHDL was well tolerated with only mild to moderate adverse events that were not significant and transient elevation of liver function tests without clinical significance.

There was no difference seen in the gene expression of thrombomodulatory proteins from samples of the plaques in both groups, likely because of the short time between infusion and harvest of the plaque. However, the rHDL group demonstrated significantly lower plasma levels of MCP-1 (a chemokine associated with atherogenesis) and MMP-9 (a proteolytic enzyme implicated in atherosclerosis and plaque stability). This effect was transient and not sustained at 48 hours. Infusion of rHDL also prevented the spike in interleukin-6 levels (a marker of inflammation) and the rise in tissue factor levels (a protein promoting thrombogenesis) seen in the placebo group at 48 hours postoperatively. These findings suggest that infusion of rHDL may play a role in stabilizing plaques and reducing the risk of undesirable perioperative cardiovascular events seen in some patients undergoing CEA.

B. Peterson, MD, FACS

Reference

1. Tardif JC, Gregoire J, L'Allier PL, et al. Effects of reconstituted high-density lipoprotein infusions on coronary atherosclerosis: a randomized controlled trial. *JAMA*. 2007;297:1675-1682.

Perivascular Adipose Adiponectin Correlates With Symptom Status of Patients Undergoing Carotid Endarterectomy

Sharma G, Tao M, Ding K, et al (Brigham and Women's Hosp, Boston, MA; et al)

Stroke 46:1696-1699, 2015

Background and Purpose.—Recent symptoms stand as a major determinant of stroke risk in patients with carotid stenosis, likely reflective of atherosclerotic plaque destabilization. In view of emerging links between vascular and adipose biology, we hypothesized that human perivascular adipose characteristics associate with carotid disease symptom status.

Methods.—Clinical history, carotid plaques, blood, and subcutaneous and perivascular adipose tissues were prospectively collected from patients undergoing carotid endarterectomy. Nine adipose-associated biological mediators were assayed and compared in patients with symptomatic ($n = 15$) versus asymptomatic ($n = 19$) disease. Bonferroni correction was performed for multiple testing ($\alpha/9 = 0.006$).

Results.—Symptomatic patients had 1.9-fold higher perivascular adiponectin levels ($P = 0.005$). Other circulating, subcutaneous, and perivascular biomarkers, as well as microscopic plaque characteristics, did not differ between symptomatic and asymptomatic patients.

Conclusions.—Symptomatic and asymptomatic carotid endarterectomy patients display a tissue-specific difference in perivascular adipose adiponectin. This difference, which was not seen in plasma or subcutaneous compartments, supports a potential local paracrine relationship with vascular disease processes that may be related to stroke mechanisms.

▶ Plaque destabilization in patients with carotid artery disease has been felt to be a major determinant of whether patients develop symptoms. Increasing data suggest a role of perivascular adipose tissue in cell-cell signaling, modulation of smooth muscle, remodeling, and inflammation. The authors hypothesized that human perivascular adipose characteristics associate with symptom status in patients with carotid artery disease.

During carotid endarterectomy, blood, subcutaneous, and perivascular tissues were harvested from 19 patients without symptoms and 15 patients with symptoms, with both groups having similar baseline characteristics. The authors found that symptomatic patients had 1.9-fold higher perivascular adiponectin ($P = .005$) compared with asymptomatic patients. Interestingly, the groups had no difference in levels of circulating adiponectin, suggesting a local effect of perivascular adipose tissue on plaque stability. Although the precise mechanism of action cannot be elucidated from this observational study, results demonstrated here should lead to further studies designed to better define the interaction between perivascular adipose tissue and vascular plaques.

B. Peterson, MD, FACS

Leg Ischemia

Atherosclerotic Plaque Analysis: A Pilot Study to Assess a Novel Tool to Predict Outcome Following Lower Limb Endovascular Intervention

Patel SD, Zymvragoudakis V, Sheehan L, et al (Guy's and St Thomas' NHS Foundation Trust, London, UK)

Eur J Vasc Endovasc Surg 50:487-493, 2015

Introduction.—Atherosclerotic plaque analysis using computed tomography angiography (CTA) has been found to be accurate and reproducible in the coronary and carotid arteries. The aim of our study was to assess the utility of this technique in predicting outcome following lower limb endovascular interventions.

Methods.—Pre-procedural CTA was retrospectively analysed in 50 patients who had undergone femoropopliteal (F—P) angioplasty (and/or stenting). Plaque analysis was performed using TeraRecon workstation by two observers blinded to the long-term outcome. Using the Hounsfield units (HU) scale atherosclerotic plaque composition was subdivided into volumes of soft (−100—100 HU) fibrocalcific (101—300 HU) or calcified (300—1000 HU) components. The relationship between plaque composition, clinical and procedural variables, and the study end points (vessel patency, binary restenosis rate, and Amputation-Free Survival [AFS]) were assessed using multivariate analysis.

Results.—The technical success rate of the endovascular procedure was 98%, with 48% of patients receiving F—P stents. The AFS was 90%, primary patency 84%, assisted primary patency 88%, and binary restenosis 44% all at 1 year. A significantly greater total volume of calcified plaque (1.1 [.01—3.2] cm^3 vs. .11 [0—1.86] cm^3, $p < .001$) was found in patients developing restenosis (>50%) compared with those who did not. Patients with a calcified plaque volume greater than 1.1 cm^3 had a significantly worse AFS than those with a volume less than 1.1 cm^3 ($p = .0038$). Multivariate analysis showed that the percentage calcified plaque ($p = .003$, HR 11.4, 95% CI 1.45—37.29) was an independent predictor of binary restenosis at 12 months, and that absolute volume of calcified plaque ($p = .001$, HR 3.56, 95% CI 1.64—7.7) was independently associated with AFS.

Conclusions.—The burden of calcified plaque, but not soft or fibrocalcific plaque is related to restenosis, reintervention, and AFS. Computed tomography plaque analysis may form an important non-invasive tool

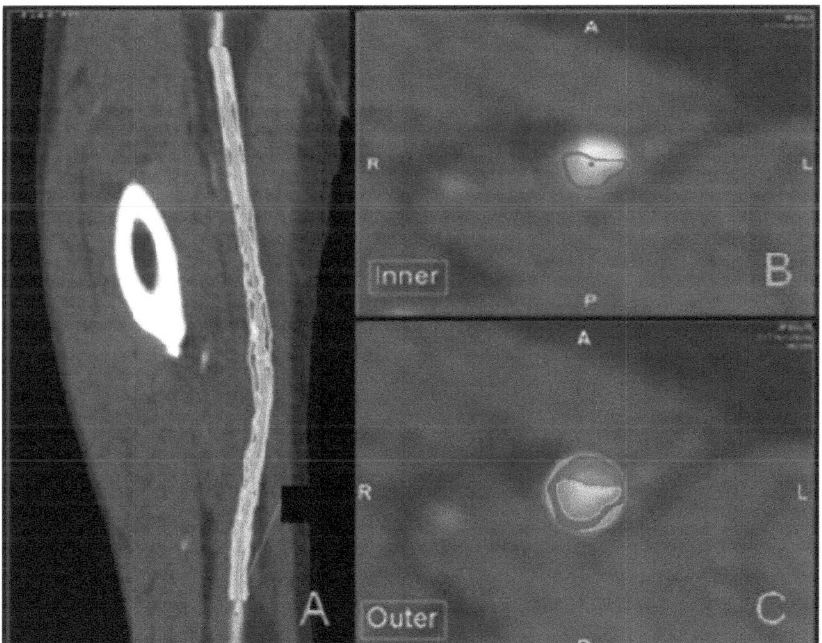

FIGURE 1.—Computed tomography angiography plaque analysis. (A) Multiplanar reformat with centerline and region of interest identified. (B) Transverse section with lumen identified. (C) Outer wall line and plaque colour map with soft (red), fibrocalcific (green), and calcified (blue) components. For interpretation of the references to color in this figure legend, the reader is referred to web version of this article. (Reprinted from Patel SD, Zymvragoudakis V, Sheehan L, et al. Atherosclerotic plaque analysis: a pilot study to assess a novel tool to predict outcome following lower limb endovascular intervention. *Eur J Vasc Endovasc Surg*. 2015;50:487-493, with permission from European Society for Vascular Surgery.)

for risk stratification in patients undergoing F–P endovascular procedures (Fig 1).

▶ CT-guided plaque analysis has been described in both coronary and carotid territories and validated as both accurate and reproducible in the identification of higher risk lesions. These authors have introduced a pilot study examining the utility of this technique in predicting outcomes following endovascular treatment of femoropopliteal disease. Two observers blinded to patient outcome independently reviewed preprocedure CT angiograms of 50 patients with Rutherford stage 3 to 6 disease and >70% femoropopliteal stenosis without coexisting significant aortoiliac or common femoral disease. All patients underwent angioplasty, the majority of whom had TASC II B disease. Selective stenting was used in approximately half of the patients for flow-limiting dissection, immediate arterial recoil and vessel rupture. Plaque composition was qualified as soft, fibrocalcific and calcific by Hounsfield Units. The authors report a strong association between the percentage of calcified plaque and binary restenosis at 12 months by both multivariate analysis and binary logistic regression and a negative correlation of total volume of calcified plaque and amputation-free survival (Fig 1).

These exciting pilot data warrant further prospective and larger scale clinical trials for validation, which not only consider those patients with multilevel disease but also corroborate plaque analysis with intravascular ultrasound or histology. The value of such a risk stratification tool may not simply aid endovascular treatment planning as the authors reference (ie, guide subintimal angioplasty, stenting, etc) but, more importantly, inform patient selection when considering open and endovascular revascularization options, guide patient education and informed consent, and dictate postintervention surveillance.

D. Coleman, MD

Local Association Between Endothelial Dysfunction and Intimal Hyperplasia: Relevance in Peripheral Artery Disease

Heinen Y, Stegemann E, Sansone R, et al (Univ Duesseldorf, Germany)
J Am Heart Assoc 4:e001472, 2015

Background.—Endothelial dysfunction is a key factor in the development of atherosclerosis. Commonly, endothelial function is determined in the brachial artery, whereas patients with peripheral artery disease (PAD) present with lower limb atherosclerosis. We hypothesized that in PAD, a segmental or local association exists between endothelial dysfunction and atherosclerotic structural changes.

Methods and Results.—We used ultrasound to study endothelial function as flow-mediated vasodilation, intima media thickness, and local stiffness of the superficial femoral artery (SFA) and brachial artery (BA). PAD patients with symptomatic SFA or below-the-knee disease were compared with age-matched patients without PAD and young healthy controls. PAD patients with SFA or below-the-knee disease exhibited endothelial dysfunction of the proximal SFA (flow-mediated vasodilation: 3.9 ± 0.6%, 3.7 ± 0.6%) compared with healthy controls (7.4 ± 1.0%) and patients without PAD (5.4 ± 0.6%). Brachial artery flow-mediated vasodilation values were not different in PAD patients with SFA or below-the-knee disease compared with patients without PAD, but they were significantly lower than those of healthy controls. Endothelial dysfunction correlated with increased intima media thickness or plaque thickness at the site of flow-mediated vasodilation measurement across vascular sites. In PAD patients with SFA disease, SFA flow-mediated vasodilation was further impaired within and distal to stenosis (prestenosis 3.9 ± 0.6%, intrastenosis 2.3 ± 0.7%, poststenosis 2.5 ± 0.6%) and recovered within 24 hours after SFA balloon angioplasty to prestenotic values but not to the brachial artery or SFA values in patients without PAD or controls.

Conclusion.—A close association exists between local endothelial function and atherosclerotic structural remodeling, suggesting that in PAD, local and segmental factors—in addition to systemic factors—influence local endothelial function. Our data point toward a pathophysiological role for lower extremity endothelial dysfunction in PAD.

▶ Patients with peripheral artery disease (PAD) have a heightened risk of major cardiovascular event. Endothelial dysfunction plays a key pathophysiologic role in the development of atherosclerosis. Several authors have previously demonstrated that systemic endothelial dysfunction in patients with cardiovascular disease (including both coronary disease and PAD) can be measured in a non-atherosclerosis-prone vessel (ie, brachial artery) as impaired flow-mediated vasodilation (FMD) and subsequently used to predict overall cardiovascular risk.

This study included well-defined inclusion criteria and methods; the investigators demonstrated an association between local endothelial dysfunction (assessed by FMD) and atherosclerotic structural remodeling (assessed by intima media thickness [IMT] and vessel stiffness). Importantly, in patients with coronary artery disease but without PAD, IMT and FMD were altered compared with younger, healthy controls, suggesting early systemic arteriosclerotic changes to both the nondiseased brachial and superficial femoral artery walls. Importantly, flow- and nitroglycerine-mediated vasodilation were significantly more altered in segments of the arterial tree compromised by clinically evident arteriosclerosis compared with both non-PAD controls with coronary artery disease and young healthy control subjects without arteriosclerosis. A significant and linear inverse correlation was identified for all study arms between IMT and FMD measurements (Fig 1 in the original article). Moreover, both intra- and poststenotic FMD increased 24 hours after percutaneous transluminal angioplasty.

Although the authors conclude that in PAD, systemic, segmental, and local features that can be either structural or functional in nature influence lower extremity endothelial function, the study is limited by several elements, including the small size (n = 10) of each study arm and confounding factors. The definition of "concomitant stable CAD" is not clarified further, and it remains unclear whether these patients suffered previous MI or had angiographic confirmation of disease burden. Although the methods suggest that participants with stable CAD and PAD were on standard optimal medical therapy, details related to medications and dosing were not included or standardized. Additionally, the incidence of diabetes is much higher in the PAD arms (60% of those with SFA PAD and 60% of those with tibial PAD compared with 0% of healthy, young controls and 20% of non-PAD controls with CAD). The author's suggestion that interventional treatment of PAD may help disrupt further development of disease progression by reestablishing better endothelial function downstream is an ambitious conclusion that is not supported by the study findings. Definition of the molecular pathways involved will be necessary, as well as demonstration of a clear benefit (and, conversely, lack of harm) through larger scale longitudinal clinical studies. Given that most patients with claudication do not experience disease progression provided that they are on appropriate medications and abstain from smoking, preemptive intervention based on the premise of halting disease progression risks "overtreatment" and potential harm.

D. Coleman, MD

Venous Disease

Growth and remodeling of canine common iliac vein in response to venous reflux and hypertension

Brass M, Berwick ZC, Zhao X, et al (Indiana Univ–Purdue Univ Indianapolis; et al)

J Vasc Surg Venous Lymphat Disord 3:303-311.e1, 2015

Objective.—The passive properties of the venous wall are important for the compliance function of the venous system. The objective of this study was to quantify the passive biomechanical response and structural growth and remodeling of veins subjected to chronic venous reflux and hypertension.

Methods.—To investigate the effects of venous reflux on venous mechanics, the tricuspid valve was injured in a canine model by disrupting the chordae tendineae. The conventional inflation-extension protocol in conjunction with intravascular ultrasound was used to investigate the passive biomechanical response of both control common iliac veins (n = 9 dogs) and common iliac veins subjected to 8 weeks of venous reflux and hypertension (n = 9 dogs). The changes in vein wall thickness and constituent composition were quantified by multiphoton microscopy and histologic evaluation.

Results.—Biomechanical results indicate that the veins became less compliant when exposed to 8 weeks of chronic venous reflux and hypertension. The mechanical stiffening was found to be associated with a significant increase in wall thickness ($P < .05$) and collagen-to-elastin ratio ($P < .05$). After 8 weeks of chronic reflux and hypertension, the circumferential vein wall stress was significantly reduced ($P < .05$) because of wall thickening, although it was not restored to control levels.

Conclusions.—The growth and remodeling of the venous wall reduces the wall stress, but the stress remains higher than at baseline at 8 weeks. The compliance of the veins also decreases because of the increase in wall thickness and remodeling of the microstructure of the venous wall. These findings provide insight into potential adaptations of the venous system in reflux and hypertension.

Clinical Relevance.—Chronic venous insufficiency (CVI) affects the venous system of the lower extremities with venous reflux and hypertension. The growth and remodeling of the venous system to the perturbed hemodynamic conditions in CVI are not well understood. The relevance of this study is to provide fundamental data on the morphologic and mechanical properties of the venous system in a translational animal model of CVI. Our findings highlight the adaptive changes of the venous system that may lead to loss of compliance and the various sequelae in CVI.

▶ Chronic venous insufficiency affects up to 35% of the US population. The underlying pathology is venous hypertension with clinical presentations of pain and swelling, skin changes, and venous leg ulceration. The pathophysiology of chronic venous insufficiency is not well understood due to a lack of adequate animal models, and no model completely represents the hemodynamic conditions seen in chronic venous insufficiency patients. The importance of this study lies in its use of a novel method to induce venous hypertension and reflux in the iliac vein, which is measured and quantified, and the chronic effects on the vein wall studied. In response to reflux and hypertension, the vein wall in this model decreases the stress and increases the wall stiffness and wall thickness, with a concomitant increase in collagen to elastin ratio. The end result is a less compliant and stiffer vein wall. The implication of this study is a better understanding of the biophysical and chemical changes that occur to the vein wall that are subjected to elevated pressures and reflux, as would be the case seen in patients with chronic venous insufficiency. Most of the vein wall remodeling occurs in the circumferential and not longitudinal directions, based on this model. These findings support the hypothesis that the composition of collagen and elastin in the wall changes and the vein stiffens when it is exposed to chronic venous reflux and hypertension. Future work in this area will be important to determine when the process is reversible when the reflux and venous hypertension is normalized and/or if pharmacologic treatments would improve vein wall stiffness and loss of compliance.

J. D. Raffetto, MD, FACS, FSVM

Morphologic changes in the vein after different numbers of radiofrequency ablation cycles

Shaidakov EV, Grigoryan AG, Korzhevskii DE, et al (Russian Academy of Med Sciences, St Petersburg; et al)

J Vasc Surg Venous Lymphat Disord 3:358-363, 2015

Objective.—It has not yet been clarified whether it is possible to decrease the percentage of recurrences after radiofrequency (RF) ablation by way of increasing the number of RF ablation cycles. The aim of this study was to assess the morphologic changes in excised vein fragments after different durations of RF ablation exposure.

Methods.—In the first part of the study, we performed a morphologic analysis of eight cases of great saphenous vein (GSV) recanalization 6 months after RF ablation. The second part was performed on a suprafascial segment of the GSV with a length of >22 cm and a minimum diameter of 5 mm in 10 patients, who had given their consent to intraoperative excision of suprafascial GSV segments after RF ablation treatment through four 1-cm-long diametrical cuts. Prior ultrasound analysis had shown an average 6.9-mm diameter of the suprafascial segments. The segment was divided into three 7-cm-long subsegments and one control segment. The first, second, and third segments were treated with three, two, and one RF ablation cycles (ClosureFast; Covidien, Mansfield, Mass), respectively; the control segment was not exposed to RF ablation at all. Morphologic study of 160 sections of the vein (five sections of each segment and 10 control specimens) was carried out. The specimens were dyed with hematoxylin and orcein. The ensuing analysis was performed by an experienced expert with the blind study method (the specimens were numbered without any hint as to the quantity of RF ablation cycles performed on them). The intergroup comparison of the depth of venous wall damage was based on comparison of the coefficient of alteration, which is calculated as the relation of damage depth to thickness of the vein.

Results.—After one RF ablation cycle, the depth of blurring of the structural elements only on some portions reached the middle of the muscle layer of the wall (coefficient of alteration, $\alpha = 26\%$). After two cycles, blurring of the structural elements on some portions extended to the adventitia ($\alpha = 53\%$). After three cycles, uniform blurring of the structural elements of all layers of the venous wall up to the adventitia was seen ($\alpha = 92\%$). The statistically significant difference in the alteration coefficient, depending on the number of cycles of RF ablation ($P < .005$), was established.

Conclusions.—The number of RF ablation cycles has an impact on the depth of vein wall damage. One and two cycles do not cause damage to all layers of the vein wall. Three cycles cause damage to all vein wall layers.

▶ Although technical outcomes of radiofrequency ablation have been mostly successful in achieving complete fibrous transformation, recurrence has been reported in a small number of cases, which may be reflective of depth of vein wall destruction with current protocols using 2 cycles at saphenofemoral junction and single cycle through the remainder of the saphenous vein. Using a protocol that included 3-, 2-, 1- radiofrequency cycles plus a controlled segment with no ablation followed by immediate segmental saphenous vein sampling, the authors show that depth of vein wall damage was affected by number of cycles, with 3- cycles causing reproducible damage to all vein wall layers. Although this observation falls in line with the study hypothesis, findings are limited by the immediate sampling of vein tissue at time zero, as opposed to a later time frame. Whether increasing the cycles for radiofrequency ablation to 3- has any effect on patient-related outcome measures, causes increased collateral damage from increased energy, or has any impact on recurrence rates are issues not addressed in this study.

M. Passman, MD

Prosthetic venous valve patient selection by validated physics-based computational models

Chen HY, Berwick ZC, Kemp A, et al (IUPUI, Indianapolis, IN; The California Med Innovations Inst, Inc, San Diego; et al)

J Vasc Surg Venous Lymphat Disord 3:75-80, 2015

Background.—There is significant interest in a venous prosthesis to replace insufficient valves. The aim of the current study was to select the patients with hemodynamic conditions most likely to benefit from a valve implant. The hypothesis is that the venous valve prosthesis is most suitable for patients with significant reflux, such as in chronic venous insufficiency (CVI), right heart hypertrophy (RHH), and right heart failure (RHF). Conversely, a prosthetic valve is likely to be of least benefit for deep venous thrombosis (DVT) patients with low flow.

Methods.—To address this hypothesis, fully coupled fluid and solid mechanics computational models were developed and validated in five acute canine implants. The animal-validated simulations were then carried out for the CVI, RHH, RHF, and DVT patients based on literature hemodynamic data. A mechanical stress ratio of leaflet wall stress to fluid wall shear stress was defined to combine the effects of both fluid mechanics and solid mechanics on leaflet function, for which a lower stress ratio is hemodynamically desirable.

Results.—The simulation results of mean valve flow velocity and percentage valve opening were found to be within 10% of the measurements in canines. The simulations show that the patients in the CVI classes 4 to 6, RHH patients, and RHF patients may have a significant reduction in stress ratio with virtual implant of a prosthetic valve. The DVT patient simulations demonstrate a minimal reduction in the stress ratio. After thrombus removal where flow is restored, however, the prosthetic valve may be helpful for post-thrombotic patients.

Conclusions.—For patient selections of the venous valve prosthesis, the most suitable patients are the CVI classes 4 to 6, RHH, and RHF patients.

The least suitable patients are the DVT patients because a valve is not effective under low-flow conditions. The present study demonstrates a physics-based approach to patient selection that can be tested in future clinical trials.

Clinical Relevance.—There is significant interest in a venous valve prosthesis to replace insufficient valves. The purpose of the current study was to select the patients with hemodynamic conditions most likely to benefit from an implant. Patients with chronic venous insufficiency classes 2 to 6, right-sided heart hypertrophy, right heart failure, and deep venous thrombosis were considered. The validated simulations found that the most suitable patients for the implant are the chronic venous insufficiency classes 4 to 6, right heart hypertrophy, and right heart failure patients. The present study demonstrates a biophysical approach to patient selection that may be useful for improving clinical outcome.

▶ Venous valves are necessary to segment the hydrostatic column of blood within the venous system and to allow prograde flow during muscular contractions, which then result in valve closure during 4 distinct phases of valve function. Venous valves become insufficient either in primary venous disease or secondary venous disease following deep venous thrombosis (DVT). Secondary venous disease results in significantly advanced clinical disease, with up to 50% of patients developing postthrombotic syndrome at 2 years. A variety of methods of valve reconstruction have been described and published, with variable results. An important aspect of venous valve repair is to select the proper patient to maximize the desired clinical outcome and resolution of symptoms. Computational modeling of valve function based on abnormal venous hemodynamics in chronic venous insufficiency (CVI) patients would be of considerable value. This is an important study because it delineates the selection of patients most likely to hemodynamically benefit from a prosthetic valve implant, with the hypothesis that the venous valve prosthesis is of most benefit when a lower stress ratio (solid wall stress/fluid wall shear stress) exists due to increased fluid shear stress and decreased solid wall stress is hemodynamically favorable. Patients with significant reflux, such as CVI clinical classes 4 to 6, should benefit. Alternatively, the valve prosthesis is likely to be of little benefit for DVT patients with low flow because valve function is dependent on blood flow. The study demonstrated that the hemodynamics of most CVI patients (clinical classes 2-6), and especially the more advanced clinical classes 4 to 6 improve with venous prosthetic valve implantation as indicated by the reduction of stress ratio and oscillatory stress index (OSI) by computational modeling. The stress ratio is more than 3 times higher for DVT patients than for the other patients after virtual placement of the prosthetic valve. After thrombus removal in a patient with DVT in whom the flow is restored, however, the prosthetic valve is found to significantly reduce the stress ratio for DVT patients. Finally, and very interestingly, the venous valve computational modeling also improved significantly the stress ratio and OSI in patients with right heart hypertrophy and right heart failure, which are conditions commonly associated with patients with chronic venous insufficiency.[1]

J. D. Raffetto, MD, FACS, FSVM

Reference

1. Lurie F, Kistner RL, Eklof B, Kessler D. Mechanism of venous valve closure and role of the valve in circulation: a new concept. *J Vasc Surg*. 2003;38:955-961.

Successful tissue engineering of competent allogeneic venous valves

Kuna VK, Rosales A, Hisdal J, et al (Sahlgrenska Academy at the Univ of Gothenburg, Sweden; Oslo Univ Hosp, Aker, Norway; et al)

J Vasc Surg Venous Lymphat Disord 3:421-430.e1, 2015

Objective.—The purpose of this study was to evaluate whether tissue-engineered human allogeneic vein valves have a normal closure time (competency) and tolerate reflux pressure in vitro.

Methods.—Fifteen human allogeneic femoral vein segments containing valves were harvested from cadavers. Valve closure time and resistance to reflux pressure (100 mm Hg) were assessed in an in vitro model to verify competency of the vein valves. The segments were tissue engineered using the technology of decellularization (DC) and recellularization (RC). The decellularized and recellularized vein segments were characterized biochemically, immunohistochemically, and biomechanically.

Results.—Four of 15 veins with valves were found to be incompetent immediately after harvest. In total, 2 of 4 segments with incompetent valves and 10 of 11 segments with competent valves were further decellularized using detergents and DNAse. DC resulted in significant decrease in host DNA compared with controls. DC scaffolds, however, retained major extracellular matrix proteins and mechanical integrity. RC resulted in successful repopulation of the lumen and valves of the scaffold with endothelial and smooth muscle cells. Valve mechanical parameters were similar to the native tissue even after DC. Eight of 10 veins with competent valves remained competent even after DC and RC, whereas the two incompetent valves remained incompetent even after DC and RC. The valve closure time to reflux pressure of the tissue-engineered veins was <0.5 second.

Conclusions.—Tissue-engineered veins with valves provide a valid template for future preclinical studies and eventual clinical applications. This technique may enable replacement of diseased incompetent or damaged deep veins to treat axial reflux and thus reduce ambulatory venous hypertension.

Clinical Relevance.—The use of natural, human scaffolds to produce tissue-engineered venous segments containing functioning valves will revolutionize the surgical correction of deep venous reflux in patients with chronic venous insufficiency and leg ulcer. Reconstructive deep venous surgery in the form of valvuloplasty, transplantation, and neovalve

construction has met limitations in the rare availability of valves to be repaired, lack of donor sites, and inadequate conditions to create new valves. This tissue-engineered procedure produces the functioning unit "valve-conduit," and surgery will be used only to implant it.

▶ Chronic venous disease is a significant disease affecting more than 25 million people in the United States, and with 6 million having advanced venous disease (clinical class 4-6). Venous leg ulcers, the most severe complication of chronic venous disease, affect 5% of patients older than 65 years. The severity of chronic venous insufficiency with higher clinical class involves both superficial and deep venous reflux. A significant proportion of patients who have had their superficial system corrected will have persistent symptoms, and about 35% of patients will have recalcitrant venous leg ulcers, increasing health care cost and decreasing quality of life. Because the deep venous system is often involved in these individuals, correcting venous hemodynamics by correcting valve dysfunction is appealing.

An ideal valve would be of autogenous tissue, durable, low morbidity, and leading to correction of the venous hemodynamics with a favorable outcome of ulcer healing. Tissue engineering utilizing living cells and appropriate biologic scaffolds are appealing as viable solutions to a difficult problem. Whole organ acellular matrices provide an attractive scaffold for the repopulation with cells for an engineered tissue or organ because of the physiologic resemblance to the original tissue, including intact 3-dimensional anatomic architecture, preserved spatial array of extracellular matrix, vascular network, and biomechanical properties. Creating regenerated donor organs by repopulating organ scaffolds with patient-specific mature or stem cell—derived populations would allow us to personalize transplantation medicine and reduce the need for long-term immunosuppressive therapy. The basis of this study is taking this concept and applying it to venous valves in the treatment of patients with chronic venous insufficiency and advanced clinical class. The interesting aspect of this study is that venous segments with an intervening valve were taken from human cadavers (femoral vein segments N = 15). The vein segments were tested for valve function and 74% were competent. The veins valve segments were decellularized and analyzed histologically by Masson trichrome demonstrating no nuclei and thus indicating lack of endothelial and smooth muscle cells, but with abundant collagen still present. In addition, the decellularized veins did not contain HLA class I or II compared with control veins. The decellularization process also led to increased elastin, same collagen, but decreased glycosaminoglycans, and a significant decrease in DNA, compared with control subjects. In all, 80% of the decellularized vein valve segments retained valve function. Recellularization was accomplished in the decellularized vein valve segments by using donor blood and a bioreactor. Immunostaining demonstrated that recellularized vein valve segments had endothelial cells and smooth muscle cells, and functional studies demonstrated that 67% had normal valve function evaluated by real-time ultrasound, with the valve opening and closing. Interestingly, the median force of first break of the valve was similar for native control valves versus the recellularized functional valves. I think that this study holds significant promise in future treatments using bioengineered tissues and regenerative medicine—in this case, venous valves that can be decellularized and then repopulated with the host cellular elements (endothelium and smooth muscle cells), retain valvular function, and utilized to treat advanced stages of chronic venous disease without the need for immunosuppressant therapy to achieve a favorable clinical outcome with venous ulcer healing and improved quality of life. Future studies will be required to determine clinical feasibility, durability, and cost-effectiveness.

J. D. Raffetto, MD, FACS, FSVM

Recanalization and flow regulate venous thrombus resolution and matrix metalloproteinase expression in vivo

Chabasse C, Siefert SA, Chaudry M, et al (Univ of Maryland, Baltimore)
J Vasc Surg Venous Lymphat Disord 3:64-74, 2015

Objective.—We examined the role of thrombus recanalization and ongoing blood flow in the process of thrombus resolution by comparing two murine in vivo models of deep venous thrombosis.

Methods.—In CD1 mice, we performed surgical inferior vena cava ligation (stasis thrombosis), stenosis (thrombosis with recanalization), or sham procedure. We analyzed thrombus weight over time as a measure of thrombus resolution and quantified the messenger RNA and protein levels of membrane-type matrix metalloproteinases (MT-MMPs) as well as effectors of the plasmin complex at days 4, 8, and 12 after surgery.

Results.—Despite similar initial thrombus size, the presence of ongoing blood flow (stenosis model) was associated with a 45.91% subsequent improvement in thrombus resolution at day 8 and 12.57% at day 12 compared with stasis thrombosis (ligation model). Immunoblot and real-time polymerase chain reaction analysis demonstrated a difference in MMP-2 and MMP-9 activity at day 8 between the two models ($P = .03$ and $P = .006$, respectively) as well as a difference in MT2-MMP gene expression at day 8 ($P = .044$) and day 12 ($P = .03$) and MT1-MMP protein expression at day 4 ($P = .021$). Histologic analyses revealed distinct areas of recanalization in the thrombi of the stenosis model compared with the ligation model as well as the recruitment of inflammatory cells, especially macrophages, and a focal pattern of localized expression of MT1-MMP and MT3-MMP proteins surrounding the areas of recanalization in the stenosis model.

Conclusions.—Recanalization and ongoing blood flow accelerate deep venous thrombus resolution in vivo and are associated with distinct patterns of MT1-MMP and MT3-MMP expression and macrophage localization in areas of intrathrombus recanalization.

Clinical Relevance.—Incomplete thrombus resolution after deep venous thrombosis is important in the development of post-thrombotic syndrome. This study directly examines the role of ongoing blood flow and recanalization in the resolution of deep venous thrombosis in vivo. We find that the presence of ongoing blood flow enhances thrombus resolution and is associated with expression of key matrix metalloproteinases in areas of recanalization within the thrombus. These findings help define the physiology of thrombus resolution and provide potential therapeutic targets to accelerate this clinically important process for patients with deep venous thrombosis.

▶ Deep venous thrombosis (DVT) is a significant problem and is associated with pulmonary embolism (PE), which together are referred as venous thromboembolism (VTE). VTE accounts for up 900 000 new cases annually, and PE is the leading preventable in-hospital cause of death with up to 300 000 patients annually. Understanding the pathophysiology of DVT and thrombus resolution is of critical importance to offer appropriate therapy to lower the risk of PE and recurrent VTE but also to understand DVT development and resolution that may offer new areas of therapeutic targets. There are various murine DVT models, and different models may provide insight into the biomolecular steps in thrombus development and resolution. This study used 2 types of models: the inferior vena cava (IVC) ligation model (stasis model) and the IVC stenosis model (stenosis). The important findings were that the stenosis model allows for recanalization and blood flow to resume, whereas the stasis model can recanalize but flow is not possible due to a completely ligated blood vessel. This study determined that the presence of ongoing blood flow enhances thrombus resolution and is associated with expression of key matrix metalloproteinases (MMP-2, MMP-9, MT-MMP-1) in areas of recanalization within the thrombus. Interestingly, there was no difference found between the 2 models for neutrophils and macrophages at day 4 and day 8, but more important is that macrophages are distributed in the areas of recanalization and flow. This was also seen with focal pattern of localized expression of MT1-MMP and MT3-MMP proteins surrounding the areas of recanalization in the stenosis model. This distinct and focal expression of these proteases around areas of endothelial recanalization suggests a potential molecular mechanism for the differences in thrombus resolution noted with the ongoing flow stenosis model. Future work will be necessary to determine how low molecular weight heparins, novel oral anticoagulants, and even statins affect recanalization in both the stasis and stenosis model with respect to thrombus weight and volume, inflammatory cells and MMPs, cytokines and chemokines, and recanalization of thrombus.

J. D. Raffetto, MD, FACS, FSVM

The soluble urokinase plasminogen activator receptor and its fragments in venous ulcers

Ahmad A, Saha P, Evans C, et al (St Thomas' Hosp, London, UK; et al)

J Vasc Surg Venous Lymphat Disord 3:190-197, 2015

Objective.—Activation of proteolytic mechanisms at the cell surface through the activity of urokinase-type plasminogen activator (uPA) bound to its receptor, uPAR, is an important process in wound healing. The soluble forms of uPAR (suPAR and its fragments I, II, and III) have nonproteolytic functions that include chemotaxis, adhesion, and proliferation, which also have a role in wound healing. The aim of this study was to determine whether suPAR and its cleaved fragments are present in venous ulcers and whether their levels are associated with healing.

Methods.—Ulcer exudates were collected from patients with venous leg ulcers (n = 30). Healing was defined as complete re-epithelialization within 6 months of compression therapy. Time-resolved fluorescence immunoassays were validated for quantification of suPAR and its fragments in ulcer exudates. The effect of exudates on keratinocyte migration was analyzed by an in vitro scratch assay.

Results.—Ulcer exudates from patients who healed (n = 9) had approximately threefold higher levels of intact suPAR (P =.005), twofold higher levels of suPARI (P =.03), and approximately threefold higher levels suPARII-III (P < .0001) compared with nonhealers (n = 21). Exudate from healing ulcers stimulated keratinocyte migration (P =.02), whereas depletion of suPAR from exudates resulted in cell apoptosis.

Conclusions.—We conclude that suPAR and its fragments are present in the environs of venous ulcers and may act as indicators of the propensity of venous ulcers to heal, with suPARII-III being the best discriminator. We speculate that suPAR and its fragments may have a role in the maintenance of an optimal ulcer-healing environment.

Clinical Relevance.—The mechanisms that regulate venous ulcer healing are still not clear, and this may be reflected in lack of ulcer healing in a significant proportion of patients treated with conventional compression therapy. Urokinase plasminogen activator (uPA) and its receptor (uPAR) are present in environs of venous ulcers, and the soluble forms of uPAR are thought to be important in wound healing. Little is known with regard to the presence of these soluble forms in the environs of venous ulcers. This study examines the levels of the soluble uPAR fragments in ulcer exudates and their potential role in ulcer healing.

▶ Venous leg ulcer (VLU) pathophysiology is complex. Further understanding of biomolecular events is important in understanding disease process and to determine possible targets for therapeutic intervention. The urokinase-type plasminogen activator (uPA) and its receptor (uPAR) have both proteolytic and nonproteolytic (cell chemotaxis, migration, adhesion, and proliferation) functions. The latter are carried out by cleavage-soluble fragments of the activated uPAR in particular uPAR fragments II and III (suPARII-III). This is an interesting well-designed study that assess healing VLU and nonhealing VLU and the suPAR fragments analyzed in the wound fluid. The important findings from this study were that suPAR and its fragments were significantly increased in the patients with healed VLU; migration of keratinocytes was significantly increased in healed VLU wound fluid; and, very interestingly, depletion of suPAR and its fragments from the wound fluid from healers (to assess whether suPAR fragments were important in promoting cell migration), caused significant decrease in keratinocyte migration, as well as cell death by apoptosis with an increase in annexin V. This study has shown that suPAR fragments suPARI and suPARII-III, with no known proteolytic activity, are present within the environment of venous ulcers and that the levels of these fragments at presentation (in particular, suPARII-III) may be informative of an ulcer that subsequently heals. suPAR and its fragments could promote cell survival, providing a putative mechanism through which these fragments might promote healing in the environs of a chronic wound. Future studies will be required to determine the mechanism of suPAR in promoting VLU wound healing, and, if possible, therapeutic intervention in the suPAR pathway for VLU that are difficult to heal.

J. D. Raffetto, MD, FACS, FSVM

2 Epidemiology

Leg Ischemia

Association between gender and outcomes of lower extremity peripheral vascular interventions

Ferranti KM, for the Vascular Study Group of New England (Penn State Hershey Med Ctr, PA; et al)

J Vasc Surg 62:990-997, 2015

Objective.—The purpose of this study was to evaluate the association of gender with outcomes of peripheral vascular intervention (PVI) for intermittent claudication and critical limb ischemia (CLI).

Methods.—We reviewed 3338 patients (1316 [39%] women) undergoing PVI for claudication (1892; 57%) or CLI (1446; 43%) in the Vascular Study Group of New England from January 2010 to June 2012. Kaplan-Meier analysis, stratified by indication, was used to assess relationships between gender and the main outcome measures of major amputation, reintervention, and survival during the first year.

Results.—Indications for PVI included claudication (n = 719 [38%] vs n = 1173 [62%]) and CLI (n = 597 [41%] vs n = 849 [59%]) in women and men, respectively ($P = .0028$). Women were older (69 vs 66 mean years; $P < .00001$), with less diabetes (43% vs 49%; $P = .01$), renal insufficiency (4.6% vs 7.3%; $P = .0029$), coronary artery disease (28% vs 35%; $P < .00001$), smoking (76% vs 86%; $P = .01$), and statin use (60% vs 64%; $P = .0058$). Technical success (95% vs 94%; $P = .11$), vascular injury (1.3% vs 1.0%; $P = .82$), and distal embolization (1.6% vs 1.3%; $P = .46$) were similar. Higher rates of hematoma (7.1% vs 3.4%; $P \leq .0001$) and access site occlusion (0.91% vs 0.24%; $P = .0085$) were observed in women compared with men. There were no differences in major amputation (0.6% vs 0.6%; $P = .81$) or mortality (2.1% vs 1.5%; $P = .20$) rates at 30 days between women and men. Reinterventions (surgical and percutaneous) were similar between genders for claudicants (log-rank test, $P = .75$) and CLI patients (log-rank test, $P = .93$). Major amputation rates during the first year were not different for women and men and with claudication (log-rank test, $P < .55$) or CLI (log-rank test, $P < .23$). One-year survival was not different between women and men with claudication (95% vs 96%; $P = .19$) or CLI (77% vs 79%; $P = .35$).

TABLE 1.—Patient Characteristics According to Gender

Variable	Women (n = 1316), No. (%)	Men (n = 2022), No. (%)	*P* Value[a]
Nonwhite race	110 (8.4)	143 (7.1)	.17
Age, mean years	69 (12.0)	66 (10.7)	
<60	301 (22.9)	534 (26.4)	<.001
60-70	335 (25.5)	691 (34.2)	
70-80	386 (29.3)	539 (26.7)	
>80	294 (22.3)	258 (12.8)	
Preoperative housing			
Home	1259 (95.7)	1959 (97.0)	.045
Skilled nursing facility	57 (4.3)	61 (3.0)	
Ambulatory status			
Independent	1038 (79.1)	1687 (83.5)	.0016
Assisted	211 (16.1)	238 (11.8)	
Wheelchair/bedridden	64 (4.9)	95 (4.7)	
Smoking status			
Never smoker	304 (23.1)	276 (13.7)	<.00001
Prior smokers	532 (40.5)	964 (47.7)	
Current smokers	479 (36.4)	781 (38.6)	
Hypertension	1136 (86.3)	1763 (87.2)	.45
Diabetes			
Nondiabetic	751 (57.1)	1034 (51.1)	.004
Non-insulin dependent	261 (19.8)	457 (22.6)	
Insulin dependent	304 (23.1)	531 (26.3)	
COPD	324 (24.6)	420 (20.8)	.007
Coronary artery disease	365 (27.7)	710 (35.1)	<.00001
Congestive heart failure	201 (15.3)	291 (14.4)	.49
Renal function			
Creatinine ≤ 1.78 mg/dL	1175 (95.4)	1736 (92.7)	.0029
Creatinine > 1.78 mg/dL	57 (4.6)	136 (7.3)	
Dialysis	71 (5.4)	115 (5.7)	.72
BMI			
<20	134 (10.5)	81 (4.1)	.08
20-29.9	709 (55.8)	1259 (64.4)	
≥30	428 (33.7)	615 (31.5)	
Indication			
Claudication	719 (54.6)	1173 (58.0)	.0028
CLI, rest pain	181 (13.8)	201 (10.0)	
CLI, tissue loss	416 (31.6)	648 (32.0)	
Prior PVI	334 (25.4)	551 (27.3)	.23
Prior LEB	196 (14.9)	374 (18.5)	.0069
Prior major amputation	56 (4.3)	101 (5.0)	.32
Preoperative medications			
Antiplatelet agent	1068 (81.2)	1686 (83.4)	.098
Anticoagulation	96 (7.3)	186 (9.2)	.055
Statin	786 (59.8)	1303 (64.5)	.0058
Beta-blocker	913 (69.4)	1520 (75.2)	.00023
Urgency			
Elective	1128 (85.8)	1721 (85.2)	.80
Urgent	181 (13.8)	288 (14.3)	
Emergent	6 (0.5)	12 (0.6)	

BMI, Body mass index; *CLI*, critical limb ischemia; *COPD*, chronic obstructive pulmonary disease; *LEB*, infrainguinal lower extremity bypass; *PVI*, peripheral vascular intervention.

[a]*P* value by χ^2 test or Kruskal-Wallis test.

(Reprinted from Ferranti KM, for the Vascular Study Group of New England. Association between gender and outcomes of lower extremity peripheral vascular interventions. *J Vasc Surg*. 2015;62:990-997, with permission from the Society for Vascular Surgery.)

Conclusions.—Whereas we observed higher rates of access site complications including hematoma and occlusion in women, we found no other evidence for gender disparity in reinterventions, major amputation, or survival rates after PVI for patients with claudication or CLI. (Table 1)

▶ Peripheral artery disease (PAD) gender disparities are a hot topic. Their etiology is poorly understood, and lack of a mechanistic explanation makes eliminating them a daunting challenge. This study from the Vascular Study Group of New England (VSGNE) observed that gender-based disparities related to lower extremity arterial intervention are primarily limited to adverse procedure-related events, the majority of which were access-site related (including access site hematoma and access vessel thrombosis). In contrast, longer term treatment outcomes (including amputation, repeat intervention, and survival) were not significantly different between men and women. Although these results should be considered encouraging in terms of outcomes other than procedure-related adverse events, it is important to avoid interpreting the absence of gender-based disparities outside the perioperative period within this analysis as confirmation that none exist. It is important to realize that all of the participants in this registry study were diagnosed with PAD, seen by a vascular specialist, and subsequently underwent a revascularization procedure. The cohort therefore represents the tip of the gender-disparity iceberg of patients who were diagnosed and received appropriate care.

Women with PAD generally present with more advanced disease later in life.[1] These observations in combination suggest that awareness of PAD among women is lacking in terms of screening timely diagnosis and related implementation of appropriate risk reduction pharmacotherapy. These notions are supported by the baseline demographic and clinical data in this analysis, which demonstrated that women were generally older at the time of presentation and had a lower prevalence of statin therapy than men (Table 1). Results from this study suggest that appropriate targets for initiatives aimed at reducing gender-based PAD disparities may include appropriate screening and risk reduction pharmacotherapy in addition to identification of specific technical modifications to endovascular procedures to decrease access site complications.

M. Corriere, MD, MS

Reference

1. Hirsch AT, Allison MA, Gomes AS, et al. on Behalf of the American Heart Association Council on Peripheral Vascular Disease, Council on Cardiovascular Nursing, Council on Cardiovascular Radiology and Intervention, Council on Cardiovascular Surgery and Anesthesia, Council on Clinical Cardiology. A call to action: women and peripheral artery disease: a scientific statement from the American Heart Association. *Circulation*. 2012;125:1449-1472.

The effect of demographic factors and lesion severity on iliac stent patency

Roach AN, Larion S, Ahanchi SS, et al (Eastern Virginia Med School, Norfolk)
J Vasc Surg 62:645-653, 2015

Objective.—The aim of our study was to perform a large multivariate analysis to identify demographic, anatomic, or procedural factors that affect iliac artery stent primary patency (PP).

Methods.—Patients receiving iliac stents from 2007 to 2013 were retrospectively reviewed. Univariate analysis assessed cohort characteristics and their effect on PP. Variables considered significant ($P < .05$) were brought forward in the multivariate analysis.

Results.—A total of 213 patients underwent primary iliac artery stenting, and 307 limbs were analyzed. The average age was 66 years (range, 38-93 years), 54% were male, and 55% were Caucasian. Indications for procedure were claudication in 68%, rest pain in 20%, and tissue loss in 12%. All TransAtlantic Inter-Society Consensus for the Management of Peripheral Arterial Disease (TASC) II classifications were included: 51% TASC II A, 25% TASC II B, 13% TASC II C, and 11% TASC II D. The treated anatomic locations were 27% isolated external iliac artery (EIA), 56% isolated common iliac artery, and 17% combined common iliac artery and EIA. Multivariate analysis found three factors were correlated with decreased PP: non-Caucasian race (hazard ratio [HR], 1.84; 95% confidence interval [CI], 1.08-3.13; $P = .025$), younger age (HR, 1.04; 95% CI, 1.01-1.08; $P = .006$), and presence of EIA occlusion (HR, 2.02; 95% CI, 1.05-3.89; $P = .036$). Overall, Kaplan-Meier analysis at 1 and 3 years revealed a PP of 86% and 53%, assisted PP of 98% and 89%, and secondary patency of 99% of 98%. Kaplan-Meier analysis showed PP at 1 year for was 91% Caucasian patients vs 77% for non-Caucasian ($P = .001$). PP was 75% in patients aged <60 years, 86% in patients aged 60-70 years, and 96% in patients aged >70 years, with a significant difference between all groups ($P < .001$). PP was significantly different for those with and without EIA occlusion ($P = .002$), with 1-year PP of 71% and 88%, respectively.

Conclusions.—In our experience with a large number of iliac interventions, younger age, non-Caucasian race, and EIA occlusion were strong predictors for loss of PP (Fig 1).

▶ This retrospective review of 307 consecutive stented iliac arteries identified external iliac artery occlusion, younger age, and non-Caucasian race as risk factors for loss of primary iliac stent patency (Fig 1). The authors have been thorough in their inclusion of demographic and anatomic factors; lesion severity has been classified by the 2007 TASC II classification system.[1] Interestingly, a large proportion of patients were female (46%) and not surprisingly the majority of patients were treated for claudication and TASC A disease. Hybrid cases were included and in total 35% of patients underwent some form of infra-inguinal intervention. Intra- and postprocedural complications were low ,and primary patency rates at 1 year appear on par with published series. As a retrospective

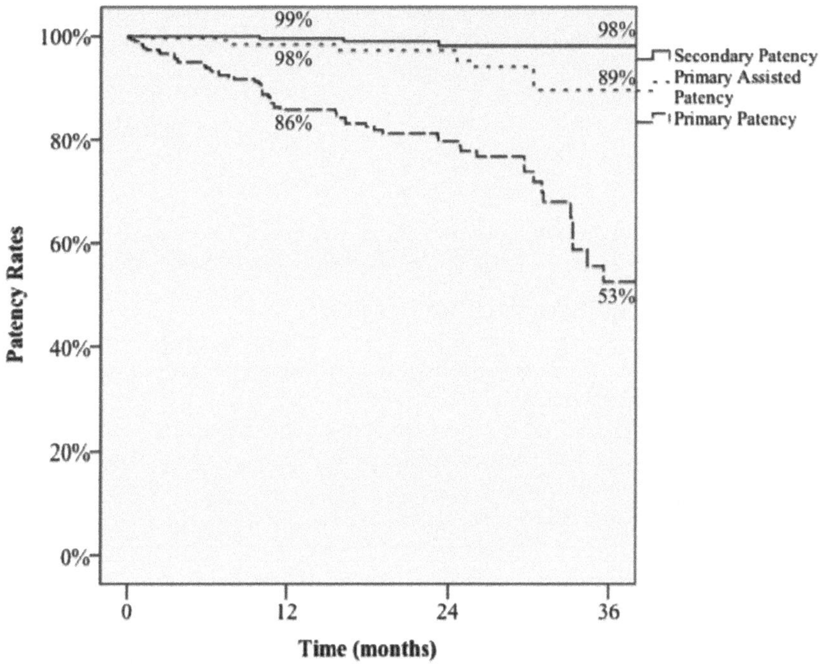

PP	306	193	90	16
PAP	286	202	99	24
SP	291	210	102	30

FIGURE 1.—Kaplan-Meier curves show rates of primary patency (PP), primary assisted patency (PAP), and secondary patency (SP) in the study cohort. (Reprinted from Roach AN, Larion S, Ahanchi SS, et al. The effect of demographic factors and lesion severity on iliac stent patency. *J Vasc Surg.* 2015;62:645-653, with permission from the Society for Vascular Surgery.)

study, lesion length could not be reliably gathered and the indication for stenting, specifically in the external iliac artery, and utilization of covered versus bare metals stents is not further distinguished. Additionally, although postoperative antiplatelet therapy is endorsed for all patients, the details of such therapy are not elaborated on. Finally, almost one-quarter of patients were lost to follow-up. Despite these study limitations, the authors bring to point a critical warning for the young patient with PAD who remains a challenge to the vascular specialist. Although interventions for lifestyle-limiting claudication may return a patient to the workforce and dramatically improve quality of life, long-term durability of both open and endovascular interventions remain limited. Because younger age predicts adverse endovascular outcomes, the selection of an "endo-first" approach for these patients (with multiple planned endovascular reinterventions to maintain patency) versus an open intervention remains debatable. More importantly, the decision to revascularize these patients should be made carefully, with clear patient education and counseling, and only after maximum medical therapy has been exhausted and patients have demonstrated a commitment to lifestyle modification (including tobacco abstinence).

D. Coleman, MD

Reference

1. Norgren L, Hiatt WR, Dormandy JA, et al. Inter-societal consensus for the management of peripheral artery disease (TASCII). *J Vasc Surg*. 2007;45:S5-S67.

Carotid and Cerebrovascular Disease

Race as a predictor of delay from diagnosis to endarterectomy in clinically significant carotid stenosis

Wise ES, Ladner TR, Song J, et al (Vanderbilt Univ Med Ctr, Nashville, TN; Vanderbilt Univ School of Medicine, Nashville, TN; Univ of Tennessee Health Sciences Ctr, Memphis)

J Vasc Surg 62:49-56, 2015

Objective.—Prompt carotid endarterectomy (CEA) in clinically significant carotid stenosis is important in the prevention of neurologic sequelae. The greatest benefit from surgery is obtained by prompt revascularization on diagnosis. It has been demonstrated that black patients both receive CEA less frequently than white patients do and experience worse postoperative outcomes. We sought to test our hypothesis that black race is an independent risk factor for a prolonged time from sonographic diagnosis of carotid stenosis warranting surgery to the day of operation (TDO).

Methods.—From 1998 to 2013 at a single institution, 166 CEA patients were retrospectively reviewed using Synthetic Derivative, a de-identified electronic medical record. Factors potentially affecting TDO, including demographics, preoperative cardiac stress testing, degree of stenosis, smoking status, and comorbidities, were noted. Multivariate analysis was performed on variables that trended with prolonged TDO on univariate analysis ($P < .10$) to determine independent ($P < .05$) predictors of TDO. Subgroup analyses were further performed on the symptomatic and asymptomatic stenosis cohorts.

Results.—There were 32 black patients and 134 white patients studied; the mean TDO was 78 ± 17 days vs 33 ± 3 days, respectively ($P < .001$). In addition to the need for preoperative cardiac stress testing, black race was the only variable that demonstrated a trend with ($P < .10$) or was an independent risk factor for ($P < .05$) prolonged TDO among all patients (B = 42 days; $P < .001$) and within the symptomatic (B = 35 days; $P = .08$) and asymptomatic (B = 35 days; $P = .003$) cohorts. On Kaplan-Meier analysis, black patients in each stratum of symptomatology (all, symptomatic, and asymptomatic patients) experienced prolonged TDO (log-rank, $P < .03$ for all three groups).

Conclusions.—Black race is a risk factor for a temporal delay in CEA for carotid stenosis. Awareness of this disparity may help surgeons avoid undesirable delays in operation for their black patients.

▶ Research into racial disparities in outcomes after carotid endarterectomy in a moderate number of retrospective studies has consistently shown a trend toward a higher rate of postoperative complications in black patients compared with white patients. A 2013 review of data involving more than 30 000 patients from the National Surgery Quality Improvement Program (NSQIP) by Brown et al,[1] cited by the authors of this study, revealed a significantly higher rate of postoperative stroke, 30-day mortality, and cardiac arrest in black patients. This retrospective study uses data from a single-center database to look specifically at the delay in surgical intervention (endarterectomy) from the time of patients' preoperative imaging that prompted the surgeon to intervene (duplex ultrasonography in all cases). Only patients who were identified as black or white race were included because there were too few numbers of other minority populations to make any statistically meaningful comparison. The patients were also stratified into symptomatic and asymptomatic subgroups. There were 166 cases randomly sampled from the database, of which the ratio of white to black patients was about 4 to 1.

The results showed a significantly longer time from sonographic diagnosis to operation for black patients overall at around 45 days difference, which was also significant when broken down into the symptomatic and asymptomatic subgroups. Although this certainly does not demonstrate a cause-and-effect relationship between delay in treatment to higher postoperative morbidity and mortality, it is an interesting trend for consideration. Previous studies have noted a higher incidence of preoperative cardiopulmonary comorbidities in black patients before carotid surgery, which could explain both a delay in time to treatment after diagnosis and a higher rate of postoperative complications. There was no difference in this study in preoperative comorbidities between white and black patients, perhaps due to the small sample size of the study, other than black patients were significantly more likely to undergo preoperative cardiac stress testing. Differences in socioeconomic factors have also been speculated to play a role in the disparity in care for black patients, but this has been challenged by several other studies as well.

M. Williams, MD

Reference

1. Brown HA, Sullivan MC, Gusberg RG, Dardik A, Sosa JA, Indes JE. Race as a predictor of morbidity, mortality, and neurologic events after carotid endarterectomy. *J Vasc Surg.* 2013;57:1325-1330.

Racial/Ethnic Variation in Carotid Artery Revascularization Utilization and Outcomes: Analysis From the National Cardiovascular Data Registry

Wayangankar SA, Kennedy KF, Aronow HD, et al (Cleveland Clinic Foundation, OH; St. Luke's Hosp, Kansas City, MO; Michigan Heart and Vascular Inst, Ypsilanti; et al)

Stroke 46:1525-1532, 2015

Background and Purpose.—It is not known whether racial or ethnic disparities observed with other revascularization procedures are also seen with carotid artery stenting (CAS) and endarterectomy (CEA).

Methods.—We compared the utilization and outcomes of CAS and CEA across racial/ethnic groups within the CARE Registry between May 2007 and December 2012.

Results.—Between 2007 and 2012, of the 13 129 patients who underwent CAS, majority were non-Hispanic whites (89.3%), followed by blacks (4.4%), Hispanics (4.3%), and other groups (2.0%). A similar distribution was observed among the 10 953 patients undergoing CEA (non-Hispanic whites, 92.6%; blacks, 3.5%; Hispanics, 2.8%; and other groups, 1.1%). During this time period, a trend toward proportionate increase in CAS utilization was observed in non-Hispanic whites and other groups, whereas the opposite was observed among Hispanics and blacks. This trend persisted even when hospitals performing both CAS and CEA were exclusively analyzed. Adherence to antiplatelet and statin therapy was significantly lower among blacks post CEA. In-hospital major adverse cardiac and cerebrovascular events remained comparable across groups post CAS and CEA. At 30 days, the incidence of stroke (7.2%) and major adverse cardiac and cerebrovascular events (8.8%) was higher among blacks post CEA ($P < 0.05$), after risk adjustment.

Conclusion.—During the study period, utilization of CAS and CEA was highest among non-Hispanic whites. There was a trend toward increased CAS utilization over time among non-Hispanic whites and other groups, and a trend toward increased CEA utilization among Hispanics and blacks. In-hospital major adverse cardiac and cerebrovascular events remained comparable between groups, whereas 30-day major adverse cardiac and cerebrovascular events were significantly higher in blacks.

▶ Several studies have shown racial and ethnic disparity in utilization of newer technology and postprocedural, in-hospital outcomes, but none have looked at the disparity of prescriptions for the postoperative period or postdischarge outcomes in patients undergoing carotid revascularization. The authors hypothesized that there are significant racial and ethnic disparities in the utilization, management, and outcomes associated with carotid revascularization.

The CARE Registry is the result of a joint effort by major medical societies and is a comprehensive national registry of patients undergoing both carotid artery stenting (CAS) and carotid endarterectomy (CEA). Using the CARE Registry in this study, the authors identified 13129 patients who underwent CAS between May 2005 and December 2012 with the following breakdown:

89.3% non-Hispanic whites, 4.4% blacks, 4.3% Hispanics, and 2.0% other racial groups (OG). There were 10 953 patients who underwent CEA during the same time period with the following breakdown: 92.6% non-Hispanic whites, 3.5% blacks, 2.8% Hispanics, and 1.1% OG. The results demonstrated a significant trend toward utilization of CAS in non-Hispanic whites and OG, with a proportionate increase in CEA utilization in blacks and Hispanics. Medication prescriptions were the same across all groups undergoing CAS, but in the CEA patients, blacks and Hispanics saw a lower rate of prescriptions for aspirin compared with whites and OG, and whites and blacks saw a lower rate of prescriptions for statins compared with Hispanics and OG. Finally, although there was no difference in in-hospital outcomes across groups and outcomes at 30 days in the CAS group, in the CEA group at 30 days, stroke and major adverse cardiac and cerebrovascular events were significantly higher among blacks compared with whites, Hispanics, and OG.

These disparate results and lack of uniform protocols to ensure patients from all ethnic groups are receiving the proper medications postoperatively are clearly disturbing, and patients from all races and ethnicities are affected. Relatively speaking, carotid artery disease is one of the most well understood disease processes in all of vascular surgery in terms of medical management. Unfortunately, this study, like many others, points out the blatant disregard for practicing evidence-based medicine, a trend that will hopefully be reversed as more articles likes this one are published.

B. Peterson, MD, FACS

Aortic Disease

A new metric for centralization of ruptured abdominal aortic aneurysm repair in large territories

Nault P, Brisson-Tessier C, Hamel D, et al (McGill Univ, Montreal, Canada; Institut national de Santé publique du Québec (INSPQ), Canada; et al)

J Vasc Surg 62:862-867, 2015

Objective.—This study proposes the DEDE (Door-from-Emergency to Door-to-EVAR [endovascular aneurysm repair]) time as a new metric for ruptured abdominal aortic aneurysm (RAAA) delay time to surgery, permitting coherent centralization in large territories. It demonstrates how the DEDE time can be applied, using data from the province of Quebec, and looks at its potential effect on 30-day mortality.

Methods.—We used the Quebec Integrated Chronic Disease Surveillance System (QICDSS), the linkage of five health administrative databases, to build a retrospective cohort of RAAA patients repaired operatively between April 1, 2006, and March 31, 2013. A validated algorithm was used to identify open surgical repair (OSR) and EVAR patients. Hospitals performing these operations were further characterized according to their location, volume of RAAA, types of surgeries (OSR vs EVAR), and surgeon's volume. Logistic and log-binomial regression analyses identified the risk of 30-day mortality with age, sex, hospital volume, and surgical groups as variables. Using the DEDE 90 metric and the attributable fraction, we projected how centralization and increasing the number of EVAR would affect the 30-day mortality.

Results.—Among patients aged ≥65 years, 895 RAAAs were identified. OSR was performed in 839 patients (93.7%) and EVAR in 56 (6.3%). The overall 30-day mortality was 34.4%, and more specifically, was 35.5% for OSR compared with 17.9% for EVAR ($P = .0046$). RAAAs were treated in 39 hospitals, including 16 centers averaging less than one RAAA repair per year. Low-volume (39.4%) vs high-volume centers (32.5%) had similar 30-day mortality ($P = .2198$). In the multivariate analysis, the relative risk for OSR was 1.95 ($P = .0211$) and was not significant for hospital volume. Applying the DEDE 90 metric and increasing access to EVAR to 50% of patients, the overall 30-day mortality would be 26.8%.

Conclusions.—DEDE 90 is a new metric for a coherent centralization model, particularly in large territories, where transport time is crucial. Increasing access to EVAR performed in high-volume centers, with consideration to transport time, could improve the 30-day mortality after a RAAA repair.

▶ An extensive review by Veith et al in 2010 suggested that endovascular aneurysm repair (EVAR) is a superior method for repair of ruptured abdominal aortic aneurysms (RAAAs) in anatomically suitable patients.[1] Our own data, referenced in this article, support this notion with eerily similar 30-day mortality statistics.[2] These authors sought to describe RAAA repair in the Canadian Province of Quebec with a view toward centralizing care in high-volume centers as a gold standard, thereby increasing access to EVAR despite geographic constraints.

Eight hundred ninety-five RAAA patients were identified in a national data set. Open repair was performed in 93.7% (n = 839) and EVAR in only 6.3% (n = 56). The overall 30-day mortality rate was respectable at only 34.4% (35.5% for open vs 17.9% for EVAR). The authors suggest that a new metric titled DEDE 90 (Door-from-Emergency to Door-to-EVAR less than 90 minutes) be used to create a standard by which all rAAA outcomes are measured. Age > 80 years, early study time period, and low surgeon volume (< 5 cases) were the only factors associated with a higher 30-day mortality suggesting that higher volume centers would have better outcomes.

I have a few criticisms of this article. First, I believe there to be a huge selection bias in the sample patient population. The authors do not report those patients who died in transport nor those who were not offered therapy and allowed to die on "comfort care." If a 90-minute metric is going to be evaluated, surely all patients should be included in the ultimate mortality statistic and this would clearly be higher in each cohort.

Second, Canada has a National Healthcare System, and it is widely known that there exists a quota for the number of medical devices that can be implanted by a given institution based on case volume. This leads to significant issues regarding the stocking of adequate inventory of aortic stent grafts to be able to address the needs of every patient with a rAAA. One cannot offer EVAR to more patients, even when those patients arrive to a high-volume center within 90 minutes, if one does not have a medical device to implant. A 6% rate of EVAR in 2016 is ridiculously low in my mind.

The authors indeed are to be congratulated, however, for attempting to lower the already impressive mortality rate by coming into the new age of endovascular first strategies in this extremely sick patient population. The DEDE 90 metric might help push the mortality lower!

B. W. Starnes, MD

References

1. Veith FJ, Powell JT, Hinchliffe RJ. Is a randomized trial necessary to determine whether endovascular repair is the preferred management strategy in patients with ruptured abdominal aortic aneurysms? *J Vasc Surg*. 2010;52:1087-1093.
2. Starnes BW, Quiroga E, Hutter C, et al. Management of ruptured abdominal aortic aneurysm in the endovascular era. *J Vasc Surg*. 2010;51:9-17.

A ruptured abdominal aortic aneurysm that requires preoperative cardiopulmonary resuscitation is not necessarily lethal

Broos PPHL, 't Mannetje YW, Loos MJA, et al (Catharina Hosp, Eindhoven, The Netherlands; Máxima Med Ctr, Veldhoven, The Netherlands; et al)
J Vasc Surg 63:49-54, 2016

Objective.—A ruptured abdominal aortic aneurysm (RAAA) is associated with a high mortality rate. If cardiopulmonary resuscitation (CPR) is required before surgical repair, mortality rates are said to approach 100%. The aim of this multicenter, retrospective study was to study outcome in RAAA patients who required CPR before a surgical (endovascular or open) repair (CPR group). RAAA patients who did not need CPR served as controls (non-CPR group).

Methods.—Over a 5-year time period, demographic and clinical characteristics and specifics of preoperative CPR if necessary were studied in all patients who were treated for a RAAA in three large, nonacademic hospitals.

Results.—A total of 199 consecutive RAAA patients were available for analysis; 176 patients were surgically treated. Thirteen of these 176 patients (7.4%) needed CPR, and 163 (92.6%) did not. A 38.5% (5 of 13) survival rate was observed in the CPR group. Thirty-day mortality was almost three times greater in the CPR group compared with the non-CPR group (61.5% vs 22.7%; $P = .005$). Both CPR patients who received endovascular aortic repair survived. In contrast, survival in 11 CPR patients who underwent open RAAA repair was 27% (3 of 11; $P = .128$). A trend for higher Hardman index was found in patients who received CPR compared with patients who did not receive CPR ($P = .052$). The 30-day mortality in patients with a 0, 1, 2, or 3 Hardman index was 16.1%, 31.0%, 37.9%, and 33.3%, respectively ($P = .093$).

TABLE 3.—Overview of Patient Characteristics, Perioperative Status, and Follow-up of Patients in the Cardiopulmonary Resuscitation (*CPR*) Group

Patient	Sex	Age, Years	CPR Location	CPR Duration, Minutes	Adrenalin,[a] mg	Defibrillation	Performed by	Narrative	Surgery	Survival, day	Status
1	F	76	ED/OT	30	NR	NR	Doctor	RR not measurable; regained blood pressure after aortic clamping.	OR	20	Dead
2	M	66	Ward/OT	20	1	NR	Doctor	CPR from ward to OT. Output in OT, RR 68/45. 8 Times ECC, 900 cc CellSaver, 6 times FFP, pH 6.98, lactate 9.9 mmol/L.	OR	2092	Alive
3	M	69	ED/OT	5 + 25	16.3	Twice	Doctor	Regained output in ED after 5 minutes. In OT again arrhythmia. CPR ceased after 25 minutes. 15 times ECC, 4 times FFP, 3.3 mg adrenaline, pH 6.8.	OR	0	Dead
4	M	79	Home	5	None	NR	Bystander	Regained output when ambulance arrived with RR 50/30. 6 Times ECC, twice FFP, 4 times colloid, pH 7.32, lactate 2.2 mmol/L.	OR	1939	Alive
5	M	78	Ward	5	None	NR	Nurse	CPR started by nurse. RR 90/40. 12 Times ECC, twice thrombocytes, 4 times FFP, pH 6.89, lactate 11.5 mmol/L.	OR	1	Dead
6	M	85	Ambulance	NR	None	Once	Paramedic	Ventricular tachycardia for which defibrillation was used. Regained output with RR 70/60. 4 Times ECC, pH 7.07, lactate 11.5 mmol/L.	EVAR	1631	Alive
7	M	76	ED	5	NR	NR	NR	Regained output in ED, remained perioperative hemodynamically unstable, RR 86/50. pH 7.21, lactate 10.8 mmol/L.	OR	21	Dead
8	M	78	ED/OT	20 + 10	3	NR	Doctor	20 minutes CPR in ED. In OT after aortic clamping 10 minutes CPR, unsuccessful. 5 Times ECC.	OR	0	Dead
9	M	83	ED	30	NR	NR	Doctor	Cardiac arrest after CTA. 11 Times ECC, 4 times FFP, pH 7.18, lactate 6.6 mmol/L.	OR	9	Dead
10	M	82	Home/ ambulance	15	None	NR	Bystander	Rib fractures with tension pneumothorax. Regained output in ambulance. 10 Times ECC, 4 time FFP, once thrombocytes, pH 7.12, lactate 7.4 mmol/L.	OR	1038	Alive
11	F	84	Home/OT	5 + 15	3	NR	Paramedic	Regained consciousness in ambulance. RR 80/64. In again OT 15 minutes CPR, however, treatment stopped because of a DNR code.	OR	0	Dead
12	M	61	ED	30	5	NR	Doctor	After CTA cardiac arrest. Adrenaline, ECC and FFPs administered, amounts unknown.	OR	0	Dead
13	M	63	ED	20	5.5	Three times	Doctor	CPR in CT room, patient regained consciousness in OT. 3 Times ECC, pH 6.90, lactate 13 mmol/L.	EVAR	432	Alive

CT, Computed tomography; *CTA*, computed tomography angiography; *DNR*, do not resuscitate; *ECC*, erythrocyte concentrate; *ED*, emergency department; *EVAR*, endovascular aortic repair; *F*, female; *FFP*, fresh frozen plasma; *M*, male; *NR*, not reported; *OR*, open repair; *OT*, operating theater; *RR*, lowest reported blood pressure.

Lactate, normal level <1.3 mmol/L; pH normal range, 7.35-7.45.

[a]Administration during CPR and intraoperative support.

Reprinted from Broos PPHL, 't Mannetje YW, Loos MJA, et al. A ruptured abdominal aortic aneurysm that requires preoperative cardiopulmonary resuscitation is not necessarily lethal. *J Vasc Surg*. 2016;63:49-54, with permission from the Society for Vascular Surgery.

Conclusions.—An RAAA that requires preoperative CPR is not necessarily a lethal combination. Patient selection must be tailored before surgery is denied (Table 3).

▶ Patients with a ruptured abdominal aortic aneurysm (RAAA) continue to be a heterogeneous group in published studies. One of the most predictable factors of mortality in these patients is the history of cardiopulmonary resuscitation before repair. The authors of this study identified 13 patients out of their cohort of 176 patients with RAAA that had undergone cardiopulmonary resuscitation (CPR) before attempted repair. Five of the 13 patients (38.5%) undergoing CPR survived and the 2 patients who underwent endovascular repair survived. The indication and location of CPR initiation is variable (Table 3). It is remarkable that 5 patients survived, and the fact that both of the endovascularly treated patients survived indicates we still have much to learn about RAAA. Of these 13 patients, 3 underwent CPR after undergoing a computed tomography, and the vital signs of the others were variable after CPR, indicating that these patients may have been severely hypotensive. Centers that have been successful in implementing RAAA protocols generally tout the concept of "directly to the operating room" and placement of an aortic occlusion balloon and subsequent repair.[1] The ability to repair these RAAAs expeditiously with endovascular techniques or gain rapid proximal control of the aorta may be the reason that the 2 patients survived in this series. In addition, identifying factors that could be predictive of mortality at high-volume centers with modern techniques could obviate the use of outdated modalities such as the Hardman index, which was developed in 1996. In an era where resource utilization and cost containment are a priority we must identify those patients who will likely survive after repair and those patients in which expensive resources are futile.

N. Singh, MD, FACS

Reference

1. Starnes BW, Quiroga E, Hutter C, et al. Management of ruptured abdominal aortic aneurysm in the endovascular era. *J Vasc Surg*. 2009;51:9-18.

Abdominal Aortic Aneurysm Genetic Associations: Mostly False? A Systematic Review and Meta-analysis

Bradley DT, Badger SA, McFarland M, et al (Queen's Univ Belfast, UK; Mater Misericordiae Univ Hosp, Dublin, Ireland; Royal Victoria Hosp, Belfast, UK)
Eur J Vasc Endovasc Surg 51:64-75, 2016

Objective/Background.—Many associations between abdominal aortic aneurysm (AAA) and genetic polymorphisms have been reported. It is unclear which are genuine and which may be caused by type 1 errors, biases, and flexible study design. The objectives of the study were to identify associations supported by current evidence and to investigate the effect of study design on reporting associations.

Methods.—Data sources were MEDLINE, Embase, and Web of Science. Reports were dual-reviewed for relevance and inclusion against predefined criteria (studies of genetic polymorphisms and AAA risk). Study characteristics and data were extracted using an agreed tool and reports assessed for quality. Heterogeneity was assessed using I^2 and fixed- and random-effects meta-analyses were conducted for variants that were reported at least twice, if any had reported an association. Strength of evidence was assessed using a standard guideline.

Results.—Searches identified 467 unique articles, of which 97 were included. Of 97 studies, 63 reported at least one association. Of 92 studies that conducted multiple tests, only 27% corrected their analyses. In total, 263 genes were investigated, and associations were reported in polymorphisms in 87 genes. Associations in *CDKN2BAS, SORT1, LRP1, IL6R, MMP3, AGTR1, ACE,* and *APOA1* were supported by meta-analyses.

Conclusion.—Uncorrected multiple testing and flexible study design (particularly testing many inheritance models and subgroups, and failure to check for Hardy—Weinberg equilibrium) contributed to apparently false associations being reported. Heterogeneity, possibly due to the case mix, geographical, temporal, and environmental variation between different studies, was evident. Polymorphisms in nine genes had strong or moderate support on the basis of the literature at this time. Suggestions are made for improving AAA genetics study design and conduct (Table 4).

► Abdominal aortic aneurysm (AAA) genetic association studies have faced multiple challenges. This is an excellent systematic review and meta-analysis of all genetic studies of AAA published between 1994 and 2014. In total, 263 genes were investigated in candidate gene studies (n = 91), genome-wide association studies (GWAS, n = 4), and genetic risk score (GRS, n = 2) studies. Of these genes, 87 genes were found to be associated with AAA at least once. Table 4 details all the genetic variants with the strength of evidence supporting the association. Meta-analyses strongly supported 6 associations: two were reported in genome-wide studies (*DAB2IP* and *LRP1*), and 4 in candidate gene studies (*9p21/CDKN2BAS, IL6R, LPA,* and *SORT1*). There was moderate evidence for associations with *LDLR, MMP3,* and *AGTR1* polymorphisms. As our interest grows in delineating the role of genetic associations with AAA pathology or the impact on outcomes, the authors offer excellent suggestions for the genetic epidemiology research community to improve the quality of reports in this field. These include prospective registration of etiological studies to avoid flexible post hoc analyses, planning for adequate power, presenting counts and risk estimates for genotypes rather than assuming models of inheritance, checking frequencies in population databases, presenting

TABLE 4.—Assessment of Evidence of Association

Gene	Polymorphism	Amount of Evidence	Replication	Protection From Bias	Overall Assessment
3p21	rs7635818	A	C	C	Weak
9p21	rs10757278	A	A	A	Strong
ACE	rs4646994	A	A	C	Weak
AGTR1	rs5186	A	B	B	Moderate
APOA1	rs964184	A	C	C	Weak
APOE	rs439401	A	C	C	Weak
APOB	rs1367117	A	C	C	Weak
CCR5	rs333	B	C	C	Weak
CRP	rs3091244	A	C	C	Weak
DAB2IP	rs7025486	A	A	A	Strong
ELN	rs2071307	B	C	C	Weak
HLA-A	A2	C	C	C	Weak
HLA-B	B61	C	C	C	Weak
HMOX1	GT(n)	C	C	C	Weak
IL6R	rs7529229	A	A	A	Strong
IL10	rs1800896	B	C	B	Weak
LDLR	rs6511720	A	B	A	Moderate
LPA	rs10455872	A	A	A	Strong
LRP1	rs1466535	A	A	A	Strong
MMP2	rs243865	B	C	B	Weak
MMP3	rs3025058	A	A	B	Moderate
MMP9	rs3918242	B	C	C	Weak
MMP13	rs2252070	C	C	C	Weak
MTHFR1	rs1801133	B	C	C	Weak
NOS3	rs1799983	B	C	B	Weak
PLA2G7	rs16874954	B	C	C	Weak
PHACTR1	rs12526453	A	C	C	Weak
SERPINE1	rs1799889	A	C	C	Weak
SORT1	rs599839	A	A	A	Strong
TGFBR1	rs10819634 rs1571590 rs1626340	A	C	C	Weak
TGFBR2	rs1036095 rs764522	A	C	B	Weak
TIMP1	rs4898	C	C	C	Weak
TIMP2	nt573G/A	C	C	C	Weak
TRIB1	rs2954029	A	C	C	Weak

Reprinted from Bradley DT, Badger SA, McFarland M, et al. Abdominal aortic aneurysm genetic associations: mostly false? A systematic review and meta-analysis. *Eur J Vasc Endovasc Surg.* 2016;51:64-75, with permission from European Society for Vascular Surgery.

analyses of Hardy-Weinberg equilibrium deviation, and correcting for multiple testing.[1,2]

S. Shalhub, MD, MPH, FACS

References

1. Little J, Higgins JP, Ioannidis JP, et al. Strengthening the reporting of genetic association studies (STREGA): an extension of the STROBE statement. *PLoS Med.* 2009;6:e22.
2. Ioannidis JP. Why most published research findings are false. *PLoS Med.* 2005;2:e124.

Geographic disparities in the burden of ruptured and unruptured abdominal aortic aneurysms

Misskey J, Osman M, Kopriva D (Univ of British Columbia, Vancouver, Canada; Saskatchewan Health Quality Council, Saskatoon, Canada; Regina Qu'Appelle Health Region, Canada)

J Vasc Surg 62:1421-1428, 2015

Background.—The province of Saskatchewan presents unique challenges for the care of ruptured abdominal aortic aneurysms (AAAs), including variable access to health care resources and long transportation distances to tertiary vascular care. This study assessed the rates of ruptured and total AAA to determine regional variations within Saskatchewan and ascertain whether there are areas of high AAA prevalence that would possibly benefit from the implementation of a targeted screening program.

Methods.—All diagnoses of AAA from 2001 to 2012 in the province of Saskatchewan were reviewed, with patients grouped by health region of residence. Diagnoses of ruptured and unruptured AAAs were obtained from the Saskatchewan Discharge Abstracts Database, Medical Services Billings Claims data, and Vital Statistics data.

Results.—During the study period, 6163 AAAs were diagnosed. The provincial age-adjusted rate of AAA was 53.0/100,000 person-years (95% confidence interval, 48.8-57.6). The highest age-adjusted rate of AAA was found in the Five Hills Health Region (FHHR), at 63.1/100,000 person-years (95% confidence interval, 57.6-69.0), which was significantly higher than the provincial average ($P < .05$). The rate of ruptured AAA in FHHR was nearly twofold higher than the provincial average (6.0 vs 2.9/100,000 person-years, respectively).

Conclusions.—There are significant geographic variations in the prevalence of AAA in the province of Saskatchewan, with the highest rate of AAA found in the FHHR (Fig 1).

▶ Environmental and genetic factors have been associated with abdominal aortic aneurysms, and the authors of this study identified a geographic variation in their province of Saskatchewan. Although large in total area (251 700 square miles), Saskatchewan has a population of slightly more than 1 million residents, and half of these people live in rural areas without a vascular specialist (Fig 1). Interestingly, the region with the highest average age-adjusted rate of abdominal aortic aneurysm (AAA) was the Five Hills Health Region (FHHR) with a 63.1 per 10000 person-years that was higher than the provincial average and the lowest was in the 3 northern regions. The FHHR was also associated with the highest rate of rupture, thus making it unlikely that the results are from detection bias; there is likely a true high prevalence in this community.

Other studies have identified regions geographic disparity; for example, a study in Sweden identified a higher incidence of AAA in the northern part of the country that was also associated with a higher incidence of coronary heart disease.[1] Identification of areas such as the FHHR could lead to further studies on this population. The FHHR is described as a rural, static, Caucasian

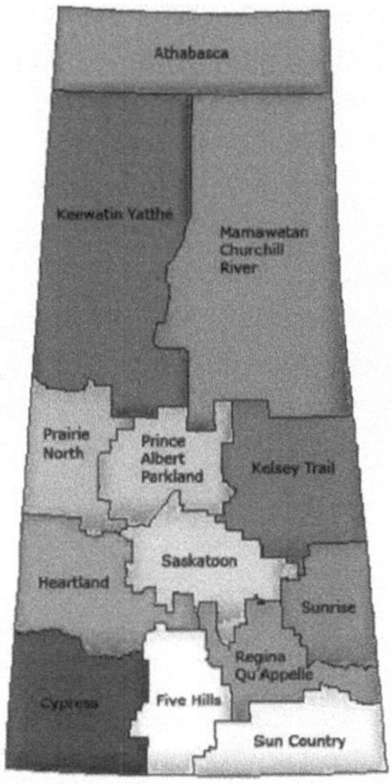

Regional Health Authority	Av. Pop
Regina	249,893.09
Saskatoon	292,557.73
Cypress	43,956.45
Five Hills	54,737.73
Heartland	45,010.55
Kelsey Trail	42,961.45
Sun County	54,243.64
Sunrise	57,846.82
Prince Albert Parkland	77,914.09
Prairie North	72,048.09
Northern Regional Health Authorities	35,579.64
Saskatchewan	1,027,347.91

FIGURE 1.—A map of the province of Saskatchewan shows the 12 Regional Health Authorities (*RHA*). The table shows the average population of each health region during the study period. (Reprinted from Misskey J, Osman M, Kopriva D. Geographic disparities in the burden of ruptured and unruptured abdominal aortic aneurysms. *J Vasc Surg*. 2015;62:1421-1428, with permission from the Society for Vascular Surgery.)

population with a pattern of net outward migration and little inward migration. An area such as this would be ideal to identify potential genetic factors that could contribute to the higher incidence of AAA here.

N. Singh, MD, FACS

Reference

1. Hultgren R, Forsberg J, Alfredsson L, Swedenborg J, Leander K. Regional variation in the incidence of abdominal aortic aneurysm in Sweden. *Br J Surg*. 2012; 99:647-653.

Venous Disease

Screening for Occult Cancer in Unprovoked Venous Thromboembolism

Carrier M, for the SOME Investigators (Ottawa Hosp Res Inst, Canada; et al)
N Engl J Med 373:697-704, 2015

Background.—Venous thromboembolism may be the earliest sign of cancer. Currently, there is a great diversity in practices regarding screening for occult cancer in a person who has an unprovoked venous thromboembolism. We sought to assess the efficacy of a screening strategy for occult cancer that included comprehensive computed tomography (CT) of the abdomen and pelvis in patients who had a first unprovoked venous thromboembolism.

Methods.—We conducted a multicenter, open-label, randomized, controlled trial in Canada. Patients were randomly assigned to undergo limited occult-cancer screening (basic blood testing, chest radiography, and screening for breast, cervical, and prostate cancer) or limited occult-cancer screening in combination with CT. The primary outcome measure was confirmed cancer that was missed by the screening strategy and detected by the end of the 1-year follow-up period.

Results.—Of the 854 patients who underwent randomization, 33 (3.9%) had a new diagnosis of occult cancer between randomization and the 1-year follow-up: 14 of the 431 patients (3.2%) in the limited-screening group and 19 of the 423 patients (4.5%) in the limited-screening-plus-CT group ($P = 0.28$). In the primary outcome analysis, 4 occult cancers (29%) were missed by the limited screening strategy, whereas 5 (26%) were missed by the strategy of limited screening plus CT ($P = 1.0$). There was no significant difference between the two study groups in the mean time to a cancer diagnosis (4.2 months in the limited-screening group and 4.0 months in the limited-screening-plus-CT group, $P = 0.88$) or in cancer-related mortality (1.4% and 0.9%, $P = 0.75$).

Conclusions.—The prevalence of occult cancer was low among patients with a first unprovoked venous thromboembolism. Routine screening with CT of the abdomen and pelvis did not provide a clinically significant benefit. (Funded by the Heart and Stroke Foundation of Canada; SOME ClinicalTrials.gov number, NCT00773448.)

▶ There is a known association of venous thromboembolism and malignancy, but performing malignancy screening upon initial diagnosis of venous thromboembolism has been debated. Based on the observation that unprovoked venous thromboembolism may be the initial sign of malignancy noted in up to 10% in other series, this study showed a lower prevalence of occult cancer in both randomized groups. With limited screening only, the addition of computed tomography scan to the screening algorithm did not add any additional benefit in earlier malignancy diagnosis. It is possible that this lower rate may also reflect a demographic in this study that was at lower risk for cancer. Although initial presentation of unprovoked venous thromboembolism could trigger malignancy screening based on the growing body of evidence, the cost-value equation of who to screen could be improved by applying additional malignancy risk profiling from patient demographic factors, which was not addressed in this study.

M. Passman, MD

3 Vascular Imaging

Carotid and Cerebrovascular

Acoustic shadowing impairs accurate characterization of stenosis in carotid ultrasound examinations

Mohebali J, Patel VI, Romero JM, et al (Harvard Med School, Boston, MA)

J Vasc Surg 62:1236-1244, 2015

Objective.—Duplex ultrasonography (DUS) has been the mainstay for diagnosing carotid artery stenosis and is often the sole diagnostic modality used prior to intervention. Highly calcified plaque, however, results in an acoustic shadow (AcS) that obscures the vessel lumen and inhibits the sonographer's ability to obtain Doppler velocity measurements. It is unknown whether DUS can accurately determine the degree of carotid stenosis in these settings.

Methods.—From July 2012 to December 2013, all patients with AcS on DUS measuring ≥5 mm in the longitudinal axis were cross-referenced with multidetector computed tomographic angiography (MD-CTA) images of the neck to define the study population. After standardizing the MD-CTA windows, percent stenosis was determined by cross-sectional area reduction using two separate previously described methods based on North American Symptomatic Carotid Endarterectomy Trial (NASCET) and European Carotid Surgery Trial (ECST) criteria. DUS waveform parameters in the internal carotid artery near the AcS were then compared with these MD-CTA measurements to determine the accuracy of DUS in characterizing the severity of carotid stenosis.

Results.—During this period, 8517 DUS studies were performed at the Massachusetts General Hospital, 550 of which had AcS, for an incidence of 6.45%. There were 92 lesions with a concomitant MD-CTA; however, seven were excluded because of poor study quality, because ≥6 months had elapsed between DUS and MD-CTA, or because the patient had undergone carotid reconstruction between studies. Of the 85 remaining lesions, DUS characterized 17 as severe (peak systolic velocity [PSV] >250 cm/s), 31 as moderate (PSV = 151-250 cm/s), and 37 as mild (PSV ≤150 cm/s) stenoses using PSV criteria. PSV weakly correlated with CTA-NASCET ($r = 0.361$; $P = .004$) and CTA-ECST ($r = 0.306$; $P = .004$) percent stenosis. Using PSV >250 cm/s as the predictor of >70% stenosis, and a ≥70% cutoff by both CTA-ECST and CTA-NASCET methods as the reference measure,

DUS sensitivity ranged from 22.7% to 32.5%, specificity from 89.4% to 91.1%, positive predictive value from 88.2% to 76.4%, and negative predictive value from 25% to 60.2%. A subgroup analysis of lesions identified as non-severe by DUS revealed that waveforms with lower deceleration were associated with severe stenosis on CTA.

Conclusions.—In the presence of AcS, DUS alone is inadequate to accurately determine the degree of carotid stenosis with sensitivity, specificity, and negative predictive values far below that needed for clinical decision-making. MD-CTA may be necessary for improved characterization of plaque in these AcS lesions. Further studies are needed to determine DUS parameters that may identify patients who should undergo further evaluation with MD-CTA to characterize the true severity of the stenosis.

▶ Carotid duplex examination has become an integral aspect of the work-up of carotid artery stenosis, with high sensitivity and specificity, and many surgeons use it as their sole imaging modality. Although it is not known how calcified vessels affect clinical aspects of carotid stenosis, their presence often creates acoustic shadows in areas of calcium in which ultrasonic waves are reflected toward the transducer. Within these areas, no Doppler spectral waveforms or velocities can be obtained, and thus true stenosis cannot be determined. The authors sought to determine the accuracy of duplex ultrasound in patients with this acoustic shadowing by retrospectively examining all patients undergoing carotid duplex identified with acoustic shadowing and corresponding computed tomographic angiography (CTA) within 6 months at a single center over an 18-month period. Both the North American Symptomatic Carotid Endarterectomy Trial and European Carotid Surgery Trial criteria for CTA stenosis were compared to the duplex findings, and duplex velocities were obtained as close as possible beyond the area of shadowing. Additionally, duplex waveforms distal to the segment of acoustic shadowing were examined to identify changes indicative of stenosis within the obscured segment. Acoustic shadowing was present in 6.5% of duplexes (n = 550) over this time period; however, only 85 had CTAs of sufficient quality to compare. Accuracy of duplex within areas of acoustic shadowing was abysmal, with a sensitivity ranging from 23% to 33% and a specificity of 89% to 91%. Patients with lower deceleration times on duplex distal to the shadowing were weakly associated with more severe stenosis on CTA. The authors concluded that use of duplex for carotid stenosis in patients with acoustic shadowing underestimates the degree of stenosis, and other imaging modalities such as CTA should be considered in these patients. Weaknesses of this study were its single nature design as well as the availability of CTA to review in only 17% of the patients with acoustic shadowing.

M. R. Smeds, MD, FACS

Common carotid artery peak systolic velocity ratio predicts high-grade common carotid stenosis

Pisimisis GT, Katsavelis D, Mandviwala T, et al (Michael E. DeBakey VA Med Ctr, Houston, TX; Creighton Univ, Omaha, NE; Baylor College of Medicine, Houston, TX)

J Vasc Surg 62:951-957, 2015

Objective.—Screening for common carotid artery (CCA) stenosis with duplex ultrasound (DUS) velocity criteria alone can be limited by within-patient and between-patients hemodynamic variability. This study aimed to evaluate inter-CCA velocity ratio criteria to predict high-grade CCA stenosis.

Methods.—This was a retrospective review of consecutive patients who underwent computed tomography angiography and DUS peak systolic velocity (PSV) measurements of bilateral CCAs, independently recorded, between 2008 and 2014. Patients with dampened CCA waveforms on DUS composed group B. The remainder without dampened waveforms constituted group A. Inter-CCA PSV ratios were calculated by dividing the higher CCA PSV by the lower one of the other side, so the ratios would always be ≥1. Ratios were subsequently paired with each respective unilateral CCA diameter stenosis and differential bilateral CCA diameter stenosis. A quadratic regression model was fitted to predict unilateral and differential stenosis. Receiver operating characteristic curve was used to determine optimal ratios for ≥50% and ≥80% CCA stenosis. The study excluded patients with carotid artery occlusion.

Results.—From a total of 201 patients, 193 patients were included in group A and 8 in group B. Within group A, 31 patients had ≥50% unilateral stenosis and 17 had ≥50% differential stenosis. All stenoses ≥50% were identified on the same side with the higher PSV. Inter-CCA PSV ratio predicted ≥50% unilateral ($r^2 = 0.536$; $P < .001$) and differential stenosis ($r^2 = 0.581$; $P < .001$). In group B, all patients had ≥60% stenosis that was near or involved the vessel origin. An increasing inter-CCA PSV ratio showed a trend toward contralateral high-grade stenosis ($r^2 = 0.596$; $P = .1$). Receiver operating characteristic curves showed an optimal threshold CCA ratio ≥2.16 for ≥50% unilateral stenosis with 92% accuracy, 62% sensitivity, and 98% specificity (area under curve = 0.854; 95% confidence interval, 0.759-0.948) and a ratio ≥2.62 for ≥50% differential stenosis with 97% accuracy, 83% sensitivity, and 98% specificity (area under curve = 0.94; 95% confidence interval, 0.835-1).

Conclusions.—DUS-based CCA PSV ratio can accurately predict unilateral and differential high-grade CCA stenosis. Also, in patients with unilateral dampened waveforms, it implied contralateral severe proximal stenosis. This parameter should be further validated in prospective studies and may serve as an adjunct screening tool to detect high-grade CCA stenosis.

▶ With regard to cerebrovascular occlusive disease, there exist several acceptable interpretive criteria guidelines for the evaluation of internal carotid artery (ICA) stenosis using duplex ultrasound (DUS). No specific evidence-based criteria exist for DUS evaluation of common carotid artery (CCA) stenosis. Although less frequently encountered in clinical practice than symptomatic internal carotid artery stenosis, severe common carotid artery stenosis is recognized as the culprit lesion responsible for ipsilateral atheroembolic stroke in a significant number of cases. In this study, the authors looked retrospectively at DUS in patients who also had computed tomographic angiography within 3 months in all-male Veterans Affairs patients to attempt to determine DUS findings predictive of significant CCA stenosis. Although previous studies looked at CCA peak systolic velocity to predict CCA stenosis, this parameter can be unreliable even within the same patient due to changes in hemodynamics. Although the impact of this study is limited by a small sample size, the authors did find evidence to suggest that the inter-CCA peak systolic velocity ratio can reliably predict significant CCA stenosis. Compared with other imaging modalities such as computed tomography, magnetic resonance, or catheter-based angiography, DUS is relatively less invasive and more cost-effective, and so further investigation into accurate interpretive criteria is certainly warranted.

M. Williams, MD

National variation in preoperative imaging, carotid duplex ultrasound criteria, and threshold for surgery for asymptomatic carotid artery stenosis

Arous EJ, on behalf of the Vascular Quality Initiative (Univ of Massachusetts Med School, Worcester; et al)

J Vasc Surg 62:937-944, 2015

Objective.—Carotid endarterectomy (CEA) for asymptomatic carotid artery stenosis is among the most common procedures performed in the United States. However, consensus is lacking regarding optimal preoperative imaging, carotid duplex ultrasound criteria, and ultimately, the threshold for surgery. We sought to characterize national variation in preoperative imaging, carotid duplex ultrasound criteria, and threshold for surgery for asymptomatic CEA.

Methods.—The Society for Vascular Surgery Vascular Quality Initiative (VQI) database was used to identify all CEA procedures performed for asymptomatic carotid artery stenosis between 2003 and 2014. VQI currently captures 100% of CEA procedures performed at >300 centers by >2000 physicians nationwide. Three analyses were performed to quantify the variation in (1) preoperative imaging, (2) carotid duplex ultrasound criteria, and (3) threshold for surgery.

Results.—Of 35,695 CEA procedures in 33,488 patients, the study cohort was limited to 19,610 CEA procedures (55%) performed for asymptomatic disease. The preoperative imaging modality used before CEA varied widely, with 57% of patients receiving a single preoperative imaging study (duplex ultrasound imaging, 46%; computed tomography angiography, 7.5%; magnetic resonance angiography, 2.0%; cerebral angiography, 1.3%) and 43% of patients receiving multiple preoperative imaging studies. Of the 16,452 asymptomatic patients (89%) who underwent preoperative duplex ultrasound imaging, there was significant variability between centers in the degree of stenosis (50%-69%, 70%-79%, 80%-99%) designated for a given peak systolic velocity, end diastolic velocity, and internal carotid artery-to-common carotid artery ratio. Although 68% of CEA procedures in asymptomatic patients were performed for an 80% to 99% stenosis, 26% were performed for a 70% to 79% stenosis, and 4.1% were performed for a 50% to 69% stenosis. At the surgeon level, the range in the percentage of CEA procedures performed for a <80% asymptomatic carotid artery stenosis is from 0% to 100%. Similarly, at the center level, institutions range in the percentage of CEA procedures performed for a <80% asymptomatic carotid artery stenosis from 0% to 100%.

Conclusions.—Despite CEA being an extremely common procedure, there is widespread variation in the three primary determinants—preoperative imaging, carotid duplex ultrasound criteria, and threshold for surgery—of whether CEA is performed for asymptomatic carotid stenosis. Standardizing the approach to care for asymptomatic carotid artery stenosis will mitigate the significant downstream effects of this variation on health care costs.

► Carotid endarterectomy has been shown to be effective in asymptomatic carotid stenosis; however, standardization of preoperative imaging and threshold for surgery does not exist. The authors aimed to examine national variation in these factors and hypothesize that this variation affects care received. This was a Society for Vascular Surgery Vascular Quality Initiative (VQI) database study looking at 19 610 carotid endarterectomies performed in patients for asymptomatic stenosis from 2003 to 2014. Preoperative imaging used, absolute peak systolic velocity (PSV), end diastolic velocity (EDV), and stenosis thresholds reported by contributing centers were obtained. Significant variation was found in selection of diagnostic tests, with 1 modality (most commonly duplex) used in 57% of patients, and the remainder undergoing multiple exams. Variation was also seen in criteria used for determination of stenosis and threshold for surgery (68% of procedures for stenosis > 80%, 26% for 70%–79% stenosis, and 4.1% for 50%–69% stenosis). Further surgeon or center-level analysis showed significant variation in proportion of patients with varying stenosis treated. The resulting conclusion was that patients receive significant differences in diagnosis and treatment recommendations depending on where they present for care. This has implications for not only care received but also costs involved with therapy. This study is limited by all inherent biases of large database studies. Additionally, imaging was not adjudicated by a core imaging laboratory, and overall risk of patients at individual centers was not determined. However, these findings suggest more stringent consensus recommendations for care of patients with carotid artery stenosis need to be developed.

M. R. Smeds, MD, FACS

The value and economic analysis of routine postoperative carotid duplex ultrasound surveillance after carotid endarterectomy

AbuRahma AF, Srivastava M, AbuRahma Z, et al (West Virginia Univ, Charleston; et al)

J Vasc Surg 62:378-384, 2015

Background.—Several studies have reported on the role of postoperative duplex ultrasound surveillance after carotid endarterectomy (CEA) with varying results. Most of these studies had a small sample size or did not analyze costeffectiveness.

Methods.—We analyzed 489 of 501 CEA patients with patch closure. All patients had immediate postoperative duplex ultrasound examination and were routinely followed up both clinically and with duplex ultrasound at regular intervals of 1 month, 6 months, 12 months, and every 12 months thereafter. A Kaplan-Meier analysis was used to estimate the rate of ≥50% and ≥80% post-CEA restenosis over time and the time frame of progression from normal to ≥50% or ≥80% restenosis. The cost of post-CEA duplex surveillance was also estimated.

Results.—Overall, 489 patients with a mean age of 68.5 years were analyzed. Ten of these had residual postoperative ≥50% stenosis, and 37 did not undergo a second duplex ultrasound examination and therefore were not included in the final analysis. The mean follow-up was 20.4 months (range, 1-63 months), with a mean number of duplex ultrasound examinations of 3.6 (range, 1-7). Eleven of 397 patients (2.8%) with a normal finding on immediate postoperative duplex ultrasound vs 4 of 45 (8.9%) with mild stenosis on immediate postoperative duplex ultrasound progressed to ≥50% restenosis ($P = .055$). Overall, 15 patients (3.1%) had ≥50% restenosis, 9 with 50% to <80% and 4 with 80% to 99% (2 of these had carotid artery stenting reintervention), and 2 had late carotid occlusion. All of these were asymptomatic, except for one who had a transient ischemic attack. The mean time to ≥50% to <80% restenosis was 14.7 months vs 19.8 months for ≥80% restenosis after the CEA. Freedom from restenosis rates were 98%, 96%, 94%, 94%, and 94% for ≥50% restenosis and 99%, 98%, 97%, 97%, and 97% for ≥80% restenosis at 1 year, 2 years, 3 years, 4 years, and 5 years, respectively. Freedom from myocardial infarction, stroke, and deaths was not significantly different between patients with and without restenosis (100%, 93%, 83%, and 83% vs 94%, 91%, 86%, and 79% at 1 year, 2 years, 3 years, and 4 years, respectively; $P = .951$). The estimated charge of this surveillance was 3.6 × 489 (number of CEAs) × \$800 (charge for carotid duplex ultrasound), which equals \$1,408,320, to detect only four patients with ≥80% to 99% restenosis who may have been potential candidates for reintervention.

Conclusions.—This study shows that the value of routine postoperative duplex ultrasound surveillance after CEA with patch closure may be limited, particularly if the finding on immediate postoperative duplex ultrasound is normal or shows minimal disease.

▶ The value of carotid duplex ultrasound (CDUS) in the diagnosis and preoperative surveillance of carotid artery disease is well established. As the medical management of carotid artery disease improves and gains favor, and while physicians, hospital administrators, and patients become more "cost-conscious," the utility of postcarotid endarterectomy (CEA) CDUS is not quite as clear. The overall incidence of recurrent stenosis after CEA is low, and the need to reintervene is even lower. Therefore, the aim of this study is to assess the utility of CDUS for surveillance after CEA with patch closure.

In this study, patients underwent CDUS within 24 hours after CEA, and this test was repeated at 1 month, 6 months, 12 months, and annually thereafter. The mean follow-up was 20.4 months with a mean number of CDUS tests in follow-up of 3.6. Overall, 2% of patients were found to have a 50% to 80% restenosis, and 1.4% of patients (4 patients) were found to have a > 80% restenosis. Mean time to restenosis was 19.3 months. Two of the 4 patients (1 symptomatic) with > 80% restenosis underwent carotid artery stenting. The remaining 2 patients were late carotid occlusions. All but 1 patient of these 15 patients with documented restenosis were asymptomatic. Freedom from > 80% restenosis at 1, 2, 3, and 4 years, respectively, was 99%, 99%, 98%, and 98%. Economic analysis estimated hospital charges for CDUS in this cohort to be \$1 408 320 and reimbursement to be \$702 400; again, with only 2 patients in this cohort undergoing reintervention for restenosis.

Clearly, the results of this study suggest that post-CEA CDUS is overutilized. This aggressive follow-up protocol is not supported by these results, especially when considering that the mean time to restenosis was over 19 months. The authors acknowledge that the 6- and 12-month CDUS tests are not supported by these results, and perhaps post-CEA surveillance CDUS should be considered at 18 months. With these results, it seems hard to justify the intense post-CEA follow-up CDUS regimen that most vascular surgeons practice. Whether our practices are based on historical protocols or are a result of practicing in a litigious environment, this study supports drastically scaling back our use of surveillance CDUS in post-CEA patients.

B. Peterson, MD, FACS

Venous Disease

Changes in the diameter and valve closure time of leg veins in primigravida women during pregnancy

Asbeutah AM, Al-Azemi M, Al-Sarhan S, et al (Kuwait Univ; Al-Ihgaqi Ctr, Kuwait City; et al)

J Vasc Surg Venous Lymphat Disord 3:147-153, 2015

Objective.—The aim of this study was to monitor the changes that develop in leg veins of primigravida women during pregnancy.

Methods.—Sixty primigravida women volunteered to undergo clinical evaluation and duplex ultrasound examination of both lower limb veins to monitor changes in vein diameter and valve closure time (VCT) during pregnancy and 3 months postpartum by duplex ultrasound. A total of four readings were taken for each subject, one reading for each trimester and the last reading at 3 months postpartum.

Results.—The mean (±standard deviation) age of participants was 26.82 ± 2.47 years; 39 limbs (32.5%) and 65 limbs (54.2%) developed C1-C3 venous changes during the second and third trimesters, respectively. Three months post partum, 36 limbs (30%) continued to have C1-C2 changes. Only four limbs in four subjects developed varicose veins along the great saphenous vein, and their VCT was more than 1 second. These subjects were found to have a family history of varicose veins. Duplex examinations showed that there was a gradual increase in the diameter and VCT from the second trimester through the third trimester of pregnancy in all examined venous segments. These changes were statistically significant by Friedman and related-samples Wilcoxon signed rank tests within the same legs ($P = .001$) but not between legs in the same subject ($P > .05$), even with adjustment for body mass index ($P = .001$-$.049$).

Conclusions.—In primigravida women, lower limb veins showed gradual increase in vein diameter and in VCT starting from the second trimester. These changes reverted to baseline in most cases 3 months after delivery.

▶ From a clinical standpoint, pregnancy has been known for some time to worsen women's symptoms of venous insufficiency, and often patients note that there is incomplete resolution of symptoms postpartum. This longitudinal study of previously "unafflicted" women shows that vein diameter and venous closure time increases steadily during pregnancy with return to baseline postpartum. The mechanisms of this are unclear: hormonal possibly in relation to increasing circulating blood volume, the equivalent of "outflow obstruction" by the gravid uterus, or some direct involvement of the venous system not yet elucidated. The unclear part, at least clinically, is that with the return of venous metrics to baseline after delivery, why then do many women note the onset of persistent venous symptoms after childbirth?

R. J. Feezor, MD, FACS

Elimination of medically unnecessary duplex venous scanning based on an established algorithm can result in significant cost savings under medicare for the institution and the taxpayer

Mouawad NJ, Go MR, Haurani MJ, et al (The Ohio State Univ Wexner Med Ctr, Columbus)

J Vasc Surg Venous Lymphat Disord 3:107-112, 2015

Objective.—The utility of duplex venous scanning (DVS) for suspected deep venous thrombosis in the emergency department (ED) remains controversial. We aimed to measure potential cost savings and economic impact in our institution and nationally for unnecessary DVS in Medicare patients seen in the ED.

Methods.—We have previously calculated that 15.3% of DVS studies can safely be avoided in patients with suspected deep venous thrombosis in our ED with adherence to our protocol. The Medicare database was queried for the number of DVS studies performed in the ED and charges/payments made in 2011. Cost savings at our institution and nationally by Medicare were computed with the 15.3% number.

Results.—In the study period, 2087 DVS studies were performed in our ED across all payers; 572 Medicare patients had 249 (43%) bilateral and 323 (57%) unilateral studies. Annual savings at our institution, with use of our protocol, were estimated at $113,778. Eliminating unnecessary after-hours DVS for 306,307 Medicare beneficiaries would result in $5,285,090 savings annually.

Conclusions.—Increasing pressure for cost containment under a value-based payment model necessitates critical evaluation of resource utilization. Applying this schema for all noninvasive vascular tests is an opportunity for responsible management of finite resources, reducing wasteful care, and significant cost containment.

▶ The elimination of medically unnecessary testing is a potential source of recapturing the profit and loss margin for institutions of all sizes and degrees of acuity. This report extrapolates a prior report indicating that use of a clinically driven protocol of a calculated Wells score and D-dimer, 15% of off-hours duplex scans could be prevented. The authors then calculate the institutional cost savings as well as the savings if extrapolated to all Medicare patients. As expected, the numbers are staggering and would easily grasp the attention of administrators and policymakers. The somewhat weak point in the argument, however, is the premise that is based on fewer than 40 patient encounters. Additionally, many institutions have the ability to perform duplex ultrasounds at night by emergency department physicians, which technically also spares the necessity and expense of an "on-call" dedicated vascular ultrasonographer. It remains to be seen whether these more crude ultrasounds have clinical validity. However, the larger practice of finding clinical data to justify a reduction in practice expenses will continue to be a lauded theme for years to come.

R. J. Feezor, MD, FACS

Quantifying saphenous reflux

Raju S, Ward M Jr, Jones TL (The Rane Ctr at St. Dominic Hosp, Jackson, MS; Univ of Tennessee Health Science Ctr, Memphis)

J Vasc Surg Venous Lymphat Disord 3:8-17, 2015

Background.—Quantification of reflux is desirable in advanced chronic venous disease as clinical features are based on its adverse impact on ambulatory venous pressure (AMVP). Prior clinical observation suggests that reflux in a saphenous vein >5 mm is likely significant. On the basis of normal calf pump mechanics, we hypothesized that a reflux volume ≥30 mL was necessary to upset pump equilibrium.

Methods.—Venous laboratory data in 119 limbs with isolated saphenous reflux were analyzed. Reflux volume was calculated by duplex ultrasound (area × velocity × duration). The relationship of reflux volume to saphenous size, calf pump function (air plethysmography, AMVP), flow resistance (Poiseuille equation), and clinical severity were examined.

Results.—Saphenous size had a bimodal relationship to reflux volume. Reflux volume of ≥30 mL occurred mostly (97% of limbs) with saphenous size of ≥5.5 mm, but 51% of saphenous veins >5.5 mm had reflux volumes <30 mL. This is because saphenous veins invariably carried less than their maximum reflux potential indicated by their size (Poiseuille equation). Variable additional focal resistance across refluxive valve cusps and narrower re-entry perforators is not taken into account when only saphenous truncal size is used for resistance calculation. Furthermore, the association of AMVP with reflux was found not to be based on a set (≥30 mL) threshold but was variable, depending on existing calf pump mechanics, compensatory in some (12% of limbs) and aggravating reflux effects in others (26%). Calf pump abnormalities were found in 70% of refluxive limbs and in 44% (n = 16) of contralateral limbs without any reflux. Reflux volume was significantly higher overall in limbs with ulcer (C6), but the range overlapped with lesser clinical classes. Seven of 14 limbs with active ulcers had reflux volume >30 mL; six of seven limbs with active ulcers and reflux volume of <30 mL had calf pump abnormalities that would be poorly tolerant of reflux even at these smaller volumes.

Conclusions.—Saphenous size alone cannot be used as an indicator of significant reflux. More than two thirds of the limbs with isolated saphenous reflux have calf pump abnormalities, which also occurred without reflux in the opposite limb—a novel finding. This means that in addition to quantification of reflux volume, calf pump assessment such as with air plethysmography and AMVP is desirable in clinical classes 3 and higher for proper assessment (Fig 8).

► This is another important article on understanding venous hemodynamics in the setting of chronic venous disease. We know that patients with chronic venous insufficiency often have reflux in the great saphenous system, and this reflux may be transmitted into the venous system via perforating veins. The fundamental question is what volume of blood refluxes into the leg and causes significant dysfunction of the calf muscle pump, due to increased ambulatory venous pressure. The important findings of this study were the following: (1) saphenous size, reflux velocity, and its duration individually are unreliable measures of reflux volume, and actual measurement of reflux volume is necessary. (2) Ninety-four percent of patients in this series with saphenous vein < 5.5 mm in size will be limited to < 30 mL. (3) Reflux in larger saphenous veins (> 5.5 mm) may be greater or lesser (49% and 51%, respectively, in this sample) than the 30-mL threshold. (4) Calf pump abnormalities (compensatory or worsening the effects of reflux) were found in 70% of refluxive limbs and in 44% of contralateral limbs without any reflux. (5) There was no correlation of reflux volume with Clinical-Etiology-Anatomy-Pathophysiology (CEAP) clinical class, and it will be will be of limited value in deciding suitability for saphenous ablation. (6) Calf pump abnormalities may be present in limbs with or without reflux.

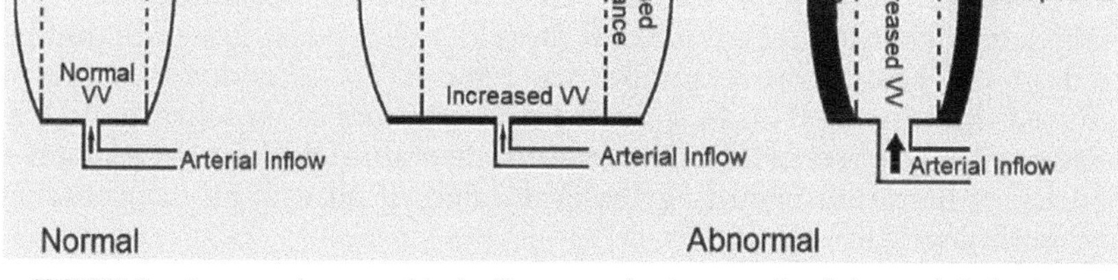

FIGURE 8.—A cartoon (not to scale) of calf pump mechanics, normal and abnormal. Reflux is extrinsic to the calf pump mechanism itself and is a major cause of its decompensation. The calf pump has a venous (bladder) component and a muscle component. Normal function is dependent on adequate priming (capacitance or venous volume [*VV*]), normal compliance, and normal ejection volume (*EV*) as shown on the *left panel*. Reflux can be buffered if the EV and compliance are increased. Increased VV can buffer reflux if EV is simultaneously increased; it can worsen the effects of reflux if EV is unchanged (*middle panel*). Most abnormalities of the calf pump involve the venous bladder component with decreased capacitance, ejection, compliance, or a combination (*right panel*). Ejection fraction (EF) and residual volume fraction (RVF) are secondary metrics of calf pump function based on interaction between primary functional parameters (VV, EV, compliance). Arterial inflow can be a source of calf pump dysfunction in some cases. See text. *GSV*, Great saphenous vein. (Reprinted from Raju S, Ward M Jr, Jones TL. Quantifying saphenous reflux. *J Vasc Surg Venous Lymphat Disord.* 2015;3:8-17, with permission from the Society for Vascular Surgery.)

Importantly, these findings are only valid for patients with isolated superficial great saphenous vein reflux because patients with any deep venous reflux were excluded. Based on this study, the best quantification of saphenous reflux is actual measurement of reflux volume. Although this study provided significant new information, especially determining that it is not the given volume of reflux but how it interacts with the calf pump that sets the clinical picture, no conclusion about selection of patients for saphenous vein ablation can be drawn from this study, and one cannot utilize this data to determine whether patients with different CEAP clinical class will benefit based on the reflux volume.

Future work in venous hemodynamics will be necessary to determine optimal therapy for patients presenting with chronic venous disease of different clinical class to better define which patients would benefit from corrective surgical procedures because the calf muscle pump has an ability to initiate compensatory mechanisms even in the face of venous reflux (Fig 8). Finally, it is interesting that a calf without reflux can have calf pump abnormalities, indicating that follow-up will be required to determine whether clinical symptoms will develop and place the limb at risk for venous disease. Identifying early disease pathology before the development of clinical signs would be ideal to prevent the consequences of advanced forms of chronic venous disease including skin changes and ulceration.

J. D. Raffetto, MD, FACS, FSVM

Venous duplex and pathologic differences in thrombus characteristics between de novo deep vein thrombi and endovenous heat-induced thrombi

Santin BJ, Lohr JM, Panke TW, et al (Ohio Vein & Vascular, Inc, Wilmington; Good Samaritan Hosp, Cincinnati, OH)

J Vasc Surg Venous Lymphat Disord 3:184-189, 2015

Objective.—Superficial venous reflux disease has been treated with endovenous ablation techniques for more than 15 years. Thrombi discovered in the postoperative period are referred to as endovenous heat-induced thrombi (EHIT). In spite of the few studies of the ultrasound differentiation between EHIT and deep vein thrombi (DVT), there remains a paucity of literature regarding the evaluation of ultrasound examination and pathologic differentiation.

Methods.—Six Yorkshire cross swine underwent femoral vein thrombosis by suture ligation or endovenous radiofrequency ablation. At 1 week after the procedure, each femoral vein was imaged by color Duplex ultrasound and sent for histologic interpretation for differentiation between EHIT and DVT. Five blinded vascular surgery faculty, two vascular surgery fellows, and three vascular surgery residents reviewed the ultrasound images.

Results.—Thrombi associated with radiofrequency ablation demonstrated a greater degree of hypercellular response, fibroblastic reaction, and edema (3.42 vs 2.92; 3.75 vs 2.42; 2.83 vs 1.33). Specimens harvested from the iatrogenic-induced DVT swine demonstrated a more prolific response to trichrome staining (3.42 vs 2.67). Evidence of revascularization was found in all of the EHIT specimens but in 33% of DVT specimens. On the basis of histologic findings, the pathologist predicted correct modality 92% of the time. Subgroup analysis comparing paired specimens from each swine failed to demonstrate any marked pathologic differences. Recorded ultrasound images from EHIT and DVT samples were reviewed by fellows, residents, and vascular surgery staff to determine whether clot was stationary or free-floating (n = 111; 93%), evidence of retracted or adherent vein (n = 105; 88%), and absence of color flow (n = 102; 85%). The degree of occlusion (partial vs total) and degree of distention of a visualized vein were least likely to be agreed on by reviewers (n = 95; 79% each, respectively). In subgroup (DVT vs EHIT) analyses, the percentage agreement was greatest among vascular surgery fellows (89% and 92%) compared with residents (82% and 79%) and faculty (78% and 77%).

Conclusions.—It is possible to differentiate the thrombus origin on pathologic examination but not clinically on ultrasound. Wide variability exists for ultrasound diagnosis of EHIT and de novo DVT. Care must be taken in evaluating post-treatment duplex scans to not assign diagnosis of EHIT when DVT may well be present and extending into the deep venous system. The modulation of collagen production in the treatment of DVT may be helpful in preventing vascular dysfunction and reducing the post-thrombotic changes. Further studies on injury after radiofrequency ablation and laser ablation are needed.

Clinical Relevance.—Care must be taken in evaluating post-treatment duplex scans to not assign a diagnosis of EHIT when DVT may well be present and extending into the deep venous system. Use of color Duplex ultrasound to establish a diagnosis of either DVT or EHIT may prove to be helpful in differentiating the most appropriate treatment for patients.

▶ Thermal ablation using laser and radiofrequency is commonly used to treat the great saphenous vein in patients with symptomatic venous insufficiency. Many studies have demonstrated thermal ablation procedure as effective and safe. Endothermal heat–induced thrombosis (EHIT) is a potential complication of venous endothermal ablation but appears to occur at a frequency of 1%. EHIT may lead to deep venous thrombosis. However, the ultrasound findings of EHIT and deep vein thrombosis (DVT) are poorly defined, as well as the chemical composition of each. In this interesting study, the authors sought to answer these questions. The authors used a swine model and caused a DVT in the femoral vein by ligation and an EHIT in the femoral vein by radiofrequency ablation. A blinded pathologist assessed the histologic characteristics of each, and vascular residents, fellows, and attendings reviewed the ultrasound imaging of the thrombosed femoral veins by each technique before histologic analysis. There were significant and distinct differences in the thrombus generated based on the modality of injury. However, the comparison analysis of ultrasound interpretation by blinded reviewers suggests that there is significant variability in characterizing acute thrombi by either forming a DVT or by EHIT. Importantly, there were no ultrasound criterion that were able to accurately differentiate the etiology of the thrombus. This study highlights the importance that when assessing postablation procedures with ultrasound, one should be cautious of assigning EHIT when in fact this could be a DVT. Further studies, and more specific means (imaging, specific markers) of determining whether a DVT is present versus a EHIT that is either significant or insignificant, are needed so that proper therapy may be provided.

J. D. Raffetto, MD, FACS, FSVM

4 Perioperative Considerations

Update in preoperative risk assessment in vascular surgery patients
Zarinsefat A, Henke P (Univ of Michigan, Ann Arbor)
J Vasc Surg 62:499-509, 2015

Multiple clinical factors and now serum biomarkers may aid with risk stratification in vascular surgical patients. Herein, we review and update the clinical risk models, biomarker data, and currently used noninvasive cardiac stress tests. We also review the most recent American Heart Association guideline changes, and suggest a pathway for risk stratification.

▶ Most peripheral artery disease patients possess concomitant coronary artery disease, and major adverse cardiac events can be see in 5% to 15% of patients undergoing vascular surgery. Modalities used to risk stratify patients undergoing vascular surgery have evolved over the past 15 years, as have the opinions regarding who needs to undergo risk stratification evaluation before surgery. Here the authors tackle the monumental task of reviewing the literature over the past 15 years with regard to clinical risk models, biomarker data, and noninvasive cardiac stress tests. The authors thoroughly review the landmark studies and pack this article with the pertinent details of each, producing a simple algorithm that will guide the preoperative work-up of complex vascular patients. Although the specific details of this algorithm may be viewed in the article, I venture to say that the authors do a phenomenal job at creating a simple algorithm that incorporates clinical risk factor models, biomarkers, and cardiovascular stress testing in a way that is easy to follow, supported by the literature, and should become part of the routine in evaluating patients preoperatively for vascular surgical procedures.

B. Peterson, MD, FACS

Prospective Randomized Double-blinded Trial Comparing 2 Anti-MRSA Agents With Supplemental Coverage of Cefazolin Before Lower Extremity Revascularization

Stone PA, AbuRahma AF, Campbell JR, et al (West Virginia Univ, Charleston; et al)

Ann Surg 262:495-501, 2015

Objective.—To compare with antibiotics with methicillin-resistant microbial coverage in a prospective fashion.

Background.—Current antibiotic prophylaxis for vascular procedures includes a first generation cephalosporin. No changes in recommendations have occurred despite changes in reports of incidence of MRSA related surgical site infections. Does supplemental anti-MRSA prophylactic coverage provide a significant reduction in Gram-positive or MRSA infections?

Methods.—Single center prospective double blinded randomized study of patients undergoing lower extremity vascular procedures from 2011 to 2014. One hundred seventy-eight (178) patients were evaluated at 90 days for surgical site infection. Infections were categorized as early infections less than 30 days of the index procedure and late after 90 days.

Results.—Early vascular surgical site infection occurred in 7 (8.24%) of patients in the Vancomycin arm, and 11 (11.83%) in the Daptomycin arm ($P = 0.43$). Gram-positive related infections and MRSA infections occurred in 1 (1.18%)/0 (0%) of Vancomycin patients and 9 (9.68%)/1 (1.08%) of Daptomycin patients, respectively ($P < 0.02$ and $P = 1.00$). Readmissions related to surgical site infections occurred in 4 (4.71%) in the Vancomycin group and 11 (11.8%) in the Daptomycin group ($P = 0.11$). Patients undergoing operative exploration occurred in 5 (5.88%) in the Vancomycin group and 10 (10.75%) of the Daptomycin group ($P = 0.17$). Late infections were reported in 3 patients, 2 of which were in the combined Daptomycin group. Median hospital charges related to readmissions due to a surgical site infection was $50,823 in the combination Vancomycin arm and $110,920 in the combination Daptomycin group; however, no statistical significance was appreciated ($P = 0.11$).

Conclusions.—Vancomycin supplemental prophylaxis seems to reduce the incidence of Gram-positive infection compared with adding supplemental Daptomycin prophylaxis. The Incidence of MRSA-related surgical site infections is low with the addition of either anti-MRSA agents compared with historical incidence of MRSA-related infection.

▶ Surgical site infections in lower extremity vascular surgery cause significant postoperative complications, including graft failure, limb loss, skyrocketing costs of treatment, and prolonged hospital stays. In recent years, drug-resistant bacteria (particularly methicillin-resistant Staphylococcus aureus [MRSA]) have played a larger role as the culprit pathogens. Despite the potential for uncleanliness in the groin region, lower extremity vascular operations still fall in the category of "clean" cases, and the recommended preoperative antibacterial prophylaxis has called for only a first-generation cephalosporin such as cefazolin. With growing concern for MRSA in postoperative infections, might patients undergoing vascular operations benefit from prophylactic anti-MRSA agents? The authors of this single-center, prospective, randomized, double blinded study pitted 2 such agents (vancomycin and daptomycin, each in combination with cefazolin) against each other as preprocedure surgical site infection prophylaxis. Two hundred patients were enrolled, and 178 eventually were included in the study, with follow-up up to 90 days examined. The majority of the operations involved a groin incision (95%), and the choice of vertical versus oblique was left to the surgeon's preference. Unfortunately, the 2 arms of the study were not compared with a control group of the current standard of care of cefazolin alone. In terms of overall surgical site infections, there was no statistically significant difference (8.24% at 30 days with vancomycin and 11.83% with daptomycin), and the incidence is in accordance with acceptable infection rates from historical data. None of the vancomycin group and only 1 in the daptomycin group developed an MRSA infection within 90 days of surgery. There was a significant difference in overall rate of Gram-positive infections in the vancomycin group compared with the Daptomycin group (1.18% vs 9.68%), but it is difficult to draw any conclusion from this finding given the relatively small sample size. A well-powered randomized study comparing the current practice recommendation of cefazolin alone with either vancomycin or daptomycin would shed more light on the subject.

M. Williams, MD

Predicting postoperative delirium after vascular surgical procedures

Visser L, Prent A, van der Laan MJ, et al (Univ of Groningen, The Netherlands)

J Vasc Surg 62:183-189, 2015

Objective.—The objective of this study was to determine the incidence of and specific preoperative and intraoperative risk factors for postoperative delirium (POD) in electively treated vascular surgery patients.

Methods.—Between March 2010 and November 2013, all vascular surgery patients were included in a prospective database. Various preoperative, intraoperative, and postoperative risk factors were collected during hospitalization. The primary outcome variable was the incidence of POD. Secondary outcome variables were any surgical complication, hospital length of stay, and mortality.

Results.—In total, 566 patients were prospectively evaluated; 463 patients were 60 years or older at the time of surgery and formed our study cohort. The median age was 72 years (interquartile range, 66-77), and 76.9% were male. Twenty-two patients (4.8%) developed POD. Factors that differed significantly by univariate analysis included current smoking ($P = .001$), increased comorbidity ($P = .001$), hypertension ($P = .003$), diabetes mellitus ($P = .001$), cognitive impairment ($P < .001$), open aortic surgery or amputation surgery ($P < .001$), elevated C-reactive protein level ($P < .001$), and blood loss ($P < .001$). Multivariate logistic regression analysis revealed preoperative cognitive impairment (odds ratio [OR], 16.4; 95% confidence interval [CI], 4.7-57.0), open aortic surgery or amputation surgery (OR, 14.0; 95% CI, 3.9-49.8), current smoking (OR, 10.5; 95% CI, 2.8-40.2), hypertension (OR, 7.6; 95% CI, 1.9-30.5) and age ≥80 years (OR, 7.3; 95% CI, 1.8-30.1) to be independent predictors of the occurrence of POD. The combination of these parameters allows us to predict delirium with a sensitivity of 86% and a specificity of 92%. The area under the curve of the corresponding receiver operating characteristics was 0.93. Delirium was associated with longer hospital length of stay ($P < .001$), more frequent and increased intensive care unit stays ($P = .008$ and $P = .003$, respectively), more surgical complications ($P < .001$), more postdischarge institutionalization ($P < .001$), and higher 1-year mortality rates ($P = .0026$).

Conclusions.—In vascular surgery patients, preoperative cognitive impairment and open aortic or amputation surgery were highly significant risk factors for the occurrence of POD. In addition, POD was significantly associated with a higher mortality and more institutionalization. Patients with these risk factors should be considered for high-standard delirium care to improve these outcomes.

▶ Postoperative delirium (POD) is a common finding after surgery and is associated with poorer outcomes compared with those of patients who do not suffer from POD. As the population continues to age and live longer, the incidence of POD is likely to increase. If recognized, the deleterious effects of POD can be lessened by prompt geriatric consultation and pharmacotherapy. Therefore, in this nonrandomized, prospective study, the authors sought to identify preoperative and intraoperative risk factors for the development of POD in vascular surgery patients.

The authors identified 463 patients over age 60 years undergoing various vascular procedures ranging from lower extremity endovascular procedures to open aortic cases and amputations. Patients were examined by nurses specially trained to recognize the signs and symptoms of delirium. Additionally, a well-established scoring system, the Delirium Observation Screening scale, was obtained in all patients 3 times per day, and a score greater than 3 prompted consultation with a geriatrician to confirm the diagnosis of POD.

Of the 463 vascular surgery patients, 22 (4.8%) developed POD. These patients had a mean age of 70, and not surprisingly, the highest incidence of POD was seen in patients undergoing amputation (16.7%) or open aortic surgery (15.1%). Multivariate analysis identified 5 independent risk factors for the development of POD: preoperative cognitive impairment, open aortic surgery or amputation, current smoking, hypertension, and age greater than or equal to 80. Using these factors, the author created a model to predict the development of POD with a sensitivity of 86% and specificity of 92%. The authors also demonstrated poorer outcomes in the POD group: more frequent intensive care unit (ICU) admission, longer length of stay in hospital and in the ICU, higher mortality, and more institutionalization after discharge. With this study, it is to be hoped that vascular patients at high risk for the development of POD can be identified, allowing for more timely diagnosis and intervention, leading to improved patient outcomes.

B. Peterson, MD, FACS

Blood Conservation Strategies Can Be Applied Safely to High-Risk Complex Aortic Surgery

Yaffee DW, DeAnda A, Ngai JY, et al (NYU Langone Med Ctr)
J Cardiothorac Vasc Anesth 29:703-709, 2015

Objective.—The present study aimed to evaluate the effect of blood conservation strategies on patient outcomes after aortic surgery.

Design.—Retrospective cohort analysis of prospective data.

Setting.—University hospital.

Participants.—Patients undergoing thoracic aortic surgery.

Interventions.—One hundred thirty-two consecutive high-risk patients (mean EuroSCORE 10.4%) underwent thoracic aortic aneurysm or dissection repair from January 2010 to September 2011. A blood conservation strategy (BCS) focused on limitation of hemodilution and tolerance of perioperative anemia was used in 57 patients (43.2%); the remaining 75(56.8%) patients were managed by traditional methods. Mortality, major complications, and red blood cell transfusion requirements were assessed. Independent risk factors for clinical outcomes were determined by multivariate analyses.

Measurements and Main Results.—Hospital mortality was 9.8% (13 of 132). Lower preoperative hemoglobin was an independent predictor of mortality ($p < 0.01$, odds ratio [OR] 1.7). Major complications were associated with perioperative transfusion: 0% complication rate in patients receiving <2 units of packed red blood cells versus 32.3% (20 of 62) in patients receiving ≥2 units. The blood conservation strategy had no significant impact on mortality ($p = 0.4$) or major complications ($p = 0.9$) despite the blood conservation patients having a higher incidence of aortic dissection and urgent/emergent procedures and lower preoperative and discharge hemoglobin. In patients with aortic aneurysms, BCS patients received 1.5 fewer units of red blood cells (58% reduction) than non-BCS patients ($p = 0.01$). Independent risk factors for transfusion were lower preoperative hemoglobin ($p < 0.01$, OR 1.5) and lack of BCS ($p = 0.02$, OR 3.6).

Conclusions.—Clinical practice guidelines for blood conservation should be considered for high-risk complex aortic surgery patients (Table 1).

▶ Blood conservation strategies (BCS) have been studied extensively in the trauma population for decades. Work has shown that not only is blood transfusion associated with complications, but, more important, that permissive anemia is not associated with increased mortality. However, many vascular and cardiac surgeons are hesitant to apply this concept to their patients because

TABLE 1.—Preoperative Patient Characteristics

Characteristic	Control (n = 75)	BCS (n = 57)	p Value
Age (years)	62.8 ± 13.8	58.0 ± 13.9	0.06
EuroSCORE(%)	10.1 ± 10.8 (5.4; 8.3; 1.1-52)	10.7 ± 9.0 (7.9; 9.0; 1.3-53.4)	0.76 (0.10)
BMI (kg/m^2)	29.1 ± 6.0	26.5 ± 4.8	0.006
Disease type			
Aneurysm	64 (85.3)	29 (50.9)	<0.001
Acute dissection	9 (12.0)	13 (22.8)	0.10
Chronic dissection	2 (2.7)	15 (26.3)	<0.001
Urgent/emergent	29 (38.7)	46 (80.7)	<0.001
Female sex	26 (34.7)	21 (36.8)	0.80
Previous cardiac surgery	19 (25.3)	9 (15.8)	0.18
Previous myocardial infarction	4 (5.3)	0 (0.0)	0.08
COPD	7 (9.3)	9 (15.8)	0.26
Diabetes	9 (12.0)	4 (7.0)	0.34
End-stage renal disease	4 (5.3)	3 (5.3)	0.99
History of endocarditis	5 (6.7)	5 (8.8)	0.65
Cerebrovascular disease	6 (8.0)	7 (12.3)	0.41
Peripheral vascular disease	33 (44.0)	40 (70.2)	0.003
Congestive heart failure	25 (33.3)	21 (36.8)	0.68

NOTE. Continuous variables presented as mean ± standard deviation (median; interquartile range; range) where applicable. *P* values for nonparametric comparison analyses performed using Mann-Whitney U test and presented in parentheses.

Abbreviations: BCS, blood conservation strategy cohort; BMI, body mass index; COPD, chronic obstructive pulmonary disease; EuroSCORE, European System for Cardiac Operative Risk Evaluation.

"vasculopaths" are older and have significantly more comorbidities than the average trauma patient.

The authors here have designed a retrospective, nonrandomized, non–case-matched cohort study to evaluate a blood conservation therapy in patients undergoing major aortic surgery. They employed the guidelines put forth by the Society of Thoracic Surgeons and the Society of Cardiovascular Anesthesiologists (STS/SCS) that involves a multidisciplinary multimodality approach. The BCS included minimization of intraoperative hemodilution, tolerance of perioperative anemia, and education of all team members. Red blood cell transfusion was triggered for asymptomatic patients with hemoglobin < 7 or symptomatic patients with hemoglobin < 8. The study group consisted of 57 consecutive patients of a single cardiac surgeon who was the primary aortic surgeon for that center. The control group comprised 75 patients undergoing aortic surgery by the remaining 8 surgeons at that institution. Interestingly (Table 1), the BCS patients had higher preoperative incidence of peripheral vascular disease, a lower mean body mass index, and a lower preoperative hemoglobin level, which are all frequently known to be associated with higher perioperative risk. Nonetheless, there was no difference in mortality or major complication for patients in the BCS group compared with the group managed by traditional methods. This is an important study to move toward compliance with transfusion guidelines because surgeons play an essential role in influencing transfusion practice in cardiac and vascular surgery, and only when surgeons actively "buy in" will BCS be achieved. Finally, preoperative adjuncts such as iron regimen, erythropoietin supplements, and even preoperative blood banking, may increase preoperative hemoglobin and, when combined with intraoperative strategies, may reset post-operative hemoglobin levels. This in turn may enable some surgeons to better resist transfusion to achieve a postoperative number.

K. C. Orion, MD

5 Abdominal Aorta

The impact of endovascular repair on specialties performing abdominal aortic aneurysm repair

Ultee KHJ, Hurks R, Buck DB, et al (Beth Israel Deaconess Med Ctr and Harvard Med School, Boston, MA; et al)

J Vasc Surg 62:562-568, 2015

Background.—Abdominal aortic aneurysm (AAA) repair has been performed by various surgical specialties for many years. Endovascular aneurysm repair (EVAR) may be a disruptive technology, having an impact on which specialties care for patients with AAA. Therefore, we examined the proportion of AAA repairs performed by various specialties over time in the United States and evaluated the impact of the introduction of EVAR.

Methods.—The Nationwide Inpatient Sample (2001-2009) was queried for intact and ruptured AAA and for open repair and EVAR. Specific procedures were used to identify vascular surgeons (VSs), cardiac surgeons (CSs), and general surgeons (GSs) as well as interventional cardiologists and interventional radiologists for states that reported unique treating physician identifiers. Annual procedure volumes were subsequently calculated for each specialty.

Results.—We identified 108,587 EVARs and 85,080 open AAA repairs (3011 EVARs and 12,811 open repairs for ruptured AAA). VSs performed an increasing proportion of AAA repairs during the study period (52% in 2001 to 66% in 2009; $P < .001$). GSs and CSs performed fewer repairs during the same period (25% to 17% [$P < .001$] and 19% to 13% [$P < .001$], respectively). EVAR was increasingly used for intact (33% to 78% of annual cases; $P < .001$) as well as ruptured AAA repair (5% to 28%; $P < .001$). The proportion of intact open repairs performed by VSs increased from 52% to 65% ($P < .001$), whereas for EVAR, the proportion went from 60% to 67% ($P < .001$). The proportion performed by VSs increased for ruptured open repairs from 37% to 53% ($P < .001$) and for ruptured EVARs from 28% to 73% ($P < .001$). Compared with treatment by VSs, treatment by a CS (0.55 [0.53-0.56]) and GS (0.66 [0.64-0.68]) was associated with a decreased likelihood of undergoing endovascular rather than open AAA repair.

Conclusions.—VSs are performing an increasing majority of AAA repairs, in large part driven by the increased utilization of EVAR for both intact and ruptured AAA repair. However, GSs and CSs still perform AAA repair. Further studies should examine the implications of these national trends on the outcome of AAA repair.

► Historically, vascular surgeons, cardiothoracic surgeons, and general surgeons treated abdominal aortic aneurysmal (AAA) disease. All of these surgical specialties originated from a common general surgery background and shared many of the surgical principles necessary to treat vascular patients. Therefore, it is plausible that these specialties managed AAAs as part of there practice. In addition, vascular surgery is a relatively young specialty that continues to increase in the number of trainees it attracts, but there is nonetheless a national shortage of these specialists that continues to grow. In the absence of vascular surgeons, other specialties have attempted to treat AAA; endovascular aneurysm repair (EVAR) has provided them with a treatment outside of surgical therapy.

In the present study, the National Inpatient Sample database is used to evaluate specialty trends over time, 2000 to 2009. As expected, vascular surgeons continue to perform the majority of AAA repairs, and as expected, vascular surgeons use EVAR to treat the majority of patients. I find it interesting that general surgeons perform 17% of aneurysm repairs and cardiothoracic surgeons perform another 13%, combined 30% nationally. General surgeons and cardiothoracic surgeons are more likely to utilize open abdominal aortic aneurysm over EVAR. As a vascular surgeon, I believe that EVAR should be performed, managed, and surveyed by a vascular surgeon, but is this unreasonable? Are 30% of aortic aneurysms treated by other specialties because we cannot provide national vascular surgery coverage? Or are providers preferentially referring AAA to general surgeons and cardiothoracic surgeons? The current article cannot answer these questions, but as vascular surgeons we should.

Z. M. Arthurs, MD, FACS

Potential clinical feasibility and financial impact of same-day discharge in patients undergoing endovascular aortic repair for elective infrarenal aortic aneurysm

Moscato VP, O'Brien-Irr MS, Dryjski ML, et al (State Univ of New York)
J Vasc Surg 62:855-861, 2015

Objective.—The purpose of this study was to evaluate the potential feasibility and financial impact of same-day discharge after elective endovascular aneurysm repair (EVAR) for abdominal aortic aneurysm.

Methods.—All elective EVARs performed between January 2012 and June 2013 were identified. Demographics, comorbidities, complications, nursing care, financial data, and length of stay were analyzed.

Results.—Sixty-seven (73%) EVARs were performed electively, 73% percutaneously. Intraoperative complications were blood loss requiring transfusion (4.5%), thrombosis (3%), femoral artery injury (1.5%), postoperative urinary retention (4.5%), myocardial infarction (3%), respiratory failure (1.5%), congestive heart failure (1.5%), and hemodynamic or rhythm alterations (37%; evident in 88% <6 hours; 13% required therapy). Monitoring only was needed in 28 patients (42%), intensive care in 15%. Seventy-two percent were discharged on postoperative day one; 6% were readmitted <30 days. Telemetry, oxygen, intravenous hydration, and urinary catheters (routine services) were used for shorter periods in uncomplicated patients and those discharged on postoperative day 1. Total hospital costs were $29,479: operating room, 80.3%; anesthesia, 2.2%; preadmission, 1%; postanesthesia unit, 3.1%; intensive care unit, 1.9%; floor, 4.7%; laboratory and diagnostic tests, 1.2%; pharmacy, 1.4%; other, 4.2%. Total cost was similar for those discharged <20 hours or $24 to 31 hours postoperatively ($P = .51$) and for monitoring only vs others ($28,146 vs $30,545; $P = .12$). Pharmacy ($351 vs $509; $P = .05$), laboratory work ($86 vs $355; $P = .01$), and diagnostic testing ($4 vs $254; $P = .02$) costs were lower for uncomplicated cases.

Conclusions.—Same-day discharge is clinically feasible in >40% of elective EVARs but requires coordination for adequate postoperative monitoring. Significant savings are unlikely as most cost is operating room and device related, and further reduction of costs in uncomplicated cases is unlikely.

► Endovascular aneurysm repair (EVAR) has revolutionized abdominal aortic aneurysm therapy. Ten to 12 years ago, our specialty was struggling with the emergence of EVAR as the primary therapy for abdominal aortic aneurysm. Today, we are struggling with the idea of making this an outpatient procedure. We have all rounded on patients in the evening after performing an EVAR and felt that the patient was ready for discharge. Identifying the pros and cons of outpatient EVAR has been more challenging. The time difference between same-day discharge and discharge on postoperative day (POD) 1 may equate to 8 to 12 hours of hospital observation.

In the current article, the authors provide a detailed analysis of 67 EVARs performed consecutively at their academic institution. Forty-two percent of patients had an uncomplicated course and would have met the criteria for same-day discharge. The remaining 58% experienced a postoperative occurrence, such as labile blood pressure or arrhythmia that demanded postoperative observation. Lachat et al found a similar pattern suggesting that 40% of EVAR patients were eligible for same-day discharge.[1]

The financial impact remains questionable. The bulk of EVAR cost is tied to device and operating room expenses. In this report, there was no overall cost advantage to same-day discharge as opposed to POD 1 discharge. There was a financial advantage to same-day discharge compared to longer hospital stays, but these are also patients who required longer stays to treat postoperative medical conditions.

Z. M. Arthurs, MD, FACS

Reference

1. Lachat ML, Pecoraro F, Mayer D, et al. Outpatient endovascular aneurysm repair: experience in 100 consecutive patients. *Ann Surg*. 2013;258:754-759.

Endovascular Versus Open Repair as Primary Strategy for Ruptured Abdominal Aortic Aneurysm: A National Population-based Study

Gunnarsson K, Wanhainen A, Djavani Gidlund K, et al (Uppsala Univ, Sweden)

Eur J Vasc Endovasc Surg 51:22-28, 2016

Objective/Background.—In randomized trials, no peri-operative survival benefit has been shown for endovascular (EVAR) repair of ruptured abdominal aortic aneurysm (rAAA) when compared with open repair. The aim of this study was to investigate the effect of primary repair strategy on early and midterm survival in a non-selected population based study.

Methods.—The Swedish Vascular Registry was consulted to identify all rAAA repairs performed in Sweden in the period 2008–12. Centers with a primary EVAR strategy (treating > 50% of rAAA with EVAR) were compared with centers with a primary open repair strategy. Peri-operative outcome, midterm survival, and incidence of rAAA repair/100,000 inhabitants aged > 50 years were assessed.

Results.—In total, 1,304 patients were identified. Three primary EVAR centers (pEVARc) operated on 236 patients (74.6% EVAR). Twenty-six primary open repair centers (pORc) operated 1,068 patients (15.6% EVAR). Patients treated at pEVARc were more often referrals (28.0% vs. 5.3%; $p < .01$), had a higher rate of respiratory comorbidity (36.5% vs. 21.9%; $p < .01$), and higher pre-operative systolic blood pressure (84.3 vs. 72.3 mmHg; $p < .01$). There was no difference in mortality based on primary treatment strategy at 30 days (pEVARc 28.0%, $n = 66$; pORc 27.4%, $n = 296$ [$p = .87$]), 1 year (pEVARc 39.9%, $n = 93$; pORc 34.7%, $n = 366$ [$p = .19$]), or 2 years (42.1%, $n = 94$; 38.3%, $n = 394$ [$p = .28$]), either overall or in subgroups based on age or referral status. Overall, patients treated with EVAR were older (mean age 76.4 vs. 74.0 years; $p < .01$), and had a lower 30 day mortality (EVAR 21.6%, $n = 74$; odds ratio 29.6%, $n = 288$ [$p = < .01$]). Incidence of rAAA repair was lower in pEVARc regions (6.07, 95% confidence interval [CI] 5.01–7.13) when compared with pORc regions (8.15, 95% CI 7.64–8.66).

Conclusion.—There was no difference in mortality after rAAA repair among centers with a primary EVAR approach when compared with a primary open repair strategy, either peri-operatively or in the midterm. The study supports the early findings of the randomized controlled trials in a national population based setting (Fig 1, Table 3).

▶ Retrospective studies have shown lower mortality after endovascular aneurysm repair (EVAR) for rupture compared with open repair, but these findings have not been replicated in randomized trials. I admit that the superior outcome of EVAR for ruptured abdominal aortic aneurysm (rAAA) seen in observational studies like our own in Seattle may be an effect of case selection, making

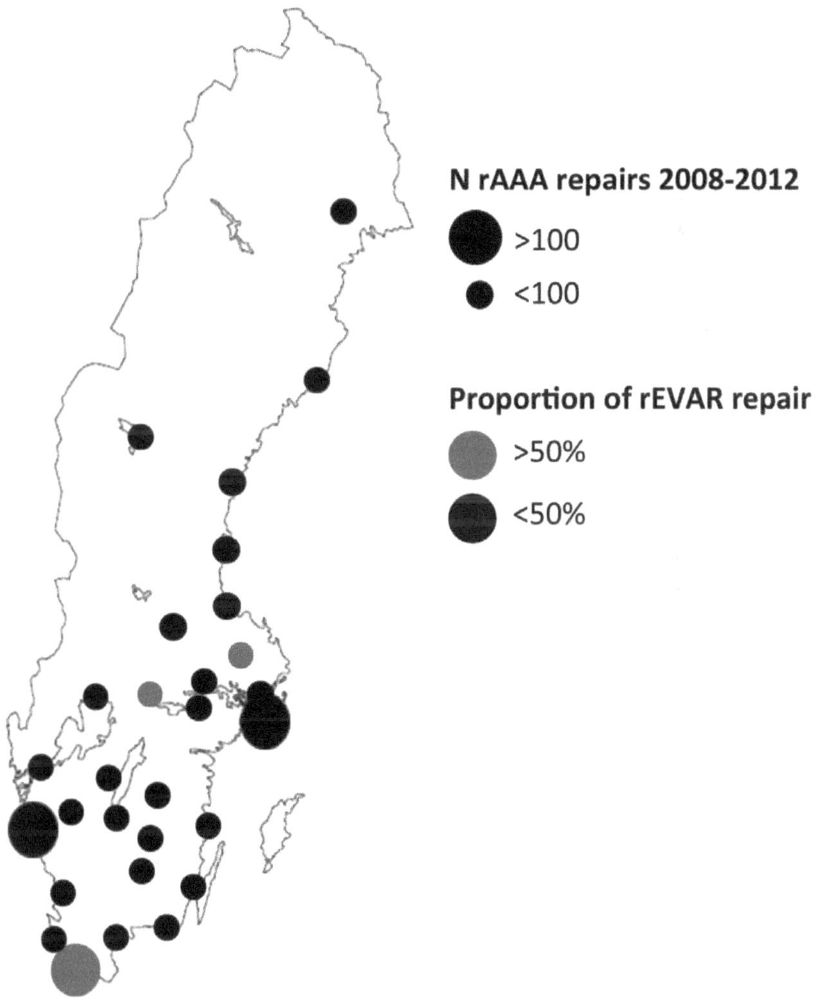

FIGURE 1.—Distribution of centers performing ruptured abdominal aortic aneurysm (rAAA) repair in Sweden, based on size and proportion of endovascular (EVAR) repair. (Reprinted from Gunnarsson K, Wanhainen A, Djavani Gidlund K, et al. Endovascular versus open repair as primary strategy for ruptured abdominal aortic aneurysm: a national population-based study. *Eur J Vasc Endovasc Surg*. 2016;51:22-28, with permission from European Society for Vascular Surgery.)

TABLE 3.—Post-operative Mortality After Ruptured Abdominal Aortic Aneurysm Repair

Mortality	pEVARc	pORc	*p*
Overall (*n*)	236	1,068	
30 days	66 (28.0)	296 (27.4)	.87
1 year	93 (39.9)	366 (34.7)	.19
2 years	94 (42.1)	394 (38.3)	.28
Excluding referrals (*n*)	170	1,011	
30 days	53 (31.2)	279 (27.6)	.36
1 year	71 (42.1)	349 (34.9)	.09
2 years	75 (45.0)	377 (38.7)	.12
Octogenarians (*n*)	69	327	
30 days	29 (42.0)	130 (39.9)	.79
1 year	41 (60.4)	161 (49.7)	.41
2 years	44 (66.6)	171 (53.9)	.68
Open repair (*n*)	60	901	
30 days	23 (38.3)	265 (29.0)	.14
1 year	29 (48.3)	322 (36.1)	.03
2 years	31 (52.4)	338 (38.6)	.02
EVAR (*n*)	176	167	
30 days	43 (24.4)	31 (18.6)	.19
1 year	64 (37.1)	44 (27.0)	.06
2 years	66 (38.6)	56 (37.4)	.40

Note. Data are *n* (%). pEVARc = primary endovascular aneurysm repair (EVAR) strategy centers; pORc = primary open repair centers.

Reprinted from Gunnarsson K, Wanhainen A, Djavani Gidlund K, et al. Endovascular versus open repair as primary strategy for ruptured abdominal aortic aneurysm: a national population-based study. *Eur J Vasc Endovasc Surg*. 2016;51:22-28, with permission from European Society for Vascular Surgery.

comparison with open repair inadequate. In Sweden, the rate of EVAR treatment of ruptures varies from 0% to 100% between centers. Thus, these authors chose to evaluate a national registry in Sweden to compare outcomes between centers having an "EVAR first" or "Open Repair first" strategy (Fig 1).

Like all other randomized trials conducted to date, the authors essentially found no difference in 30-day mortality rates based on primary method of repair: EVAR 28.0% versus open repair 27.4%. The authors essentially concluded that their study confirmed there was no early or midterm survival difference between primary open and endovascular operative strategies for ruptured AAA. What was most unusual in my mind about this study was that if an EVAR was performed for rAAA in a Swedish hospital with an "EVAR first" strategy, the 30-day mortality was 24.4%, whereas if an EVAR was performed in a Swedish hospital with an "open repair first" strategy, the 30-day mortality was only 18.6% (Table 3). This obviously demonstrates the huge selection bias based on hemodynamic stability and anatomic suitability.

It is well known that our institution was an early adopter of EVAR first for rAAA, and I remain a firm believer that it is better for these patients than attempts at open repair. Because only 25% of all rAAAs were repaired using EVAR in Sweden over the study period, I am certain that as experience is gained and protocols are solidified, the data will change as these late adopters become more proficient.

B. W. Starnes, MD

Aortic neck enlargement after endovascular aneurysm repair using balloon-expandable versus self-expanding endografts

Savlovskis J, Krievins D, de Vries J-PPM, et al (Pauls Stradins Clinical Univ Hosp, Riga, Latvia; St. Antonius Hosp, Nieuwegein, The Netherlands; et al)

J Vasc Surg 62:541-549, 2015

Objective.—This study evaluated changes in aortic neck diameter after endovascular aneurysm repair (EVAR) using a balloon-expandable stent (BES) endograft compared with a commercially available self-expanding stent (SES) endograft. We hypothesized that forces applied to the aortic neck by SES endografts may induce aortic neck enlargement over time and that such enlargement may not occur in aneurysm patients treated with a device that does not use a proximal SES.

Methods.—This was a retrospective quantitative computed tomography (CT) image analysis of patients treated with the Nellix (Endologix, Irvine, Calif) BES (n = 49) or the Endurant II (Medtronic, Minneapolis, Minn) SES (n = 56) endograft from 2008 to 2010. Patients with preimplant, post-implant, and at least 1-year serial CT scans underwent quantitative morphometric assessment by two independent vascular radiologists blinded to the outcome results. Changes in the infrarenal neck over time were compared with the suprarenal aorta for each patient.

Results.—Follow-up extended to 4.8 years for the BES and to 4.6 years for the SES, with no significant difference in median follow-up time (34 months for BESs and 24 months for SESs; $P = .06$).There were no differences in preimplant neck diameter (25.2 ± 0.9 mm vs 25.7 ± 1.1 mm; $P = .54$) or length (27.7 ± 3.7 mm vs 23.6 ± 3.7 mm; $P = .12$) between BESs and SESs at baseline. After implantation, neck diameter increased by 1.1 ± 0.5 mm in BES patients and 2.6 ± 0.5 mm in SES patients ($P = .07$) compared with the preoperative diameter. At 3 years, neck diameter increased by 0.5 ± 0.9 mm in BES patients and by 3.8 ± 1.0 mm in SES patients ($P = .0002$) compared with the first postoperative CT scan. The annual postimplant rate of increase in the infrarenal neck diameter was fivefold greater in SES patients (1.1 ± 0.1 mm/y) than in BES patients (0.22 ± 0.04 mm/y; $P < .0001$). There were no significant differences in the diameter of the suprarenal aorta at baseline or at 3 years and no differences in the annual rate of change in suprarenal aortic diameter between BES and SES endografts.

Conclusions.—EVAR using SES endografts resulted in progressive infrarenal aortic neck enlargement, whereas EVAR using BES endografts resulted in no neck enlargement over time. These data suggest that infrarenal neck enlargement after EVAR with SES endografts is likely related to the force exerted by SES elements rather than disease progression in the infrarenal neck.

▶ Aortic neck dilation has been a debated topic since the advent of endovascular aneurysm repair (EVAR). With open repair, we observed proximal anastomosis degeneration in 5% to 8% of patients over 10 years. In the case of EVAR, the aortic neck generally dilates to the nominal size of the device implanted over 1 to 3 years. It is clear that 1 etiology of late endograft failure is neck degeneration. The current article examines 2 endografts, Nellix (Endologix, Irvine, CA) and Endurant II (Medtronic, Minneapolis, MN). The Nellix device uses 2 balloon expandable stents (BES) that deliver no outward radial force on the aortic neck, whereas the Endurant II utilizes a self-expanding stent (SES) to deliver continual radial force against the aortic neck.

The 2 cohorts are matched well. Both endografts treated similar anatomies, with similar neck lengths, neck diameters, and abdominal aortic aneurysm sizes. Over a 3-year follow-up period, there is no demonstrable aortic neck dilation within the BES patients; however, the SES patients demonstrated neck dilation that equated to 1 mm per year. At 3 years, the SES patients experienced a 25% increase in aortic neck diameter. Despite neck dilation, no type Ia endoleaks or migration was detected.

Many surgeons have felt that a self-expanding prosthesis would hasten aortic degeneration over time and lead to late failures. Advocates of self-expanding sealing stents argued that aortic neck dilation is an expression of ongoing aneurysm degeneration of the infrarenal segment. This article adds to the increasing body of literature associating aortic neck dilation with self-expanding stent designs.

Z. M. Arthurs, MD, FACS

Aortic neck evolution after endovascular repair with TriVascular Ovation stent graft

de Donato G, Setacci F, Bresadola L, et al (Univ of Siena, Italy; Sapienza Univ of Rome, Italy; et al)

J Vasc Surg 63:8-15, 2016

Objective.—Aortic neck dilation has been reported after endovascular aneurysm repair (EVAR) with self-expanding devices. With a core laboratory analysis of morphologic changes, this study evaluated midterm results of aortic neck evolution after EVAR by endograft with no chronic outward force.

Methods.—This was a multicenter registry of all patients undergoing EVAR with the Ovation endograft (TriVascular, Santa Rosa, Calif). Inclusion criteria were at least 24 months of follow-up. Standard computed tomography (CT) scans were reviewed centrally using a dedicated software with multiplanar and volume reconstructions. Proximal aortic neck was segmented into zone A (suprarenal aorta/fixation area), zone B (infrarenal aorta, from lowest renal artery to the first polymer-filled ring), and zone C (infrarenal aorta, at level of the first polymer-filled ring/sealing zone). Images were analyzed for neck enlargement (≥2 mm), graft migration (≥3 mm), endoleak, barb detachment, neck bulging, and patency of the celiac trunk and superior mesenteric and renal arteries.

Results.—Inclusion criteria were met in 161 patients (mean age, 75.2 years; 92% male). During a mean follow-up period of 32 months (range, 24-50), 17 patients died (no abdominal aortic aneurysm-related death). Primary clinical success at 2 years was 95.1% (defined as absence of aneurysm-related death, type I or type III endoleak, graft infection or thrombosis, aneurysm expansion >5 mm, aneurysm rupture, or conversion to open repair). Assisted primary clinical success was 100%. CT scan images at a minimum follow-up of 2 years were available in 89 cases. Patency of visceral arteries at the level of suprarenal fixation (zone A) was 100%. Neither graft migration nor barb detachment or neck bulging was observed. None of the patients had significant neck enlargement. The mean change in the diameter was 0.18 ± 0.22 mm at zone A, −0.32 ± 0.87 mm at zone B, and −0.06 ± 0.97 mm at zone C. Changes at zone B correlated significantly with changes at zone C (correlation coefficient, 0.183; $P = .05$), whereas no correlation was found with zone A (correlation coefficient, 0.000; $P = 1.0$).

Conclusions.—No aortic neck dilation occurred in this series at CT scan after a minimum 24-month follow-up. This may suggest that aortic neck evolution is not associated with EVAR at midterm follow-up when an endograft with no chronic outward radial force is implanted.

▶ Self-expanding stents used in endovascular aneurysm repair engineering have demonstrated aortic neck dilation over 1 to 3 years. To date, we have no longitudinal database demonstrating causation for late endograft failures that occur 5 to 10 years after implant. Late Type Ia endoleak does account for a large number of late reinterventions, late ruptures, and late graft explants. However, there has been no association with these clinical events and endograft design. This year, the LEOPARD trial (Looking at EVAR Outcomes by Primary Analysis of Randomized Data) has been designed to provide a randomized, unbiased assessment of endograft performance.

This article examines neck morphology over time using the Ovation Endograft (TriVascular, Santa Rosa, CA). A multicenter registry was queried to include 161 patients with at least 2 years of follow-up; however, only 89 patients had computed tomography scans available for core lab review. The Ovation device has a suprarenal self-expanding stent anchored to the proximal portion of the fabric, but the primarily endograft sealing mechanism is based on 2 polymer-filled rings. These rings do not exert radial force on the aorta, differentiating this design from other self-expanding stent designs. Not surprisingly, the authors found no aortic neck dilation over time.

I suspect that this device has minimal effects on the aortic neck morphology; they have shown us that there is little to no change over 2 years. However, it will take 5 to 10 years to determine whether this equates to improved clinical outcomes.

Z. M. Arthurs, MD, FACS

Endovascular Treatment of Ruptured Abdominal Aortic Aneurysms with Hostile Aortic Neck Anatomy

Broos PPHL, 't Mannetje YW, Cuypers PhWM, et al (Catharina Hosp, Eindhoven, The Netherlands)

Eur J Vasc Endovasc Surg 50:313-319, 2015

Objective.—To compare the mid-term results of endovascular aortic aneurysm repair (EVAR) for ruptured abdominal aortic aneurysms (RAAAs) in patients with favourable aortic neck anatomy (FNA) and hostile aortic neck anatomy (HNA).

Methods.—Patients treated for a RAAA in a high volume endovascular centre in the Netherlands between February 2009 and January 2014 were identified retrospectively and divided into two groups based on aortic neck anatomy, FNA and HNA. HNA was defined as RAAA with a proximal neck of <10 mm, or a proximal neck of 10–15 mm with a suprarenal angulation (α) >45° and/or an infrarenal angulation (β) >60°, or a proximal neck of >15 mm combined with α >60° and/or β >75°. Patient demographics, procedure details, 30 day and 1 year outcomes were recorded.

Results.—Of 39 included patients, 17 (44%) had HNA. Technical success was 100% for FNA and 88% for HNA ($p = .184$). There were no type IA endoleaks on completion angiography in either group; however, more adjunctive procedures were necessary for intra-operative type IA endoleaks in the HNA group (24% vs. 0%, $p = .029$). Thirty day mortality rates were comparable, FNA 14% vs. HNA 12% ($p = 1.000$). There were no statistically significant differences at 1 year follow up in type I endoleaks, secondary endovascular procedures, or all cause mortality.

Conclusion.—Emergency EVAR provides excellent results for treatment of RAAA patients with both FNA and HNA. EVAR in RAAAs with HNA is technically feasible and safe in experienced endovascular centres.

▶ Historically, ruptured abdominal aortic aneurysms (RAAA) have carried a mortality rate of 50% to 100%. Several factors can be attributed to such an ominous outcome, but none is more important than rapid control of hemorrhage. For these reasons, endovascular aneurysm repair (EVAR) in this setting has been challenged by the fundamental concern for ongoing hemorrhage. Today, many centers offer EVAR as the primary therapy for RAAA. Advocates for this approach taught the benefits of avoiding laparotomy and the ability to avoid general anesthesia. Critics claim this approach delays operative control and that not all patients can be treated with EVAR.

In the present study, authors from a single center report their experience utilizing EVAR for RAAA. The authors specifically examine outcomes of EVAR in RAAA with hostile neck anatomy versus favorable neck anatomy. In general, larger aortic neck diameters, angulated necks, and short necks are associated with early, intermediate, and long-term technical failures. Like most retrospective analyses, the current report is plagued by selection bias. Twenty percent of patients were treated with open repair, due to juxtarenal AAA. The definition of a juxtarenal aneurysm is not provided. In many instances, the definition of juxtarenal AAA and a hostile neck may overlap. For instance, a 4-mm neck was treated with EVAR in the current report and labeled a hostile neck; this case could have been classified as a juxtarenal AAA and directed toward open repair. The 20% of patients directed toward open repair cannot be overlooked. Despite this limitation, the authors demonstrate good clinical and technical outcomes of EVAR for RAAA with both favorable and hostile neck anatomy.

It is not surprising that excellent early outcomes (9–12 months of follow-up) were achieved. Currently, our specialty struggles to identify the patients at risk for intermediate and late failures. I pose the question, which RAAA with hostile neck anatomy should be bridged to either elective open repair or fenestrated stent grafting to prevent late failures?

Z. M. Arthurs, MD, FACS

Evaluation of the Zenith low-profile abdominal aortic aneurysm stent graft

Sobocinski J, Briffa F, Holt PJ, et al (Centre Hospitalier Régional Universitaire de Lille, France; Univ of London, UK)

J Vasc Surg 62:841-847, 2015

Background.—Low-profile (LP) stent grafts are now commercially available in Europe for endovascular aortic aneurysm repair (EVAR). In this study the midterm outcomes and characteristics of patients treated with this last generation of stent grafts were compared with a cohort of patients treated with "standard-profile" (SP) stent grafts.

Methods.—The current study enrolled all patients treated for elective EVAR by the SP Zenith Flex stent graft (Cook Medical, Bloomington, Ind) between March 2010 and November 2011 and patients treated for elective EVAR by the Zenith LP stent graft (Cook Medical) between November 2011 and March 2013. All patients had a follow-up >18 months. Preoperative computed tomography angiograms were analyzed on a dedicated three-dimensional workstation. All data were prospectively collected in an electronic database and retrospectively analyzed. A comparative study was conducted.

Results.—The present study included 208 patients (107 SP and 101 LP). Patients' physiologic characteristics were similar in both groups. The iliac anatomy was considered "more challenging" in LP patients: respectively, 7% and 22% ($P = .002$) of SP and LP patients had bilateral external iliac diameter <7 mm; and 16% and 34% ($P = .005$) had a combination of an external iliac diameter <7 mm and an iliac tortuosity ratio index >1.5. No 30-day deaths were documented. The 24-month freedom from reintervention and overall survival rates after SP and LP were, respectively, 88% and 91% ($P = .450$) and 92% and 96% ($P = .153$). The 24-month rates for freedom from sac expansion and from limb occlusion were 96.4% and 98.7% ($P = .320$) and 92% and 95% ($P = .293$), respectively. One patient in each group presented with a type I endoleak during follow-up, and two LP patients presented with a type III endoleak ($P = .235$).

TABLE 4.—Adjuncts at the Time of Index Procedure

Variable	SP, No.	LP, No.	*P*
Kissing iliac stent	7	6	
Unilateral iliac stenting			
Right	2	1	
Left	5	2	
Subtotal for iliac axis	14	9	.382
Proximal aortic extension (ESBE)	2	0	
Total	16	9	.205

ESBE, Main Body Extension Graft; *LP*, low profile; *SP*, standard profile.

Reprinted from Sobocinski J, Briffa F, Holt PJ, et al. Evaluation of the Zenith low-profile abdominal aortic aneurysm stent graft. *J Vasc Surg*. 2015;62:841-847, with permission from by the Society for Vascular Surgery.

Conclusions.—This study demonstrates that the last-generation LP stent grafts have favorable midterm outcomes similar to SP stent grafts despite being used to treat more patients with unfavorable iliac anatomy (Table 4).

▶ The search for a lower profile endograft to treat abdominal aortic aneurysm continues. As more devices have been developed, the profile of these devices has decreased. The first US Food and Drug Administration–approved stent-graft was the Ancure device (Guidant Corporation), which was 25 Fr. Over the ensuing time, the profile of most devices has become smaller. The Cook (Bloomington, IN) Zenith low-profile stent graft described in this publication has been able to be compressed into a 16-Fr delivery system. This change was accomplished by changing the metal from stainless steel to nitinol as well as modifications of the suprarenal stent and elimination of the top cap many are familiar with when deploying the Zenith device. The goal of this movement is to be able to offer endovascular aortic aneurysm repair to patients with compromised iliac access and avoid invasive surgery. The authors compared their experience with the standard and low-profile device and identified significant difference in patients treated with smaller external iliac diameter (<7 mm) in the LP group (22.2% vs 6.9% in the SP group) as well as more patients with a higher tortuosity index in the LP group (22 patients vs 7 in the SP group). The adjunctive procedures used in this series at the time of the index procedure are seen in Table 4 and are comparable between the 2 devices.

Evolving technology continues to be a paramount, but in this quest for lower profile, we should not compromise the device integrity. This study demonstrates that in this cohort of patients, the technology works, but the median follow-up for the LP was 24 months. Time will tell if this device change has compromised an already effective design of the SP device.

N. Singh, MD, FACS

Patients with familial abdominal aortic aneurysms are at increased risk for endoleak and secondary intervention following elective endovascular aneurysm repair

Ryer EJ, Garvin RP, Thomas B, et al (Geisinger Med Ctr, Danville, PA)
J Vasc Surg 62:1119-1124, 2015

Objective.—A recent investigation has documented an increased risk of aneurysm-related complications after endovascular aneurysm repair (EVAR) of familial abdominal aortic aneurysms (fAAAs). We hypothesized that fAAA patients are not at increased risk for complications following open AAA repair or EVAR when compared with sporadic abdominal aortic aneurysm (spAAA) patients. To this end, we performed a single institution retrospective review.

Methods.—Epidemiologic data were collected through the electronic medical record. Family history data were obtained from a questionnaire administered at the initial vascular surgery consultation. Major adverse events were defined as myocardial infarction, respiratory failure, renal failure, bowel ischemia, limb ischemia, multisystem organ failure, intracranial hemorrhage, paraplegia, hemorrhage, or death. Endoleaks were classified in accordance with the standardized reporting practices of the Society for Vascular Surgery. AAA-related complications were defined as the need for a secondary intervention due to endoleak, limb ischemia, or postimplantation rupture.

Results.—A total of 392 patients with complete clinical data underwent elective AAA repair from 2004 to 2014. Of these 392 patients, 89 (23%) were classified as fAAA patients and 303 (77%) were classified as spAAA patients. With the exception of increased rates of chronic obstructive pulmonary disease ($P = .0009$) and pack-years smoked ($P = .03$) in spAAA patients, demographics did not differ. Sixty-two percent ($n = 55$) of fAAA patients and 68% ($n = 205$) of spAAA patients underwent EVAR ($P = .30$). fAAA patients did not incur any significant difference in major adverse events following open AAA repair (fAAA, 9% vs spAAA, 11%; $P = .75$). Additionally, fAAA patients did not incur any significant difference in major adverse events following EVAR (fAAA, 4% vs spAAA, 5%; $P = .70$). Patients with fAAA did have a significantly increased rate of endoleak (fAAA, 24% vs spAAA, 12%; $P = .03$) and secondary intervention following EVAR (fAAA, 21% vs spAAA, 12%; $P = .04$).

Conclusions.—The current study shows that patients with fAAA do not have increased perioperative morbidity following open or endovascular AAA repair. However, patients with fAAA do have an increased risk of endoleak and secondary intervention following EVAR. These findings suggest that EVAR and open AAA repair are both safe and effective for fAAA patients. The increased rate of endoleak and secondary intervention in patients with fAAA suggests that this subpopulation may benefit from

TABLE 7.—Complications Following Endovascular Aneurysm Repair (EVAR)

Variable	fAAA (n = 55)	spAAA (n = 205)	P
Follow-up, months	52 ± 33	49 ± 31	.54
Total acute major adverse events	2 (4)	10 (5)	.70
ICH	1	0	
Paraplegia	1	0	
Colonic ischemia	0	2	
Renal failure	0	3	
Limb ischemia	0	3	
MI	0	1	
Iliac artery rupture	0	1	
Total endoleaks	13 (24)	25 (12)	.03
Type I	3 (6)	2 (1)	.03
Type II	10 (18)	23 (11)	.17
Secondary interventions	12 (21)	23 (12)	.04
Proximal stent/cuff	3	2	.03
Limb extension	1[a]	0	.05
Embolization	4	16	.90
Conversion to open	1	1	.32
Limb ischemia	4	4	.04
Time to secondary intervention, months	28 ± 33	23 ± 22	.57
Post repair rupture	1	0	.05

fAAA, Familial abdominal aortic aneurysm; *ICH*, intracranial hemorrhage; *MI*, myocardial infarction; *spAAA*, sporadic abdominal aortic aneurysm. Data are presented as mean ± standard deviation or number (%).

[a]One patient underwent proximal aortic cuff placement and iliac limb extension for type Ia and type Ib endoleaks.

Reprinted from Ryer EJ, Garvin RP, Thomas B, et al. Patients with familial abdominal aortic aneurysms are at increased risk for endoleak and secondary intervention following elective endovascular aneurysm repair. *J Vasc Surg*. 2015;62:1119-1124, with permission from the Society for Vascular Surgery.

closer post-EVAR surveillance or open surgical repair in good risk patients (Table 7, Supplementary Table).

▶ This is a single institution retrospective review to assess repair outcomes and the significance of having a familial abdominal aortic aneurysm (fAAA). The review included 392 patients who underwent elective open and endovascular AAA repair from 2004 to 2014. Endovascular aneurysm repair (EVAR) was performed in 260 (55 fAAA, 205 sporadic AAA [spAAA]) cases. Family history of aortic or cerebral aneurysms was present in 23% of patients after excluding those with syndromic familial aortic diseases. The authors are to be congratulated at the level of detail involved in obtaining this family history. Unexpectedly, patients with fAAA were comparable in age to those with spAAA. It is not expected that fAAA places one at a higher risk of surgical complications, but it is interesting that there was a higher percentage of late type I endoleaks (fAAA, 24% vs spAAA, 12%) in 5 patients total (Supplementary Table) despite adherence to the manufacturer's instructions for use. These patients did require secondary interventions (proximal stent/cuff extension; Table 7). Although these findings do not change current practice in regard to EVAR in patients with fAAA, they do raise awareness of the need

SUPPLEMENTARY TABLE.—Details of Patients with Type I Endoleak Following Endovascular Aneurysm Repair (EVAR)

spAAA	AAA Size, cm	Time to Endoleak	Proximal Neck Diameter, mm	Proximal Neck Length, mm	Neck Thrombus	Neck Calcification	Iliac Tortuosity	Iliac Aneurysms	Endograft
1	5.6	6 years	25	16	Minimal	None	None	No	Cook Zenith
2	5.8	17 months	25	25	None	None	None	No	Cook Zenith
fAAA	AAA size, cm	Time to endoleak	Proximal neck diameter, mm	Proximal neck length, mm	Neck thrombus	Neck calcification	Iliac tortuosity	Iliac aneurysms	Endograft
1	5.1	7 years	19	36	None	Minimal	None	No	Medtronic Aneurx
2	5.2	22 months	22	20	None	Minimal	None	No	Cook Zenith
3	5.7	18 months	22	17	None	None	None	No	Gore Excluder

AAA, Abdominal aortic aneurysm; *fAAA*, familial AAA; *spAAA*, sporadic AAA.

Reprinted from Ryer EJ, Garvin RP, Thomas B, et al. Patients with familial abdominal aortic aneurysms are at increased risk for endoleak and secondary intervention following elective endovascular aneurysm repair. *J Vasc Surg*. 2015;62:1119-1124, with permission from the Society for Vascular Surgery.

to tailor postoperative surveillance to detect early endoleaks that warrant repair.[1]

S. Shalhub, MD, MPH, FACS

Reference

1. van de Luijtgaarden KM, Bastos Goncalves F, Hoeks SE, et al. Familial abdominal aortic aneurysm is associated with more complications after endovascular aneurysm repair. *J Vasc Surg*. 2014;59:275-282.

Outcomes of endovascular aneurysm repair with contemporary volume-dependent sac embolization in patients at risk for type II endoleak

Piazza M, Squizzato F, Zavatta M, et al (Padova Univ School of Medicine, Italy; et al)

J Vasc Surg 63:32-38, 2016

Objective.—The aim of this study was to evaluate outcomes of intraoperative aneurysm sac embolization during endovascular aneurysm repair (EVAR) in patients considered at risk for type II endoleak (EII), using a sac volume-dependent dose of fibrin glue and coils.

Methods.—Between January 2012 and December 2014, 126 patients underwent EVAR. Based on preoperative computed tomography evaluation of anatomic criteria, 107 patients (85%) were defined as at risk for EII and assigned to randomization for standard EVAR (group A; n = 55, 44%) or EVAR with intraoperative sac embolization (group B; n = 52, 42%); the remaining 19 patients (15%) were defined as at low risk for EII and excluded from the randomization (group C). Computed tomography scans were evaluated with OsiriX Pro 4.0 software to obtain aneurysm sac volume. Freedom from EII, freedom from EII-related reintervention, and aneurysm sac volume shrinkage at 6, 12, and 24 months were compared by Kaplan-Meier estimates. Patients in group C underwent the same follow-up protocol as groups A and B.

Results.—Patient characteristics, Society for Vascular Surgery comorbidity scores (0.99 ± 0.50 vs 0.95 ± 0.55; $P = .70$), and operative time (149 ± 50 minutes vs 157 ± 39 minutes; $P = .63$) were similar for groups A and B. Freedom from EII was significantly lower for group A compared with group B at 3 months (58% vs 80%; $P = .002$), 6 months (68% vs 85%; $P = .04$), and 12 months (70% vs 87%; $P = .04$) but not statistically significant at 24 months (85% vs 87%; $P = .57$). Freedom from EII-related reintervention at 24 months was significantly lower for group A compared with group B (82% vs 96%; $P = .04$). Patients in group B showed a significantly overall mean difference in aneurysm sac volume shrinkage compared with group A at 6 months ($-11 \pm 17\ cm^3$ vs $-2 \pm 14\ cm^3$; $P < .01$), 12 months ($-18 \pm 26\ cm^3$ vs $-3 \pm 32\ cm^3$; $P = .02$), and 24 months ($-27 \pm 25\ cm^3$ vs $-5 \pm 26\ cm^3$; $P < .01$). Patients in group C had the lowest EII rate compared with groups

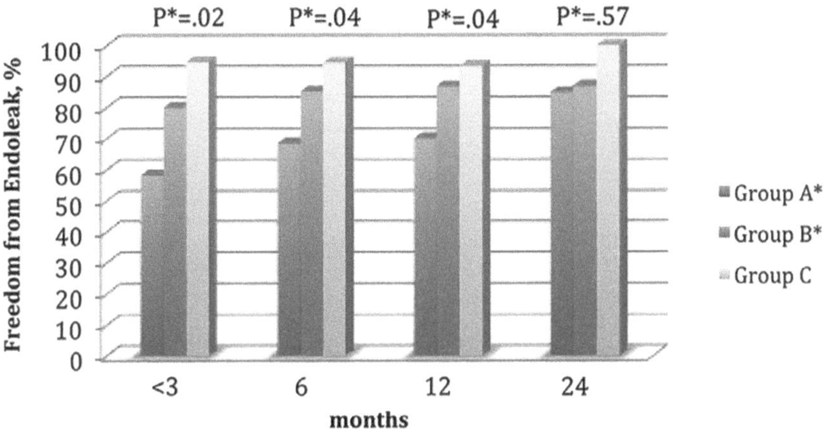

FIGURE 2.—Descriptive analysis of freedom from type II endoleaks (EIIs) during early and midterm follow-up in groups A, B, and C. (Reprinted from Piazza M, Squizzato F, Zavatta M, et al. Outcomes of endovascular aneurysm repair with contemporary volume-dependent sac embolization in patients at risk for type II endoleak. *J Vasc Surg*. 2016;63:32-38, with permission from the Society for Vascular Surgery.)

A and B (6 months, 5%; 12 months, 6%; 24 months, 0%) and no EII-related reintervention.

Conclusions.—This randomized study confirms that sac embolization during EVAR, using a sac volume-dependent dose of fibrin glue and coils, is a valid method to significantly reduce EII and its complications during early and midterm followup in patients considered at risk. Although further confirmatory studies are needed, the faster aneurysm sac volume shrinkage over time in patients who underwent embolization compared with standard EVAR may be a positive aspect influencing the lower EII rate also during long-term follow-up (Fig 2, Table 4).

▶ Type II endoleaks continue to be a vexing problem for patients as well as their surgeons. It is a pathology that has been created because of endovascular aneurysm repair (EVAR) that has no open surgical equivalent and has variable outcomes. What we do understand is that it generally leads to more intense surveillance and more reinterventions that do not have great success rates. The authors attempted to solve this problem by treating at the time of the EVAR. Randomizing patients to standard EVAR versus EVAR with embolization based on those characteristics that predict high risk for a type II endoleak (inferior mesenteric artery > 3 mm; patency of at least 3 pairs of lumbar arteries, etc). Some details are worth mentioning: during the procedure, they used a standardized technique with an additional access below their large sheaths, leaving this 5-FR sheath in the aorta during the procedure. After performing the EVAR, they would place a catheter through the smaller sheath and inject a standard amount of fibrin glue based on sac volume as well as coils. Balloon occlusion was maintained during injection, and they had a 100% technical success rate without an increase in mean operative time between the 2 groups. I believe this fact is important because most surgeons would be somewhat hesitant to employ

TABLE 4.—Aneurysm Sac Volume Variation Compared with the Preoperative Volume

Variable[a]	Group A	Group B	P
CTA ≤3 months			
Volume variation			
cm^3	+2.7 ± 12.8	−1.2 ± 5.8	.05
%	+2.3 ± 11.1	−0.9 ± 4.3	.05
CTA at 6 months			
Volume variation			
cm^3	−2.2 ± 14.2	−10.6 ± 17.1	.007[b]
%	−1.7 ± 15.3	−7.5 ± 10.6	.02[b]
CTA at 12 months			
Volume variation			
cm^3	−2.9 ± 32.2	−18.9 ± 26.6	.02[b]
%	−2.1 ± 26.8	−14.2 ± 16.7	.02[b]
CTA at 24 months			
Volume variation			
cm^3	−4.6 ± 25.9	−27.3 ± 24.7	.008[b]
%	−2.9 ± 21.5	−21.6 ± 17.2	.005[b]

CTA, Computed tomography angiography.
[a]Data are presented as the mean ± standard deviation (cm^3 and %).
[b]Statistically significant.
Reprinted from Piazza M, Squizzato F, Zavatta M, et al. Outcomes of endovascular aneurysm repair with contemporary volume-dependent sac embolization in patients at risk for type II endoleak. *J Vasc Surg*. 2016;63:32-38, with permission from the Society for Vascular Surgery.

this technique if associated distal embolization or significant increase in operative times were noted. Freedom of type II endoleaks was higher in the embolization group as was the aneurysm sac shrinkage rate (Fig 2, Table 4). In addition, the cost in patients undergoing upfront embolization was less than those who required reintervention.

Most surgeons would agree that a standardized, safe technique that decreases future reintervention rates after EVAR would be ideal. This study is important because it describes a technique of sac embolization that could prevent future procedures for the patient as well as influence the overall cost.

N. Singh, MD, FACS

Type Ia endoleaks after fenestrated and branched endografts may lead to component instability and increased aortic mortality

O'Callaghan A, Greenberg RK, Eagleton MJ, et al (Cleveland Clinic Foundation, OH)
J Vasc Surg 61:908-914, 2015

Objectives.—Fenestrated and branched endografts allow for proximal sealing zone extension into or above the visceral aorta to optimize landing in healthy aorta. We describe the incidence, causes, and implications of proximal endoleak development in patients undergoing complex endovascular aortic aneurysm repair.

Methods.—All patients undergoing a fenestrated/branched repair were entered onto a prospective database, and this analysis included all those with at least one postoperative contrast computed tomography scan. Preoperative and postoperative three-dimensional imaging was reanalyzed to characterize morphology and identify endoleak. A blinded assessor used the preoperative imaging to resize the repairs in the endoleak group and a matched cohort of patients without endoleak. The outcome measures were proximal endoleak development, mortality, and component stability, and a comparison was made with all patients undergoing complex aortic repair.

Results.—From 2001 to July 2013, 969 patients underwent repair in a physician-sponsored investigational device exemption trial. Excluded were 24 emergency patients and 21 patients without requisite imaging, leaving 924 available for analysis. A proximal type Ia endoleak developed in 26 patients (2.8%). Poor choice of landing zone was implicated in most cases, with an area of sealing in the visceral aorta, compared with the thoracic aorta, being significantly associated with endoleak development ($P < .01$). Aortic-related mortality was significantly higher in the endoleak group (26.9%) than in the group without endoleak (6.2%; $P = .001$). These patients also experienced a higher incidence of component instability of 30.8% compared with 9.6% in patients without type Ia endoleak ($P < .01$).

Conclusions.—Fenestrated/branched endovascular repair has a low incidence of sealing zone failure despite the increased complexity. However, development of a proximal endoleak destabilizes the repair and leads to increased mortality. Increasing complexity of design seems to improve the long-term outcome for patients requiring complex aortic repair (Figs 2 and 3).

▶ Fenestrated and branched endografts have allowed vascular surgeons to treat increasingly complex aortic aneurysms. As we approach 20 years of experience, many wonder what the durability of these reconstructions will be. The group at Cleveland Clinic has led the country in their skill and knowledge in these approaches. In that following, they now begin to evaluate outcomes and how to improve. Here, they present a tremendously large series of patients undergoing fenestrated or branched repair as part of a physician-sponsored, single-center, investigational device exemption trial. Type Ia endoleaks were associated with increased aortic-related mortality (Fig 2). The authors found that juxtarenal repairs using the visceral aorta as a sealing location were significantly more likely to develop a type Ia endoleak than those with sealing zones in the distal thoracic aorta. Therefore, the choice of landing zone can be implicated as a cause for future endoleak. This reasoning follows our previous experience from infrarenal EVARs. Type Ia endoleaks were more common with difficult landing zones: short neck lengths, severe angulation, conical geometry, calcification, and thrombus. The authors propose that parallel (<10% change in diameter over the course of the neck) is important when selecting a landing zone. Angulation may be less of an issue within the perivisceral aorta compared

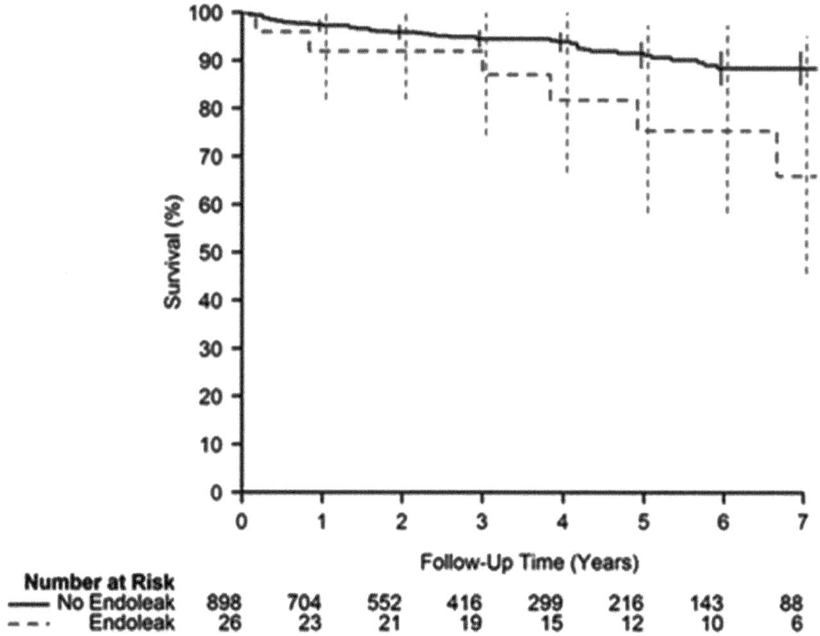

FIGURE 2.—Aortic-related survival by endoleak group. The *range bars* show the standard error. (Reprinted from O'Callaghan A, Greenberg RK, Eagleton MJ, et al. Type Ia endoleaks after fenestrated and branched endografts may lead to component instability and increased aortic mortality. *J Vasc Surg*. 2015;61:908-914, with permission the Society for Vascular Surgery.)

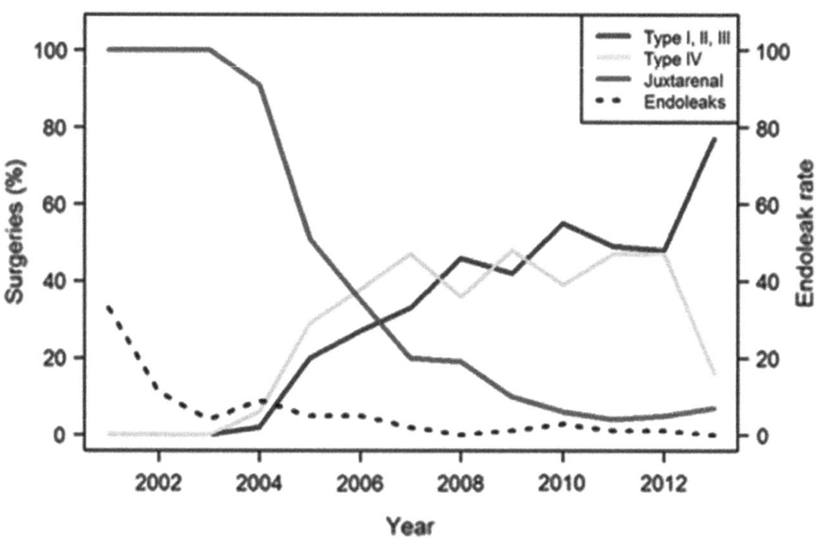

FIGURE 3.—This line graph shows how our practice has changed over the life of the study to include more of the visceral aorta in the repair to achieve a healthier sealing zone. There has been a consequent decrease in the number of juxtarenal repairs. (Reprinted from O'Callaghan A, Greenberg RK, Eagleton MJ, et al. Type Ia endoleaks after fenestrated and branched endografts may lead to component instability and increased aortic mortality. *J Vasc Surg*. 2015;61:908-914, with permission the Society for Vascular Surgery.)

with the infrarenal aorta. Fig 3 demonstrates their change in practice over time. In essence, they moved up to include more of the visceral and thoracic aorta in the repair to achieve a higher sealing zone. The repairs are categorized not on the type of the original classification of the aneurysm but rather by the extent of the repair. As a result, the number of type IV repairs have dramatically decreased. What the group hopes to accomplish is a decreased rate of type Ia endoleaks with this technique. However, as aortic coverage changes, so increases the risks of that coverage. What is not evaluated here, but is certainly an important part of aortic surgery is the risk of spinal ischemia. As we move higher and higher in the thoracic aorta, not only do we exclude more native aorta, which is a known risk of spinal ischemia, but we may also encroach the crucial artery of Adamkiewicz. We look forward to continued reports of outcomes with higher sealing zones in complex aortic endografting.

K. C. Orion, MD

Incidence and Outcomes of Severe Renal Impairment Following Ruptured Abdominal Aortic Aneurysm Repair

Ambler GK, Coughlin PA, Hayes PD, et al (Cambridge Univ Hosps NHS Foundation Trust, UK)

Eur J Vasc Endovasc Surg 50:443-449, 2015

Introduction.—Acute kidney injury (AKI) following ruptured abdominal aortic aneurysm (rAAA) repair is common and multifactorial. A standard definition of AKI after endovascular repair (EVAR), the Aneurysm Renal Injury Score (ARISe), has been proposed to facilitate standardised reporting and thus improve understanding of this issue.

Methods.—Data were collected retrospectively on AKI in a prospectively maintained database of all patients treated for rAAA in a single tertiary referral centre since the availability of routine out of hours emergency EVAR. The ARISe score was used to describe the degree of AKI and factors which correlated with poor renal outcomes were assessed.

Results.—Two-hundred and five patients were treated between January 2006 and April 2014. Of these, 125 were treated with open repair (OSR) and 80 were treated with EVAR. Severe AKI (defined as ARISe score ≥ 3) occurred in 36% of patients. After correction for confounders, patients treated with OSR were significantly more likely to develop severe AKI (43% vs. 26%, $p = .02$). There was no significant difference in preoperative serum creatinine between groups, but increased preoperative serum creatinine was strongly associated with severe AKI postoperatively ($p < .001$). Age, sex, endograft type, and preoperative CT scanning were not associated with differences in renal outcomes. Clamp position above renal arteries was predictive of severe AKI in patients treated with OSR ($p < .01$). Patients suffering severe AKI had significantly higher mortality at 30 days and 12 months (28% vs. 5% and 44% vs. 13%, $p < .001$ for both comparisons).

Conclusion.—Severe AKI is common following successful repair of rAAA. In this large case series of high-risk patients, OSR was associated with significantly higher rates of severe AKI compared with EVAR, despite the increased dose of contrast involved in EVAR and the older age of these patients. In turn, severe AKI was associated with higher mortality rates (Tables 1, 3 and 4).

► Renal failure after vascular procedures has been demonstrated to contribute to morbidity as well as mortality. In ruptured abdominal aortic aneurysm (rAAA), many factors contribute to renal impairment—namely, hypotension, potential for preoperative chronic kidney disease, contrast utilization during endovascular aneurysm repair (EVAR) and suprarenal clamp placement with open repair. The authors of this study reviewed their experience with rAAA and the incidence of renal impairment postoperatively. To measure renal impairment, they employed the Aneurysm Renal Injury Score (ARISe, Table 1), which is based on the RIFLE classification (Risk, Injury, Failure, Loss, End-stage) and tailored toward EVAR but applicable to open repair as well. They defined severe AKI as ARISe ≥3 AKI and found that it occurred in 36% of all patients surviving at least 24 hours. Fifty-four of these patients required temporary renal replacement therapy and 3 required permanent renal replacement therapy. More patients that underwent open repair suffered AKI than those treated with EVAR (43% vs 26%). Contrast volume in EVAR patients was correlated with AKI but did not reach statistical significance despite the median volume of contrast that was an astonishing 200 cc. In the open group, the authors studied the level of the proximal aortic clamp and scored it from infrarenal to supraceliac (Table 3) and found that when they excluded the clamp level above the infrarenal position, no statistical difference in the incidence of severe AKI between EVAR, and the open group was noted. Those patients suffering from severe AKI had an expected higher mortality versus those patients not having the condition (Table 4).

Again, this study underscores the importance of renal failure on vascular surgery patient outcomes particularly those with rAAA. We must strive to incorporate aspects of this study to avoid this added risk to a vulnerable population. In addition, when publishing experiences, a standardized method of describing

TABLE 1.—Aneurysm Renal Injury Score (ARISe) classification[11]

Score	Definition
1	Rise in serum creatinine > 26 μmol/L but < 50% increase from baseline or urine output < 0.5 mL/ kg/h for 6 hours within 7 days
2	Rise in baseline serum creatinine 50–99% within 7 days
3	Rise in baseline serum creatinine ≥ 100% within 7 days
4	Requirement for temporary renal replacement therapy
5	Permanent renal replacement therapy

Editor's Note: Please refer to original journal article for full references.

TABLE 3.—Effect of Severe AKI or Requirement for RRT (Renal Replacement Therapy) on Mortality and Length of Stay

Outcome	ARISe < 3	Severe AKI (ARISe 3–5)	RRT	p (Severe AKI)	p (RRT)
30-day mortality (%)	5	28	33	<.001	<.001
12-month mortality	13	44	52	<.001	<.001
Length of stay: median (IQR)	10 (7–18)	26 (13–40)	25 (11–44)	<.001	<.001

Reprinted from Ambler GK, Coughlin PA, Hayes PD, et al. Incidence and outcomes of severe renal impairment following ruptured abdominal aortic aneurysm repair. *Eur J Vasc Endovasc Surg*. 2015;50:443-449, with permission from European Society for Vascular Surgery.

TABLE 4.—Effect of Aortic Clamp Level on Acute Renal Outcomes

LOC Score During Anastomosis	Number of Patients	Incidence of Severe AKI (%)	Need for RRT (%)
0 (infra-renal)	94	37	30
1 (trans-renal)	9	44	44
2 (supra-renal)	15	80	64
3 (higher level clamp)	5	-	-

LOC = Level of Clamp.
Percentages in columns 3 and 4 are based on the 112 patients treated with OSR who survived at least 24 hours.
No patients with LOC score = 3 survived 24 hours.
Reprinted from Ambler GK, Coughlin PA, Hayes PD, et al. Incidence and outcomes of severe renal impairment following ruptured abdominal aortic aneurysm repair. *Eur J Vasc Endovasc Surg*. 2015;50:443-449, with permission from European Society for Vascular Surgery.

renal impairment should be undertaken as well as accurate measurement of contrast used during an EVAR. In this study, contrast was estimated based on the number of 50-mL vials opened. More accurate means are available and necessary to truly identify factors that can lead to renal impairment.

N. Singh, MD, FACS

Postoperative renal dysfunction independently predicts late mortality in patients undergoing aortic reconstruction

Patel VI, Lancaster RT, Ergul E, et al (Vascular Study Group of New England (VSGNE), Boston, MA)
J Vasc Surg 62:1405-1412, 2015

Objective.—Preoperative chronic kidney disease (CKD) has been shown to predict postoperative renal complications and mortality after open aortic surgery; the impact of postoperative renal complications less severe than permanent dialysis are unknown. We evaluated the impact of postoperative renal dysfunction severity on survival using a regional quality improvement registry.

Methods.—Patients undergoing intact open aortic reconstruction in the Vascular Study Group of New England registry (2003-2012) were stratified by severity of postoperative renal complications; none, creatinine increase of greater than 0.5 mg/dL (incCr), or any hemodialysis (HD). Predictors of renal dysfunction and impact of renal complications on survival were analyzed using multivariable methods.

Results.—We included 2695 patients, of which 65% (n = 1733) underwent open abdominal aortic aneurysm repair, and 35% (n = 962) open aortoiliac reconstruction. At baseline, 15% of patients had preoperative moderate CKD and 1.2% had severe CKD. Postoperative renal complications of incCr occurred in 8.5% of patients, and 1.5% required HD. Multivariable cumlogit regression identified severe baseline CKD (odds ratio [OR], 15; 95% confidence interval [CI], 6.4-34; $P < .001$, moderate CKD (OR, 2.8; 95% CI, 1.9-3.3; $P < .001$), suprarenal clamp use (OR, 2.2; 95% CI, 1.6-2.9; $P < .001$), perioperative vasopressor requirements (OR, 2.2; 95% CI, 1.6-2.9; $P < .001$), operating time (OR, 1.004 per minute; 95% CI, 1.003-1.006; $P < .001$), and chronic obstructive pulmonary disease (OR, 1.5; 95% CI, 1.2-1.8; $P < .001$) as independent predictors of worsening strata of postoperative renal dysfunction. Multivariable logistic regression analysis showed that patient age (OR, 1.06 per year; 95% CI, 1.01-1.1; $P = .01$), baseline chronic obstructive pulmonary disease (OR, 1.6; 95% CI, 1.2-2.2; $P < .01$), incCr (OR, 3.7; 95% CI, 1.8-7.4; $P = .009$), and HD (OR, 4.8; 95% CI, 1.8-12.7); $P = .009$) independently increased 30-day mortality. Risk-adjusted multivariable Cox regression showed that incCr (hazard ratio, 1.8; 95% CI, 1.3-2.6; $P < .001$) and HD (hazard ratio, 4.4; 95% CI, 2.8-6.9; $P < .001$) increased risk of late death independent of a variety of other clinical variables, including baseline CKD. The 5-year survival was lower (log-rank $P < .001$) in patients with incCr (66% ± 4%), and HD (38% ± 10%) compared with those with no renal complications (77% ± 1%).

Conclusions.—Increasing severity of postoperative renal dysfunction independently predicts increased risk of late mortality after open aortic surgery. Perioperative measures to decrease renal complications may potentially prolong the survival of patients after open aortic surgery (Fig 1, Tables 4 and 5).

▶ Postoperative renal dysfunction is a known contributor of increased morbidity and mortality in patients undergoing aortic reconstruction. The authors of this study used the Vascular Study Group of New England (VSGNE) registry to identify clinical and technical predictors of increasing severity of renal dysfunction and its impact on both perioperative and long-term mortality. By using this large database, they were able to identify that progression to any hemodialysis increased mortality to 23%. In addition to severe chronic kidney disease (CKD), moderate CKD, chronic obstructive pulmonary disease, procedure time, and vasopressor use were all independent predictors of renal complications (Table 4). The modeling the authors performed also indicated that an increased creatinine level leads to late mortality as well as early mortality (Figure 1). Many of the same factors that predict renal complications also predict late mortality (Table 5).

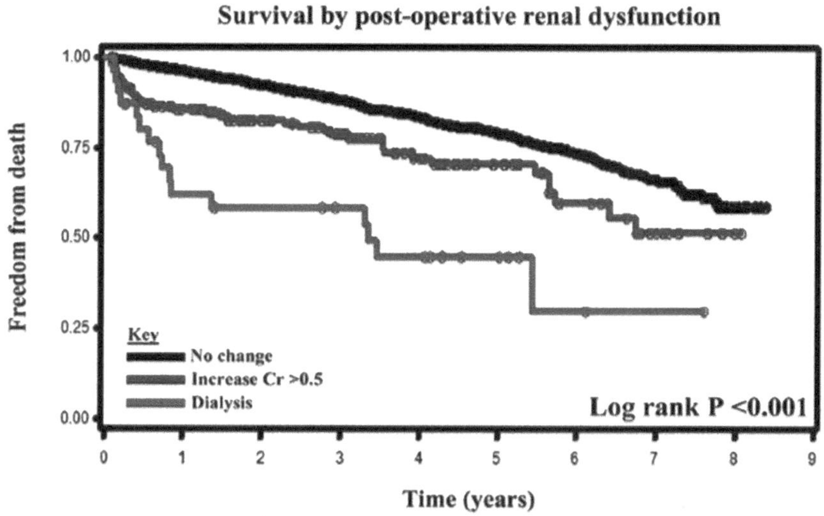

YEAR:	0	1	2	3	4	5
No renal complication						
Survival (%)	100	96	91	87	82	77
Number at risk	2062	1517	1107	869	668	485
Standard error (%)	0	0	1	1	1	1
Increase in creatinine > 0.5 mg/dL						
Survival (%)	100	84	80	75	70	66
Number at risk	229	161	115	96	66	41
Standard error (%)	0	2	3	3	4	4
Any post-operative dialysis						
Survival (%)	100	65	58	54	47	38
Number at risk	47	26	22	16	14	4
Standard error (%)	0	6	7	8	8	10

FIGURE 1.—Survival. Kaplan-Meier curves plotting the fraction of the study population alive over time for patients with no postoperative renal dysfunction, increase in creatinine >0.5 mg/dL, or dialysis dependent renal failure. The standard error of the curve representing postoperative hemodialysis (HD) is greater than 10% beyond 5 years, and may be an unreliable estimate of survival beyond that time point. (Reprinted from Patel VI, Lancaster RT, Ergul E, et al. Postoperative renal dysfunction independently predicts late mortality in patients undergoing aortic reconstruction. *J Vasc Surg.* 2015;62:1405-1412, with permission from the Society for Vascular Surgery.)

Postoperative renal dysfunction leads to worse outcomes in aortic surgery and those with severe preoperative renal insufficiency have 15 times the risk of postoperative renal dysfunction that leads to significant perioperative and long-term mortality. When considering an open aortic reconstruction on these

TABLE 4.—Independent Predictors of Renal Complications*

Outcome	HR	95% CI	*P* Value
Severe CKD	15	6.4-34	<.001
Moderate CKD	2.8	1.9-3.8	<.001
Suprarenal clamp	2.2	1.6-2.9	<.001
Chronic obstructive pulmonary disease	1.5	1.2-1.8	.02
Procedure time, minutes	1.004	1.003-1.006	<.001
Vasopressor requirement	2.2	1.6-2.9	<.001

CI, Confidence interval; *CKD*, chronic kidney disease; *HR*, hazard ratio.

*Multivariable cumlogit regression model for increase in creatinine or postoperative dialysis.

Reprinted from Patel VI, Lancaster RT, Ergul E, et al. Postoperative renal dysfunction independently predicts late mortality in patients undergoing aortic reconstruction. *J Vasc Surg*. 2015;62:1405-1412, with permission from the Society for Vascular Surgery.

TABLE 5.—Independent Predictors of Late Mortality*

Outcome	HR	95% CI	*P* Value
Increased creatinine >0.5 mg/dL	1.8	1.3-2.6	<.001
Any postoperative dialysis	4.4	2.8-6.9	<.001
Severe CKD	2.1	1.1-3.9	.03
Age (per year)	1.07	1.05-1.08	<.001
Urgent operation	1.7	1.4-2.1	<.001
Chronic obstructive pulmonary disease	1.5	1.2-1.8	<.001
Postoperative MI	1.7	1.2-2.4	<.001
CHF	1.5	1.2-1.8	<.001

CHF, Any degree of congestive heart failure; *CI*, confidence interval; *CKD*, chronic kidney disease; *HR*, hazard ratio; *MI*, myocardial infarction.

*Model risk adjusted for gender, moderate CKD, postoperative MI, and gender.

Reprinted from Patel VI, Lancaster RT, Ergul E, et al. Postoperative renal dysfunction independently predicts late mortality in patients undergoing aortic reconstruction. *J Vasc Surg*. 2015;62:1405-1412, with permission from the Society for Vascular Surgery.

patients, significant counseling should include the higher rate of mortality and any means to optimize renal function before the procedure.

N. Singh, MD, FACS

Renal Outcomes Following Fenestrated and Branched Endografting

Martin-Gonzalez T, Pinçon C, Maurel B, et al (CHRU Lille, France; Université Lille Nord de France; et al)

Eur J Vasc Endovasc Surg 50:420-430, 2015

Objective.—The purpose of this study was to analyze immediate and long-term renal outcomes (renal function and renal events) after fenestrated (FEVAR) and branched endovascular aortic aneurysm repair (BEVAR).

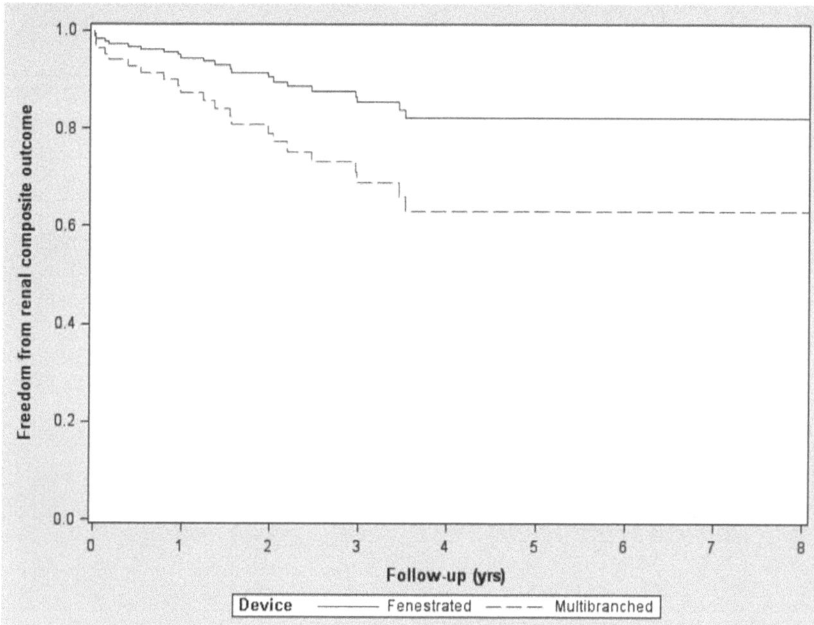

Year of follow-up	0	1	2	3	4	5	6	7	8
Patients at risk Fen device	186	149	109	73	39	23	8	3	2
Patients at risk Branch device	38	24	19	13	8	4	1	1	1

FIGURE 2.—Freedom from renal composite outcome as estimated by the multivariate Cox model. (Reprinted from Martin-Gonzalez T, Pinçon C, Maurel B, et al. Renal outcomes following fenestrated and branched endografting. *Eur J Vasc Endovasc Surg*. 2015;50:420-430, with permission from European Society for Vascular Surgery.)

Methods.—All FEVAR and BEVAR performed between October 2004 and October 2012 were included in this study. Post-operative acute renal failure (ARF) was defined according to the RIFLE criteria. Renal volume (calculated with a 3D workstation) and estimated glomerular filtration rate (GFR) (estimated with the Modification of Diet in Renal Disease [MDRD] formula) were evaluated before the procedure, before discharge, 12 months after, and yearly thereafter. Renal stent occlusion, dissection, fracture, stenosis, kink, renal stent related endoleak, and renal stent secondary intervention were all considered "renal composite events" and analyzed. A time to event analysis was performed for renal events and secondary renal interventions.

Results.—225 patients were treated with FEVAR and BEVAR. Renal target vessels ($n = 427$) were perfused by fenestrations ($n = 374$), or branches ($n = 53$). Median follow up was 3.1 years (2.9–3.3 years). Technical success was achieved in 95.5% of patients. Post-operative ARF was

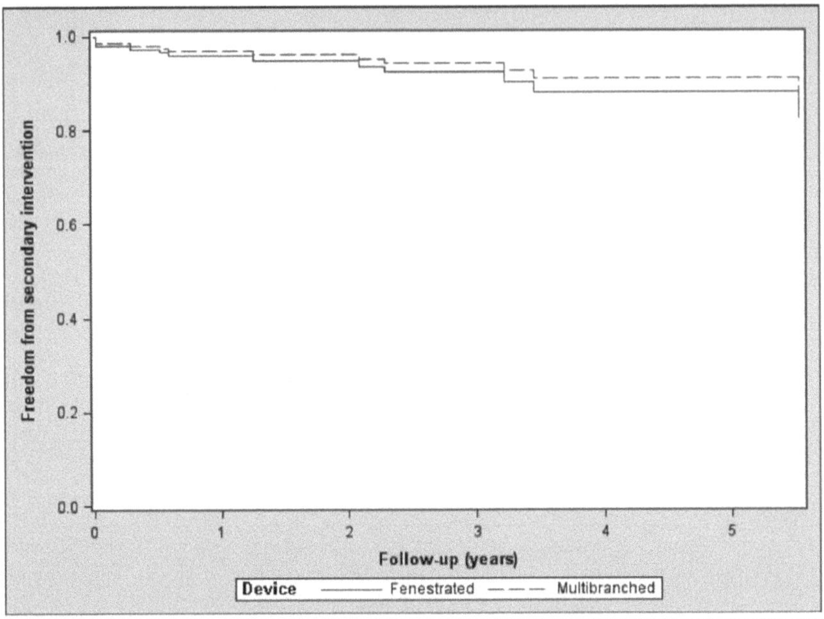

Year of follow-up	0	1	2	3	4	5	6	7	8
Patients at risk Fen device	180	153	115	77	41	25	8	3	2
Patients at risk Branch device	33	24	19	13	8	3	0	0	0

FIGURE 3.—Freedom from secondary renal intervention as estimated by the multivariate Cox model. (Reprinted from Martin-Gonzalez T, Pinçon C, Maurel B, et al. Renal outcomes following fenestrated and branched endografting. *Eur J Vasc Endovasc Surg*. 2015;50:420-430, with permission from European Society for Vascular Surgery.)

seen in 64 patients (29%). Mean total renal volume and eGFR at 1 year, 2 year, and 3 year follow up were significantly lower when compared with pre-operative levels (after BEVAR and FEVAR); the decrease at 3 years was 14.8% (6.7%; 22.2%) ($p = .0006$) for total renal volume and 14.3% (3.1%; 24.3%) ($p = .02$) for eGFR. The 30 day and 5 year freedom from renal composite event was 98.6% (95.8–99.6%) and 84.5% (76.5–89.9%) after FEVAR and BEVAR (NS). The 30 day and 5 year freedom from renal occlusion was 99.5% (96.7–99.9%) and 94.4% (89.3–97.1%) after FEVAR and BEVAR (NS).

Conclusion.—FEVAR and BEVAR are durable options for the treatment of complex aortic aneurysms and are associated with low renal morbidity, without differences between device types. The clinical impact of decreasing renal volume over time in these patients is yet to be fully understood (Figs 2 and 3).

▶ Postoperative renal impairment is one of the most frequent major complications after treatment of complex aneurysms using any modality. Using systematic reviews, previous authors have described an incidence of early transient renal failure of 15% after fenestrated endovascular aortic aneurysm repair (FEVAR) compared with 20% after open repair.[1] These authors used the RIFLE criteria to determine the incidence of postoperative acute renal failure and used a "renal composite endpoint" along with renal volumes and renal lengths to determine postoperative outcomes at a single high-volume center.

Two hundred twenty-five patients were included in the study group. Renal target vessels were perfused by either fenestrations (n = 374) or branches (n = 53). Postoperative acute renal failure (as defined by the RIFLE criteria) was seen in 64 patients (29%). Preoperative chronic kidney disease, procedure time, and preoperative metformin use were identified as risk factors for acute renal failure. Not surprisingly, freedom from the renal composite outcome (renal stent occlusion, dissection, fracture, stenosis, kink, renal stent-related endoleak, and renal stent secondary intervention) were worse in the branched cases (Fig 2), but this was not statistically different from FEVAR cases, probably due to small numbers of branches. Freedom from secondary renal intervention was equivalent between groups, and branch vessel patency was excellent (Fig 3).

This study highlights the durability of modern endovascular repair of complex aneurysmal disease. It is clear that this is where the future of aortic aneurysm repair lies. We do, however, need better tools to assess outcomes and to help guide better stent designs that improve branch vessel patency over the long term.

B. W. Starnes, MD

Reference

1. Nordon IM, Hinchliffe RJ, Holt PJ, Loftus IM, Thompson MM. Modern treatment of juxtarenal abdominal aortic aneurysms with fenestrated endografting and open repair: a systematic review. *Eur J Vasc Endovasc Surg*. 2009;38:35-41.

Renal outcomes analysis after endovascular and open aortic aneurysm repair

Martin-Gonzalez T, Pinçon C, Hertault A, et al (CHRU Lille, France)
J Vasc Surg 62:569-577, 2015

Objective.—The purpose of this study was to compare renal outcomes (glomerular filtration rate [GFR] and renal volume) after endovascular aneurysm repair (EVAR) and open repair (OR) of abdominal aortic aneurysm (AAA).

Methods.—All AAA repairs performed between November 2009 and July 2011 were included in this retrospective study. Patients requiring suprarenal clamping and renal bypass or reimplantation and patients requiring fenestrated endografting were excluded from the OR and EVAR groups, respectively. All EVARs were performed with transrenal proximal fixation. Renal volume (calculated with a three-dimensional workstation) and GFR(estimated with the Modification of Diet in Renal Disease formula) were evaluated before the procedure, at 12 months after the procedure, and yearly thereafter.

Results.—The study included 90 patients (41 ORs and 49 EVARs). Both groups were comparable except for age at intervention, body mass index, smoking, peripheral arterial disease, arrhythmia, and vitamin K antagonist treatment. Median follow-up was 2.8 years for OR (2.5-2.9 years) and 3.2 years for EVAR (3.0-3.4 years). In both groups, we found a significant decrease when comparing postoperative estimated GFR with 1-year (14.4% decrease [3.8%-23.8%]; $P = .002$) and 3-year (12.8% decrease [3.8%-20.9%]; $P = .0007$) levels. In both groups, total renal volumes significantly diminished. Median preoperative total renal volume (372 cm^3 [311-349]) significantly decreased (6.7% [2.8%-10.5%]; $P = .008$) between 1 year and 2 years of follow-up.

Conclusions.—Renal function impairment is similar after open and endovascular AAA repair. It is associated with a decrease in total renal volume, which seems to be an early and constant marker of postoperative renal impairment.

▶ In the present series, the authors examine the impact of open infrarenal aneurysm repair and endovascular aneurysm repair (EVAR) on renal function over time. The group provides a retrospective evaluation of 90 patients treated over a 20-month period. The group used 1 stent-graft manufacturer with suprarenal struts for all EVAR patients, and the group excluded suprarenal clamps in the open cohort. The follow-up regimen was also similar in that the open repair group also received computed tomography angiogram surveillance at 1 and 3 years. During the 2.8 years of follow-up, both open aneurysm repair and EVAR patients suffered progressive renal function decline as measured by glomerular filtration rate (GFR) and renal volume. However, there was not significant difference between the 2 groups. On average, GFR decreased 12.8% over the follow-up period and does not appear to be related to endovascular aneurysm repair.

Z. M. Arthurs, MD, FACS

F-EVAR does not Impair Renal Function more than Open Surgery for Juxtarenal Aortic Aneurysms: Single Centre Results

Shahverdyan R, Majd MP, Thul R, et al (Univ Hosp of Cologne, Germany)
Eur J Vasc Endovasc Surg 50:432-441, 2015

Objective.—To compare the results of elective open surgical repair (OSR) and total endovascular repair of juxtarenal aortic aneurysms (JAA), with either the Cook Zenith or the Vascutek Anaconda fenestrated stent grafts (F-EVAR) in a university hospital setting.

Patients and Methods.—Between April 1999 and July 2014, of 926 patients with an abdominal aortic aneurysm, 69 were juxtarenal, where 34 had an elective OSR and 35 had F-EVAR. A post-operative rise of baseline creatinine by >50% and/or deterioration of estimated glomerular filtration rate by 25% were defined as renal failure.

Results.—The demographics of the patients were similar except for heart insufficiency, peripheral arterial disease, and pre-existing renal artery stenosis ($p < .05$). Median aneurysm diameters were 57 mm (range 50–80 mm) and 56 mm (range 36–64 mm) ($p = .194$), respectively, and the median pre-operative serum creatinine levels were 94 µmol/L (range 65–286 µmol/L) and 96 µmol/L (range 57–333 µmol/L) ($p = .871$) with median estimated glomerular filtration rate of 68 mL/min (range 21–117 mL/min) and 70 mL/min (range 18–114 mL/min) ($p = .308$) in the open and endovascular groups, respectively. The technical success (OSR versus F-EVAR) was 100% versus 94.3% with complete exclusion

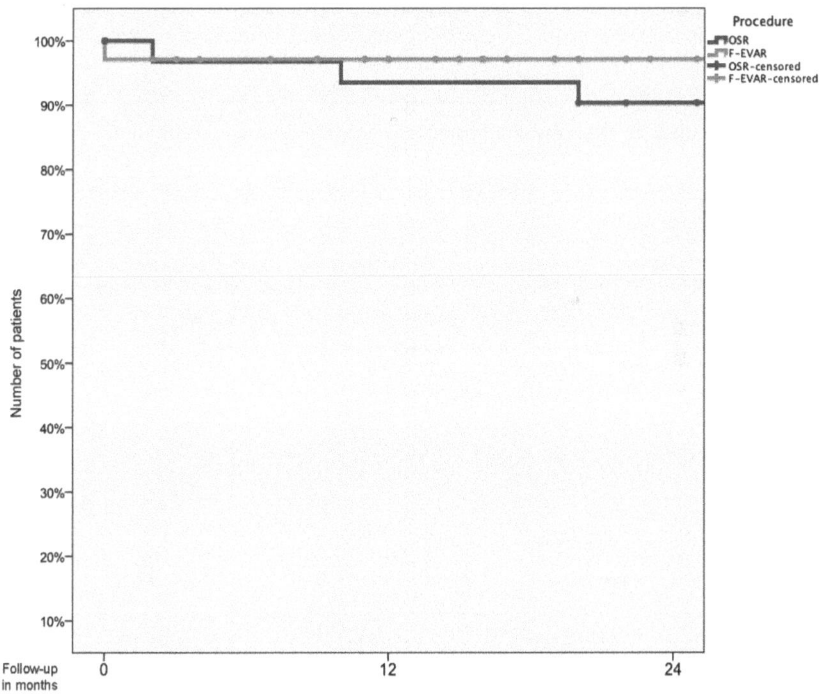

Numbers at risk

OSR	34	29	26
F-EVAR	35	25	11

FIGURE 5.—Kaplan-Meier curve, demonstrating estimated long-term survival rates after OSR and F-EVAR within the follow up period of 24 months. (Reprinted from Shahverdyan R, Majd MP, Thul R, et al. F-EVAR does not impair renal function more than open surgery for juxtarenal aortic aneurysms: single centre results. *Eur J Vasc Endovasc Surg.* 2015;50:432-441, with permission from European Society for Vascular Surgery.)

of the aneurysms in all cases. Median procedure time was 171 versus 188 min. During median in hospital stay of 11 versus 7 days ($p = .05$), mortality was 0 versus 2.9% and new onset of post-operative renal insufficiency was detected in 26.5% versus 8.5% patients ($p = .05$), although with 11.8% versus 5.7% being persistent ($p = .428$). During follow up, statistically similar new (late or persistent post-operative) renal insufficiency was detected in 14.7% versus 8.8% with dialysis in 3% of patients in each group with similar mortality within the 24 months.

Conclusions.—This retrospective analysis demonstrates that OSR might be combined with more acute postoperative renal impairment than F-EVAR for JAA, but with similar intermediate term procedure related mortality and renal outcomes (Fig 5, Table 1).

▶ To my knowledge, no study has been published reporting a direct comparison of open surgical repair and fenestrated endovascular aneurysm repair (FEVAR) for juxta-renal abdominal aortic aneurysms. The present study is a single-institution retrospective analysis of all aortic aneurysm repairs done between April 1999 and July 2014. Of 926 repairs, only 69 were considered juxta-renal which, at the outset seems to be a low percentage to me. Thirty-four underwent

TABLE 1.—Patients' Pre-operative Demographics and Comorbidities

	OSR	F-EVAR	*p*
No. of patients	34	35	
Gender, M:F	26:8	30:5	.371
Age, median in y (range)	72 (57–83)	72 (60–84)	.938
Aneurysm dd in mm, median (range)	57 (50–80)	56 (36–64)	.194
Comorbidities			
Previous MI	9 (26%)	8 (23%)	.785
Hypertension	26 (76%)	30 (85%)	.371
Coronary heart disease	18 (53%)	16 (45%)	.633
Heart insufficiency	20 (59%)	2 (5%)	.001[a]
COPD	13 (38%)	7 (20%)	.117
PAD	5 (15%)	16 (45%)	.008[a]
Smoking (current or past)	23 (67%)	27 (77%)	.405
Diabetes	5 (14%)	2 (5%)	.259
Chronic renal insufficiency	2 (6%)	4 (11%)	.673
Dialysis prior to procedure	1 (3%)	0	.493
Creatinine, µmol/L, median (range)	94 (65–286)	96 (57–333)	.871
eGFR, mL/min, median (range)	68 (21–117)	70 (18–114)	.308
Haemoglobin, g/dL, median (range)	14.2 (9.1–18.2)	14.4 (11–17.8)	.414
Renal artery stenosis	6 (17%)	0	.010[a]
ASA			
ASA I	2 (6%)	0	.239
ASA II	13 (38%)	15 (43%)	.808
ASA III	16 (47%)	18 (51%)	.811
ASA IV	3 (9%)	2 (5%)	.673
ASA V	0	0	

ASA = American Society of Anesthesiologists; COPD = chronic obstructive pulmonary disease; dd = diameter; eGFR = estimated glomerular filtration rate; MI = myocardial infarction; PAD = peripheral arterial disease; y = years.

[a]Significant.

Reprinted from Shahverdyan R, Majd MP, Thul R, et al. F-EVAR does not impair renal function more than open surgery for juxtarenal aortic aneurysms: single centre results. *Eur J Vasc Endovasc Surg*. 2015;50:432-441, with permission from European Society for Vascular Surgery.

open surgical repair, and 35 underwent FEVAR; these were the groups that were directly compared with regard to mortality and renal events (Table 1).

The important point in this study was that new-immediate onset of renal insufficiency after open surgical repair was 26.5% versus only 8.5% after FEVAR, which, the authors surmised, could be explained by the suprarenal cross-clamp in the open group. Although I agree with the conclusion based on my own experience, I think that this finding is a little bit of a stretch because of the profound selection bias. Early in the FEVAR experience, patients with existing renal artery stenosis were excluded from treatment due to fear of inability to cannulate the vessel. There were no patients with renal artery stenosis in the FEVAR group and 6 in the open group. This finding alone could have changed the outcomes in this small series, even though the baseline characteristics were no different. Outcomes for the FEVAR group were better at 2 years (Fig 5).

In my opinion, FEVAR will eventually replace open surgical repair for juxtarenal aortic aneurysms and the durability of renal stenting will prove to be strong. It is also my opinion that as technical expertise improves, the majority of patients with any hint of a diseased or short infrarenal aortic neck will be offered this therapy. This article is one more level of support for this concept.

B. W. Starnes, MD

Chimney Grafts in Aortic Stent Grafting: Hazardous or Useful Technique? Systematic Review of Current Data

Lindblad B, Bin Jabr A, Holst J, et al (Skåne Univ Hosp, Malmö, Sweden)

Eur J Vasc Endovasc Surg 50:722-731, 2015

Background.—The chimney graft (CG) technique was introduced to rescue accidentally covered aortic branches during aortic endovascular repair. It extends the sealing zone. There is concern about "gutter" type I endoleak (EL-I) and about the durability of CGs. The aim of the present report was to analyze the rapidly increasing existing data.

Methods.—A search was performed (PRISMA criteria) for all studies of visceral and thoracic/arch chimney grafts. Technical and clinical details and outcome were assessed.

Results.—The present review includes 831 patients who underwent EVAR/TEVAR (endovascular aneurysm repair/thoracic endovascular aneurysm repair) with one or more chimney, periscope, or sandwich grafts. For aortic visceral vessels 517 patients received 911 visceral CGs and 314 patients received 364 arch CGs. Most procedures (81% visceral and 69% arch CGs) were elective. Thirty day mortality was 4% for both groups. The rate of early EL-I was 13% (visceral CGs) and 11% (arch CGs). Most EL-I were handled conservatively (observation: 70% for visceral CG and 45% for arch CG). Early CG patency was high (97–99%) and remained high during follow up (median 17 months). Late (after 30 days) EL-I was reported in nine visceral (2%) and 12 arch (4%) CG cases. Few other late complications were reported, but those losing a kidney at the initial repair seemed to have a high risk of requiring permanent hemodialysis.

Conclusion.—Increasing amounts of data support the benefit of visceral and arch chimney graft techniques. In particular, the low early mortality and complication rates and high long-term patency seem advantageous; however, the majority of cases have been treated electively, and there is a high risk of bias in all studies. Mid- to long-term data suggest few late complications, except in cases where one renal artery was sacrificed. The CG technique is valuable for complex urgent patients and needs further documentation for other patient groups.

▶ The principle of chimney graft techniques has emerged in the past several years as an option for complex aneurysm from the arch to the aortic and even iliac bifurcations. Heterogeneity of the reports in terms of setting (urgent/elective) as well as the substantially different risk profile of comparative aortic territories (arch vs thoracoabdominal aortic aneurysm) had led to great skepticism of the validity of the approach. The authors seek to derive a review of the published literature and have reported 911 chimneys among 517 patients, culled from case reports and series of 3 to 43 patients.

The authors correctly cite a publication bias inherent to the reporting of early mortality, which was only 4% among visceral chimney and arch chimney patients. Technical failures were often handled with extra-anatomic bypass, although some were reported as asymptomatic. Certainly, the latter would be typical of a late failure of the renal chimney, whereas loss of a superior mesenteric artery chimney is routinely devastating. Ultimately, sac regression is the true test of reassurance that an endovascular repair has "shut the door" on an aneurysm, and these data are absent from most series. Major endoleaks remain problematic and interestingly, among arch chimneys, are associated with the diameter of the brachiocephalic; this would suggest the array of endovascular devices is not suitable for some patients' anatomy.

A fair assessment of the "state of the art" for the chimney approach is offered as suitable for emergent cases not fit for open repair or those who cannot have a fenestrated or branched technology and restricted use for elective cases.

M. Arnold, MD

Debate: Whether branched/fenestrated endovascular aneurysm repair procedures are better than snorkels, chimneys or periscopes in the treatment of most thoracoabdominal and juxtarenal aneurysms

Hertault A, Haulon S, Lee JT (CHRU, Lille, France; Stanford Univ Med Ctr, CA)

J Vasc Surg 62:1357-1365, 2015

Vascular surgeons are an innovative group, and during the last decade, we have seen unparalleled advances in the endovascular treatment of extensive aortic pathologies. Collaborative efforts between surgeons and industry have introduced fenestrated and branched devices that are becoming more widely used, with wider regulatory approval, availability, and less need for customization. Prior to this, parallel stent approaches had been developed to fill the void where this technology was not available or for urgent cases. A separate and distinct body of evidence and expertise subsequently developed for both strategies. This debate explores where these approaches now sit in the armamentarium of vascular surgeons (Tables 1 and 2).

▶ As the endo-revolution continues, vascular surgeons have continued to innovate and expand indications and treatment options for complex juxtarenal and thoracic-abdominal aneurysms. Two separate approaches have emerged as options for maintaining branch patency. One approach is the layering of side branch stents alongside the endograft, the so-called chimney, snorkel, or periscope type repairs (ch-EVAR). The other is a fused device with fenestrations or side branches attached (F-EVAR). The superiority of one technique over the other is hotly debated. This article sought to delineate the pros and cons of each repair.

The argument favoring ch-EVAR sites the universal availability of the technique. Surgeons use various combinations of covered stents and grafts depending on the situation. These are all things that are readily available at a large endovascular center and thus making this technique suitable for emergent type repairs. Although direct side-to-side comparisons are not available, there is a significant amount of data that shows no significant difference between ch-EVAR and F-EVAR with regard to technical success, target branch vessel patency, early mortality, type I endoleak, postoperative renal dysfunction, or need for secondary intervention. In addition, those who are pro ch-EVAR point to the fact that one of the biggest pieces of the data favoring F-EVAR comes from a single center, the Cleveland Clinic, which has extensive experience. They note that these data do not reflect "real-world" practice. Tables 1 and 2 summarize some of the most recent data on ch-EVAR and F-EVAR.

Proponents of the F-EVAR technique point to the gutters formed in the ch-EVAR repair as the "Achilles heel" of the technique. They site a type Ia endoleak rate of up to 10.2%. In addition, because of the extensive manipulation that occurs in the arch during this repair, a recent meta-analysis demonstrated a 3.2% stroke rate with ch-EVAR compared with 0.3% with F-EVAR ($P = 0.012$). F-EVAR advocates note that because the ch-EVAR repair allows the surgeon to use myriad combinations of stents and endografts, standardization of the data for reporting and evaluation is problematic. To the question of lack of availability of the F-EVAR device, supporters note that "off-the-shelf" devices are in the pipeline and should be available soon for general use.

The authors on both sides of the debate make excellent points. Although there are excellent data supporting either technique, what is lacking is a "head-to-head" trial evaluating both in a prospective fashion. The feasibility of this may make it prohibitive. What is most likely is that as F-EVAR becomes

TABLE 1.—Early Results of Chimney Endovascular Aneurysm Repair (ch-EVAR) for Juxtarenal Aortic Aneurysms (JAAs) and Pararenal Aortic Aneurysms (PAAs)

First Author, Year	No.	Number of Target Vessels	Number of Emergency Cases	Technical Success[a]	Endoleaks I	II	III	UK	Primary Branch Patency	Early Reintervention	30-Day Mortality
Ohrlander, 2008[3]	6	11	5	6/6	—	—	—	—	11/11	None	0/6
Hiramoto, 2009[2]	29	31	-	29/29	3	8	—	—	31/31	None	1/29
Donas, 2010[4]	15	15	5	15/15	—	1	—	—	15/15	None	0/15
Bruen, 2011[5]	21	37	-	20/21	1	—	—	—	36/37	NR	1/21
Coscas, 2011[6]	16	26	4	14/16	2		—	1	25/26	5/16	2/16
Lee, 2012[7]	28	57	-	56/57	NR	NR	NR	NR	56/57	None	2/28
Schiro, 2013[8]	9	9	2	9/9	2	—	—	—	9/9	None	0/9
Lachat, 2013[9]	77	169	NR	53/77	19	14	1	—	165/170[a]	NR	NR (at least 2/77)
Ducasse, 2014[10]	22	22	-	21/22	1	4	—	—	22/22	1/22	1/22
Scali, 2014[11]	41	76	8	38/41	1	—	—	—	76/76	2/41	2/41

Editor's Note: Please refer to original journal article for full references.

NR, Not reported; *UK*, unknown.

[a]As defined by reporting standards.[13]

Reprinted from Hertault A, Haulon S, Lee JT. Debate: Whether branched/fenestrated endovascular aneurysm repair procedures are better than snorkels, chimneys, or periscopes in the treatment of most thoracoabdominal and juxtarenal aneurysms. *J Vasc Surg*. 2015;62:1357-1365, with permission from Elsevier.

TABLE 2.—Midterm Outcomes of Chimney Endovascular Aneurysm Repair (ch-EVAR) for juxtarenal Aortic Aneurysms (JAAs) And Pararenal Aortic Aneurysms (PAAs)

First Author, Year	No.	Number of Target Vessels	Mean Follow-up, Months	Endoleaks I	II	III	UK	Primary Branch Patency	Reintervention	Chronic Dialysis	Aneurysm-Related Death[a]
Follow-up <12 months Ohrlander, 2008[3]	6	11	NR (0-24)	–	–	–	–	10/11	–	1/6	1/6
Hiramoto, 2009[2]	29	31	12.5 (0-74.7)	–	NR	NR	NR	31/31	- 1 renal additional stenting for stenosis (9 months)	0/29	1/29
Bruen, 2011[5]	21	37	NR	–	1	–	–	1 SMA occlusion 1 SMA stenosis	- repeated angioplasties	0/21	1/21
Coscas, 2011[6]	16	26	10.5 (2-19)	1	–	–	1	25/26	25/26	0/14	2/16
Donas, 2012	72	127	12.1 (1-26) - 15.9 (1-29)	1	6	–	–	1 left renal occlusion (J45) 1 renal stenosis	- 1 iliorenal bypass- Repeated renal angioplasties - 1 proximal cuff for persistent type Ia	0%	0%
Lee, 2012[7]	28	57	10.7 (3-25)	2	3	1	–	56/57	- 1 extender cuff for treatment of type III endoleak	1/28	2/28
Schiro, 2013[8]	9	9	12 (5-24)	2	–	–	–	9/9	None	0/9	2/9
Follow-up >12 months Lachat, 2013[9]	77	169	25.5 (±16)	3	Type	I/III		165/170	12/77	NR	NR
Ducasse, 2014[10]	22	22	18 (7-35)	–	3	–	–	22/22	None	0/22	1/22
Scali, 2014[11]	41	76	18.2[b] (1.4-41.5)	3	4	–	3	76/76	3/41	2/41	NR

Editor's Note: Please refer to original journal article for full references.
NR, Not reported; *UK*, unknown.
[a]Including 30-day mortality.
[b]Median.
Reprinted from Hertault A, Haulon S, Lee JT. Debate: Whether branched/fenestrated endovascular aneurysm repair procedures are better than snorkels, chimneys, or periscopes in the treatment of most thoracoabdominal and juxtarenal aneurysms. *J Vasc Surg*. 2015;62:1357-1365, with permission from Elsevier.

available as an off-the-shelf device, ch-EVAR will remain a bail-out of emergency technique.

M. Arnold, MD

A Single Center Experience of Aortic and Iliac Artery Aneurysm Treated with Multilayer Flow Modulator

Pane B, Spinella G, Perfumo C, et al (Univ of Genoa, Italy)

Ann Vasc Surg 30:166-174, 2016

Background.—The aim of this study was to analyze our series of endovascular treatments using a multilayer flow modulator (MFM) and to show the midterm results.

Methods.—At our institution, 8 patients were treated with an MFM. Four patients presented with an aortic aneurysm (2 type II thoracoabdominal aortic aneurysms [TAAAs], 1 type IV TAAA, and 1 juxtarenal abdominal aortic aneurysm) and 4 with an aneurysm involving the common iliac artery. Mortality, rupture and secondary intervention, major complications, patency of collateral vessels, and volume analysis were evaluated. Treated patients were followed up with computed tomography angiography at 1, 3, 6, and 12 months.

Results.—Results showed no 30-day mortality or major complications; technical success was achieved in 87.5% of patients, patency of collateral vessels was reached in all cases at intraoperative completion angiography. Mean follow-up was 22.1 months (range, 18–30), survival rate was 87.5%, and one case of death unrelated to MFM treatment was reported. During follow-up, MFM and collateral vessel patency were observed in all cases. Secondary endovascular or open surgical procedures were not needed during follow-up. Volume analysis showed a slight increase in patients with aortic aneurysm, and an overall trend to increase in thrombosis was observed in all cases.

Conclusions.—Endovascular treatment of aneurysms with MFM seems to have encouraging midterm results. Should our results be confirmed by larger series and longer follow-up studies, MFM may become a viable alternative to other endovascular approaches (Fig 3).

▶ The authors present a single-center experience of 8 patients who underwent multilayer flow modulator (MFM) implants for treatment of complex aneurysmal disease. I agree with the authors that these results are encouraging because, of the 8 patients treated, only 1 patient sustained a non–aneurysm-related death; however, it is not clear that these particular patients are "out of the woods" because follow-up mean is 22 months. The technology is interesting, and the authors present a nice review of limited peer-reviewed articles available for MFM. One ongoing question is whether the newly created laminar flow still creates the same pulsatile pressure on the aortic wall as turbulent flow. In Fig 3A and B, flow is clearly seen outside the stent with perfusion of the branched vessel. One must consider that arterial pressure is still transmitted through the

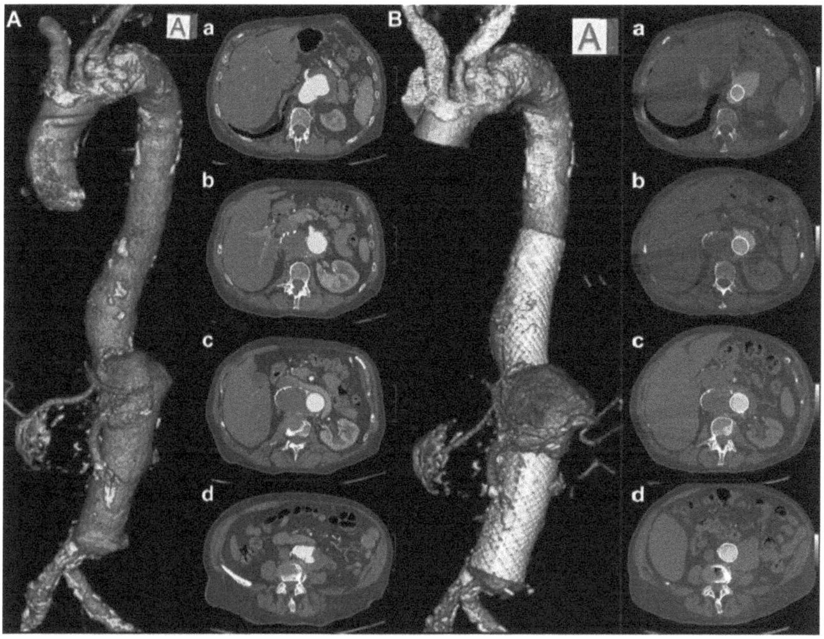

FIGURE 3.—Patient 3. (A) Volume rendering of type IV thoracoabdominal aortic aneurysm before endoprosthesis deployment. (a–d) Contrast-enhanced computed tomography slices showing aortic aneurysm before treatment. (B) Volume rendering after endoprosthesis deployment. (a–d) Contrast-enhanced computed tomography slices showing aortic aneurysm treatment with endoprosthesis. Notice sac thrombosis and collateral vessel patency. (Reprinted from Pane B, Spinella G, Perfumo C, et al, A single center experience of aortic and iliac artery aneurysm treated with multilayer flow modulator. *Ann Vasc Surg.* 2016;30:166-174, with permission from Elsevier.)

interstices of the stent graft, and rupture risk would seem to be present. Whether laminar flow reduces the risk is unclear, and studying this long term will be challenging. Additionally, there are other technical considerations not addressed. For example, is laminar flow maintained if the device requires advanced angulation, or is laminar flow maintained solely through inline stent grafts. Future work is needed, and this article is an excellent description of a single-center experience with promising midterm results.

B. Propper, MD, FACS

6 Thoracic Aorta

Presentation, Diagnosis, and Outcomes of Acute Aortic Dissection: 17-Year Trends From the International Registry of Acute Aortic Dissection

Pape LA, Awais M, Woznicki EM, et al (Univ of Massachusetts Hosp, Worcester; Univ of Michigan, Ann Arbor; et al)

J Am Coll Cardiol 66:350-358, 2015

Background.—Diagnosis, treatment, and outcomes of acute aortic dissection (AAS) are changing.

Objectives.—This study examined 17-year trends in the presentation, diagnosis, and hospital outcomes of AAD from the International Registry of Acute Aortic Dissection (IRAD).

Methods.—Data from 4,428 patients enrolled at 28 IRAD centers between December 26, 1995, and February 6, 2013, were analyzed. Patients were divided according to enrollment date into6equalgroups and by AAD type: A (n = 2,952) or B (n = 1,476).

Results.—There was no change in the presenting complaints of severe or worst-ever pain for type A and type B AAD (93% and 94%, respectively), nor in the incidence of chest pain (83% and 71%, respectively). Use of computed tomography (CT) for diagnosis of type A increased from 46% to 73% ($p < 0.001$). Surgical management for type A increased from 79% to 90% ($p < 0.001$). Endovascular management of type B increased from 7% to 31% ($p < 0.001$). Type A in-hospital mortality decreased significantly (31% to 22%; $p < 0.001$), as surgical mortality (25% to 18%; $p = 0.003$). There was no significant trend in in-hospital mortality in type B (from 12% to 14%).

Conclusions.—Presenting symptoms and physical findings of AAD have not changed significantly. Use of chest CT increased for type A. More patients in both groups were managed with interventional procedures: surgery in type A and endovascular therapy in type B. A significant decrease in overall in-hospital mortality was seen for type A but not for type B.

▶ The authors present a 17-year review of International Registry of Acute Aortic Dissection (IRAD) data broken down by date of enrollment. They separate the patient population into 6 groups and evaluate a variety of parameters with regard to acute aortic dissection. What is clear from this report is that mortality from AAD is decreasing, while use of CT scan and endovascular therapy for type B dissections are increasing. One could guess that the decreased mortality for type A dissections is 2-fold. First, more CT scan is being used, so diagnosis and treatment can occur earlier; second, with early diagnosis, more patients are transferred to IRAD centers, as noted by the authors. Additionally, the data show less medical treatment in the more recent patients with type A dissection, presumably getting these patients to definitive surgical repair. Other advances in cardiac surgery have likely contributed to decreased surgical mortality. Despite these advances, surgical mortality still hovers around 20% for those who survive long enough to undergo surgery and the overall morbidity and mortality should not be underestimated. In terms of type B dissections, endovascular therapy has become the mainstay for treatment. Open surgical interventions are occurring in only 10% of cases, and these likely have some other complicating factor (eg, malperfusion). Interestingly mortality for type B dissections has not changed. The exact etiology of this is unknown, but one could guess that mortality secondary to type B dissection in the acute setting is likely related to organ failure from malperfusion. Although endovascular therapy has advanced the repair and seal of the initial tear, cases in which visceral or peripheral malperfusion exists are still highly mortal.

B. Propper, MD, FACS

Routine Genetic Testing for Thoracic Aortic Aneurysm and Dissection in a Clinical Setting

Ziganshin BA, Bailey AE, Coons C, et al (Yale Univ School of Medicine, New Haven, CT)

Ann Thorac Surg 100:1604-1611, 2015

Background.—Hereditary factors play an important etiologic role in thoracic aortic aneurysm and dissection (TAAD), with a number of genes proven to predispose to this condition. We initiated a clinical program for routine genetic testing of individuals for TAAD by whole exome sequencing (WES). Here we present our initial results.

Methods.—The WES was performed in 102 patients (mean age 56.8 years; range 13 to 83; 70 males [68.6%]) with TAAD. The following 21-gene panel was tested by WES: ACTA2, ADAMTS10, COL1A1, COL1A2, COL3A1, COL5A1, COL5A2, ELN, FBLN4, FLNA, FBN1, FBN2, MYH11, MYLK, NOTCH1, PRKG1, SLC2A10, SMAD3, TGFB2, TGFBR1, TGFBR2.

Results.—Seventy-four patients (72.5%) had no medically important genetic alterations. Four patients (3.9%) had a deleterious mutation identified in the FBN1, COL5A1, MYLK, and FLNA genes. Twenty-two (21.6%) previously unreported suspicious variants of unknown significance were identified in 1 or more of the following genes: FBN1 (n = 5); MYH11 (n = 4); ACTA2 (n = 2); COL1A1 (n = 2); TGFBR1 (n = 2); COL3A1 (n = 1); COL5A1 (n = 1); COL5A2 (n = 1); FLNA (n = 1);

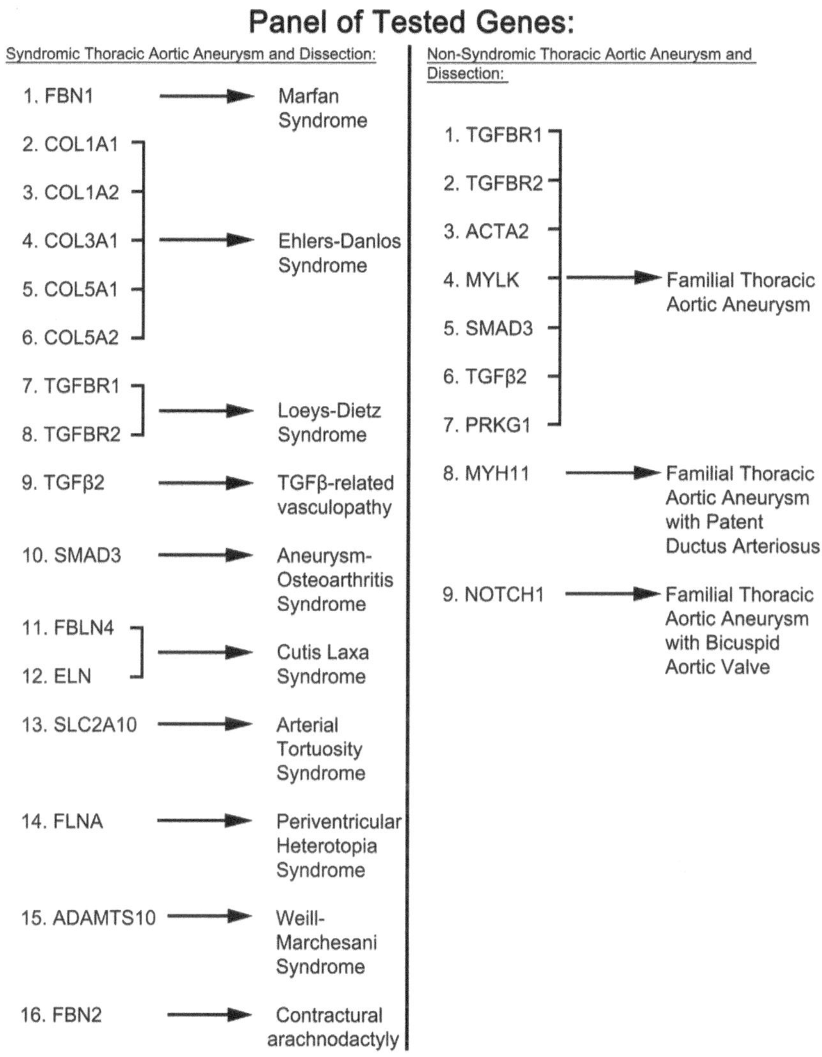

FIGURE 1.—Panel of 21 tested genes. Note that TRFBR1, TGFBR2, SMAD2, and TGBβ2 genes appear in both lists (syndromic on the left, and nonsyndromic on the right), so that the total number of genes tested is 21. (TAAD = thoracic aortic aneurysm and dissection.) (Reprinted from Ziganshin BA, Bailey AE, Coons C, et al. Routine genetic testing for thoracic aortic aneurysm and dissection in a clinical setting. *Ann Thorac Surg*. 2015;100:1604-1611, with permission from The Society of Thoracic Surgeons.)

NOTCH1 (n = 1); PRKG1 (n = 1); and TGFBR3 (n = 1). Identified mutations had implications for clinical management.

Conclusions.—Routine genetic screening of patients with TAAD provides information that enables genetically personalized care and permits identification of novel mutations responsible for aortic pathology. Analysis of large data sets of variants of unknown significance that include associated clinical features will help define the mutational spectrum of known genes underlying this phenotype and potential identify new candidate loci (Fig 1).

▶ Advances in genetic medicine have paved the way for a deeper understanding of the events that perturb aortic homeostasis and result in the development of aortic dissection and aortic aneurysm. Furthermore, advances in the techniques related to genetic testing have also opened the door to diagnosis a bit wider, as previously it was thought that 10% of mutations would be missed. The authors initiated whole exome sequencing, which is a newer technique. In this technique, the entire exome is examined, unlike previous testing directed at particular conditions. In this article, the results for 102 patients are reported.

Whole exome sequencing revealed new mutations or suspicious variants in 28 of 102 patients. Although counseling of those patients with known mutations and downstream syndromes is well understood, a greater question arises in how to manage those patients in which a suspicious variant is identified. Indeed, should those patients initiate lifelong medical therapies, restrict lifestyle from competitive sports, and give careful consideration to reproduction? These are weighty questions and should be fielded by an experienced cardiovascular geneticist. Thus, practically, it is best for patients to have counseling before testing, and not as a routine order by a surgeon when confronted with thoracic aortic disease alone.

J. H. Black III, MD, FACS

The Risk for Type B Aortic Dissection in Marfan Syndrome

den Hartog AW, Franken R, Zwinderman AH, et al (Academic Med Ctr, Amsterdam, the Netherlands; Interuniversity Cardiology Inst of the Netherlands, Utrecht; et al)

J Am Coll Cardiol 65:246-254, 2015

Background.—Aortic dissections involving the descending aorta are a major clinical problem in patients with Marfan syndrome.

Objectives.—The purpose of this study was to identify clinical parameters associated with type B aortic dissection and to develop a risk model to predict type B aortic dissection in patients with Marfan syndrome.

Methods.—Patients with the diagnosis of Marfan syndrome and magnetic resonance imaging or computed tomographic imaging of the aorta were followed for a median of 6 years for the occurrence of type B dissection or the combined end point of type B aortic dissection, distal aortic surgery, and death. A model using various clinical parameters as well as genotyping was developed to predict the risk for type B dissection in patients with Marfan syndrome.

Results.—Between 1998 and 2013, 54 type B aortic dissections occurred in 600 patients with Marfan syndrome (mean age 36 ± 14 years, 52% male). Independent variables associated with type B aortic dissection were prior prophylactic aortic surgery (hazard ratio: 2.1; 95% confidence interval: 1.2 to 3.8; $p = 0.010$) and a proximal descending aorta diameter ≥27 mm (hazard ratio: 2.2; 95% confidence interval: 1.1 to 4.3; $p = 0.020$). In the risk model, the 10-year occurrence of type B aortic dissection in low-, moderate-, and high-risk patients was 6%, 19%, and 34%, respectively. Angiotensin II receptor blocker therapy was associated with fewer type B aortic dissections (hazard ratio: 0.3; 95% confidence interval: 0.1 to 0.9; $p = 0.030$).

Conclusions.—Patients with Marfan syndrome with prior prophylactic aortic surgery are at substantial risk for type B aortic dissection, even when the descending aorta is only slightly dilated. Angiotensin II receptor blocker therapy may be protective in the prevention of type B aortic dissections.

▶ The authors present a nice review of a large group of patients being tracked within the Dutch Medical System. The review gives us a 15-year look at patients with known Marfan syndrome. The purpose of this review was to identify factors that may contribute to type B dissections in the patient subset. The authors conclude that prior prophylactic aortic surgery is a risk factor for development of a type B dissection. The size and longevity of this study allows for access to a large repository of data about those with Marfan syndrome. What remains unknown and continues to be a topic of interest is the differences among Marfan patients with regard to vessel dilation and changes in morphology. We still do not know whether patients who required prophylactic surgery did so because of a more aggressive Marfan presentation, hence predisposing them to dissection. This theory also holds true for the enlarged descending proximal aorta. Although the authors conclude that these 2 factors increase the risk of dissection, I would argue that these factors, including dissection, are identifying a more aggressive form of the genetic mutation.

The other conclusion reached from this study is that the use of angiotensin II receptor blocker medications is protective. Although this has been shown in other studies and I concur with the authors conclusion, I do not see evidence from the data presented to make that conclusion from this particular study.

For physicians who treat patients with Marfan syndrome, this report provides a few areas that can be targeted when evaluating long-term risk for a patient. For those with prior aortic surgery or enlarged descending aorta, the physician should consider that this may impart higher long-term risk for aortic complications.

B. Propper, MD, FACS

Endovascular Simulation Leads to Efficiency and Competence in Thoracic Endovascular Aortic Repair Procedures

Kendrick DE, Gosling AF, Nagavalli A, et al (Univ Hosps—Case Med Ctr, Cleveland, OH)

J Surg Educ 72:1158-1164, 2015

Objective.—Endovascular interventions such as thoracic endovascular aortic repair (TEVAR) have largely replaced invasive open procedures, and have been demonstrated to be effective in treating patients. Our study used endovascular simulation to assess the effect of TEVAR rehearsal on surgical trainees at different levels in training.

Design.—Participants were oriented on an endovascular simulator and subsequently a simulated TEVAR was performed during 4 separate sessions over a 1-month period. Metrics included total procedure/fluoroscopy time and volume of contrast used. Likert scale qualitative analysis evaluated participant's skills involving major procedural steps. Analysis of data across cohorts included 1-way analysis of variance, Kruskal-Wallis, and paired *t*-tests.

Setting.—All data were collected at University Hospitals—Case Medical Center, Cleveland, OH.

Participants.—In all, 12 trainees in 3 cohorts (student, surgery resident postgraduate year [PGY] 1-3, surgery resident/fellow PGY 4-7, $n = 4$ each) were recruited.

Results.—All trainees reduced total procedure time (mean = 537 ± 148 vs 269 ± 66 s, first session vs fourth, $P < 0.05$, CI: 195-341) and fluoroscopy time (mean = 201 ± 74 vs 110 ± 37 s, $P < 0.05$, CI: 51-132) with TEVAR case progression. The student cohort decreased procedure time from 551 ± 84 s to 313 ± 65 s ($P < 0.05$, CI: 189-287) whereas PGYs 1 to 3 decreased procedure time from 591 ± 149 s to 264 ± 29 s ($P < 0.05$, CI: 113-541). Use of contrast decreased over time, but the difference was not significant. Participants acquired proficiency after a few runs in most steps of the procedure. The average qualitative score for all groups combined improved significantly ($P < 0.03$). PGY 4 to 7 trainees had higher technical scores but this was not statistically significant. The initial gap in junior vs senior trainee performance narrowed after a few practice sessions in all aspects evaluated.

Conclusions.—TEVAR rehearsal on an endovascular simulator can reduce overall procedure and fluoroscopy time, independent of trainee skill level or experience, as well as improve subjective measures of technical success. Further studies are needed to compare simulator performance to outcomes in live cases.

▶ Simulation has become a cornerstone in surgical training over the past 10 years. General surgery residents must now pass a laparoscopic simulation before graduation. As work hours diminish, many senior integrated vascular residents report decreased confidence in performing low-volume cases even after a 6- or 7-year training program dedicated to vascular procedures. The authors at Case Medical Center sought to evaluate whether endovascular simulation may be a helpful adjunct to their vascular residency. They divided 12 trainees into 3 groups: students, junior residents (postgraduate year 1–3), and senior residents or fellows. They performed a thoracic endovascular aortic repair (TEVAR) simulation case on 4 separate occasions. The results showed marked improvements in all 3 groups. Not surprisingly, the greatest amount of progress was found in junior residents because senior residents were likely exposed to TEVARs previously in their training. This lends credence that the benefit of simulation favors those with less experience and in fact may be helpful as a steppingstone by practicing basic catheter and guidewire skills before live endovascular cases. However, everyone would agree that although simulation can provide preparation of the resident to entering an operating room, it cannot and should not replace their operative experience overall.

K. C. Orion, MD

Late aortic remodeling persists in the stented segment after endovascular repair of acute complicated type B aortic dissection

Conrad MF, Carvalho S, Ergul E, et al (Harvard Med School, Boston, MA)
J Vasc Surg 62:600-605, 2015

Objective.—Thoracic endovascular aortic repair (TEVAR) for acute complicated type B aortic dissection (AD) promotes early positive aortic remodeling. However, little is known about the long-term effect of TEVAR on the dissected aorta, which is the goal of this study.

Methods.—Between August 2005 and August 2009, 31 patients with complicated type B AD were treated with TEVAR and had >1-year follow-up imaging. Computed tomography angiograms obtained at 1 month, 1 year, and long term (average, 42 months) were compared with baseline scans. The largest diameters of the stented thoracic aorta, stented true lumen, and stented false lumen were recorded at each time point, as were the values in the unstented distal thoracic aorta and the abdominal aorta. Changes over time were evaluated by a mixed effect analysis of variance model of repeated measures.

Results.—The average age of the cohort was 56 years, and 74% were male. Indications for TEVAR were as follows: 61% malperfusion, 32% refractory hypertension, 45% impending rupture, and 32% persistent pain; 58% had more than one indication. All patients were treated in the acute phase within 7 days of the initial presentation. The average length of aorta covered was 19 cm. Observation of the stented segment over time showed that the maximum diameter of the stented thoracic aorta was stable ($P = \text{NS}$), the diameter of the stented true lumen increased ($P < .001$), and the diameter of the stented false lumen decreased ($P < .001$); 84% had complete false lumen obliteration across the stented aortic segment. Observation of the uncovered thoracic aorta over time showed that the maximum diameter increased ($P = .014$), as did the visceral segment of the aorta ($P < .001$). The average growth of the visceral segment was 31% in patients with a patent false lumen vs 3% in those with a thrombosed false lumen ($P = .004$). One patient had aneurysmal degeneration of the false lumen and required an additional endograft at 18 months.

Conclusions.—TEVAR of acute AD promotes long-term remodeling across the stented segment, with false lumen obliteration in 84% of patients. However, false lumen obliteration beyond the stented segment appears necessary to prevent late aneurysmal degeneration of the distal aorta (Fig 4).

▶ The management of acute type B aortic dissection (TBAD) continues to evolve. This is a retrospective natural history study on the longer term outcomes of 31 patients with complicated TBAD who were treated with thoracic endovascular aortic repair (TEVAR) coverage of the proximal entry tear between 2005 and 2009. Complicated TBAD was defined as malperfusion syndrome, refractory hypertension, rupture or impending rupture, or intractable pain. The study adds to the body of contemporary literature by helping us understand the aortic remodeling after TEVAR for acute TBAD. The average follow-up was 42 months (range, 14–98 months). The average length of aorta covered was 19 cm and resulted in complete false lumen obliteration across the stented aortic segment in 84% of the cases. However, just as others have previously demonstrated, late aneurysmal degeneration of the distal aorta in the uncovered regions does occur, as demonstrated in Fig 4. False lumen thrombosis was

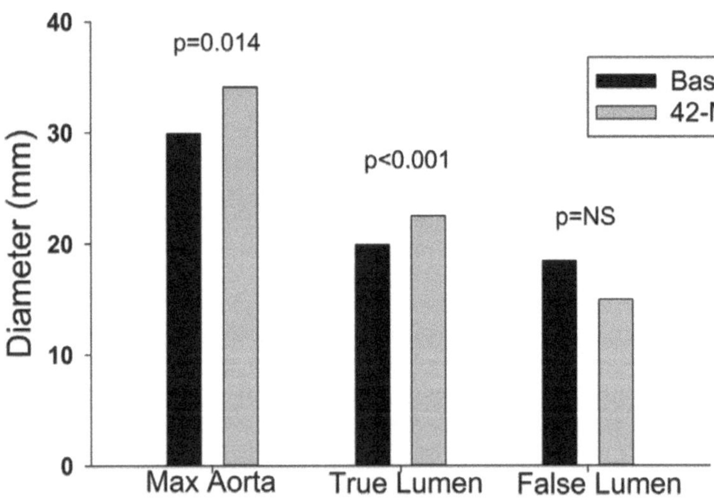

FIGURE 4.—Changes in the maximum aortic, true lumen, and false lumen diameters in the unstented segment of the aorta from baseline to 42-month follow-up. (Reprinted from Conrad MF, Carvalho S, Ergul E, et al. Late aortic remodeling persists in the stented segment after endovascular repair of acute complicated type B aortic dissection. *J Vasc Surg.* 2015;62:600-605, with permission from the Society for Vascular Surgery.)

identified as an imaging marker associated with reduction of aortic growth, supporting the observation that total obliteration of the false lumen is key factor in the prevention of long-term aneurysmal degeneration of the dissected aorta. Data from this study and others serve as a preliminary data for future prospective studies assessing the role of TEVAR in the altering the natural history of TBAD.[1-3]

S. Shalhub, MD, MPH, FACS

References

1. White RA, Miller DC, Criado FJ, et al. Multidisciplinary Society for Vascular Surgery Outcomes Committee. Report on the results of thoracic endovascular aortic repair for acute, complicated, type B aortic dissection at 30 days and 1 year from a multidisciplinary subcommittee of the Society for Vascular Surgery Outcomes Committee. *J Vasc Surg*. 2011;53:1082-1090.
2. Nienaber CA, Kische S, Rousseau H, et al. INSTEAD-XL Trial. Endovascular repair of type B aortic dissection: long-term results of the randomized investigation of stent grafts in aortic dissection trial. *Circ Cardiovasc Interv*. 2013;6:407-416.
3. Cambria RP, Crawford RS, Cho JS, et al. A multicenter clinical trial of endovascular stent graft repair of acutecatastrophes of the descending thoracic aorta. *J Vasc Surg*. 2009;50:1255-1264.e1-4.

Left Subclavian Arterial Coverage and Stroke During Thoracic Aortic Endografting: A Systematic Review

Waterford SD, Chou D, Bombien R, et al (Cedars-Sinai Med Ctr, Los Angeles, CA)

Ann Thorac Surg 101:381-389, 2016

Stroke is a devastating complication of thoracic endovascular aortic repair (TEVAR). Whether left subclavian artery (LSA) coverage and LSA revascularization affect stroke rate is debated. Whether patients with aneurysms or dissections undergoing TEVAR have higher stroke rates is also debated. We report a systematic review of 63 studies comprising more than 3,000 patients. We conclude that stroke risk after TEVAR is increased by LSA coverage, and that LSA revascularization reduces stroke risk. LSA revascularization may lower the rate of posterior stroke. TEVAR for aneurysm is associated with increased stroke risk compared to TEVAR for dissection (Fig 2, Table 1).

▶ Stroke is one of the most devastating complications after thoracic aortic surgery. With the advent of thoracic aortic endograft repair (TEVAR), the question of whether to revascularize the left subclavian artery (LSA) has been debated for decades. Originally, the artery was covered indiscriminately because the effects were thought to be of little consequence. However, as an increasing number of procedures are performed, the incidence of stroke became evident. The authors here perform an extensive review of 63 articles with the question of whether LSA coverage increases the risk of stroke, what kind of stroke occurs (anterior or posterior), and whether this risk is

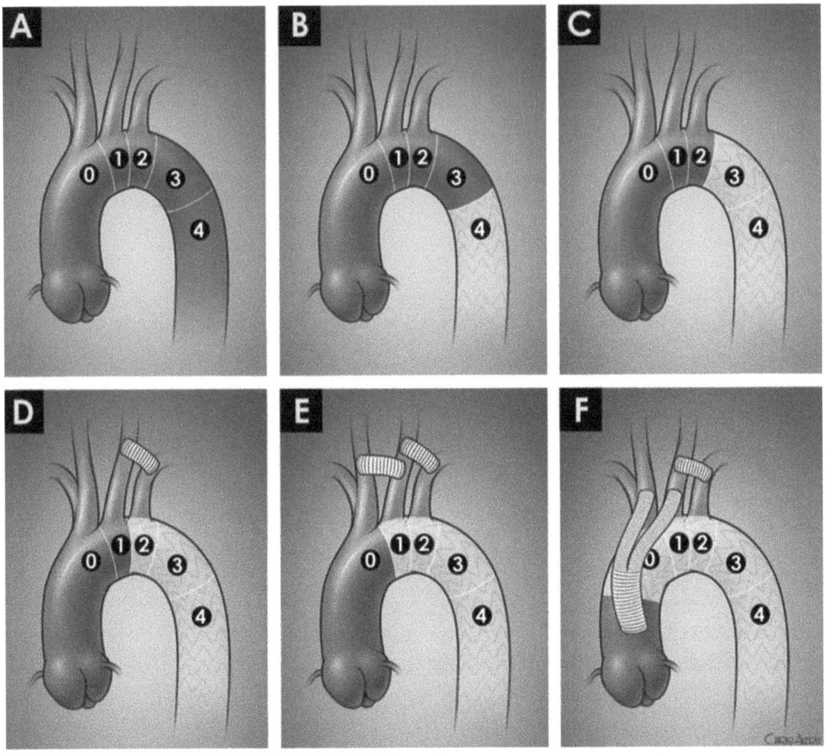

FIGURE 2.—TEVAR zones and corresponding hybrid strategies. (A) Distribution of landing zones for thoracic endovascular aortic repair. (B and C) Placement of a device in zones 3 or 4 does not require any revascularization. (D) Revascularization of covered left subclavian artery with a left carotid-subclavian bypass. (E) Revascularization of covered left carotid and subclavian arteries with a carotid-carotid and carotid subclavian bypass. (F) Complete revascularization of all aortic arch vessels with aorto-innominate and left carotid bypass as well as carotid-subclavian bypass. (Reprinted from Waterford SD, Chou D, Bombien R, et al. Left subclavian arterial coverage and stroke during thoracic aortic endografting: a systematic review. *Ann Thorac Surg*. 2016;101:381-389, with permission from The Society of Thoracic Surgeons.)

different in aneurysmal disease or dissection. In Table 1, a series of 25 studies show that the risk for stroke with LSA coverage is 7.4% versus 4.0% for distal deployment. Moving further, one would expect that revascularization of the LSA would markedly reduce stroke rate. Indeed, carotid-subclavian bypass or transposition reduced overall stroke rate from 5.6% to 3.1%. What is interesting is the high rate of stroke without the coverage of LSA, suggesting that either intercostal artery coverage or atheromatous debris during the procedure may play a role. The authors address this concern by evaluating the anatomic distribution of strokes. In the entire review, 26.2% of strokes following LSA coverage were in fact posterior strokes, a result of vertebrobasilar compromise. Moreover, TEVAR for aneurysmal disease is associated with a higher stroke rate, thereby confirming the multifactorial etiology of stroke. As a result of the studies in this review, many vascular and thoracic surgeons have modified

TABLE 1.—Description of Studies

First Author, Year	Number of Patients	Stroke Rate With LSA Coverage	Stroke Rate With LSA Coverage With Prior Revascularization	Stroke Rate With LSA Coverage Without Prior Revascularization	Stroke Rate With Deployment Distal to LSA
Antonello 2013 [11]	31	0/31 (0%)	NA	0/31 (0%)	NA
Attia 2007 [12]	2	0/2 (0%)	NA	0/2 (0%)	NA
Böckler 2006 [13]	30	0/13 (0%)	0/1 (0%)	0/12 (0%)	0/17 (0%)
Buth 2007 [9]	606	5/159 (3.1%)	0/40 (0%)	5/119 (4.2%)	14/447 (3.1%)
Chaikof 2009 [14]	197	5/42 (11.9%)	NR	NR	1/155 (0.6%)
Chiesa 2010 [15]	65	1/65 (1.5%)	NR	NR	NA
Chung 2011 [16]	733	24/279 (8.6%)	NR	NR	18/454 (4.0%)
Desai 2011 [17]	502	11/141 (7.8%)	NR	NR	36/361 (10.0%)
Ehrlich 2009 [18]	41	0/8 (0%)	NA	0/8 (0%)	0/33 (0%)
Fairman 2012 [19]	157	2/51 (3.9%)	0/22 (0%)	2/29 (6.9%)	2/106 (1.9%)
Feezor 2009 [20]	33	4/22 (18.2%)	0/3 (0%)	4/19 (21.1%)	0/11 (0%)
Guangqi 2009 [21]	121	2/37 (5.4%)	0/1 (0%)	2/36 (5.6%)	2/84 (2.4%)
Holt 2010 [22]	52	5/52 (9.6%)	0/13 (0%)	5/39 (12.8%)	N/A
Kaya 2009 [23]	113	2/14 (14.3%)	0/1 (0%)	2/13 (15.4%)	3/99 (3.0%)
Khoynezhad 2007 [24]	180	2/39 (5.1%)	NR	NR	6/141 (4.3%)
Kotelis 2009 [25]	220	3/88 (3.4%)	1/22 (4.5%)	2/66 (3.0%)	5/132 (3.8%)
Lee 2011 [26]	145	5/145 (3.4%)	1/32 (3.1%)	4/113 (3.5%)	NA
Makaroun 2005 [27]	142	4/28 (14.3%)	4/28 (14.3%)	NA	1/114 (0.9%)
Marcheix 2006 [28]	45	1/6 (16.7%)	NA	1/6 (16.7%)	5/39 (12.8%)
Mariscalco 2012 [29]	76	4/27 (14.8%)	1/12 (8.3%)	3/15 (20%)	4/49 (8.2%)
Melissano 2012 [30]	139	4/139 (2.9%)	2/73 (2.7%)	2/66 (3.0%)	NA
Oberhuber 2010 [31]	48	0/35 (0%)	NA	0/35 (0%)	0/13 (0%)
Orend 2007 [32]	34	0/23 (0%)	NA	0/23 (0%)	0/11 (0%)
Parsa 2010 [33]	55	0/38 (0%)	0/13 (0%)	0/25 (0%)	0/17 (0%)
Patel 2006 [34]	73	0/16 (0%)	0/3 (0%)	0/13 (0%)	5/57 (8.8%)
Peterson 2006 [35]	70	4/30 (13.3%)	0/22 (0%)	4/8 (50%)	1/40 (2.5%)
Preventza 2008 [36]	69	2/69 (2.9%)	0/13 (0%)	2/56 (3.6%)	NA
Reece 2007 [37]	64	3/27 (11.1%)	1/7 (14.3%)	2/20 (10%)	0/37 (0%)
Riesenman 2007 [38]	108	3/24 (12.5%)	NA	3/24 (12.5%)	2/84 (2.4%)
Shu 2011 [39]	45	0/7 (0%)	NA	0/7 (0%)	0/38 (0%)
Spiliotopoulos 2014 [40]	76	0/76 (0%)	0/65 (0%)	0/11 (0%)	NA
Stone 2006 [41]	105	8/21 (38.1%)	NR	NR	2/84 (2.4%)
Woo 2008 [42]	70	6/70 (8.6%)	3/42 (7.1%)	3/28 (10.7%)	NA

LSA = left subclavian artery; NA = not applicable; NR = not reported.

Editor's Note: Please refer to original journal article for full references.

their practice. There are many ways to revascularize the LSA, as shown in Fig 2, and the Society for Vascular Surgery has issued guidelines recommending LSA revascularization in all elective TEVAR cases and consideration in acute aortic syndromes, either before or after emergent intervention. In our practice, we routinely revascularize in elective cases and even expand our prophylaxis against stroke by placing spinal drains in elective TEVARs to decrease the risk of spinal ischemia.

K. C. Orion, MD

Long-Term Changes in Aortic Length after Thoracic Endovascular Aortic Repair

Naguib NNN, Zima B, Nour-Eldin N-EA, et al (Frankfurt Univ Hosp, Frankfurt am Main, Germany; et al)

J Vasc Interv Radiol 27:181-187, 2016

Purpose.—To study long-term changes to the thoracic aorta following thoracic endovascular aortic repair (TEVAR) for treatment of different aortic pathologic conditions.

Materials and Methods.—This retrospective study included 53 consecutive patients (mean age, 58.8 y ± 14; 13 female and 40 male) in whom TEVAR was performed between October 2002 and May 2010. The mean duration of follow-up was 21.1 months (range, 0.5–96 mo). Statistical analysis was performed with the Friedman test and Conover–Iman test.

Results.—Nineteen patients with aortic aneurysm (group 1), 25 patients with type B dissection (group 2), and 9 patients with other pathologic conditions (group 3) were treated with TEVAR. The mean overall aortic lengths (from the origin of the left subclavian artery to the origin of the celiac trunk) before TEVAR were 271.4 mm, 268.6 mm, and 233.6 mm in groups 1, 2, and 3, respectively. At 12-month follow-up, the lengths were 282.8 mm, 294.4 mm, and 237.5 mm in groups 1, 2, and 3, respectively. The changes in aortic lengths following TEVAR were statistically significant ($P < .001$). A second intervention was required in 14 patients, and 6 patients died during follow-up.

Conclusions.—A significant change in the overall aortic length was observed following TEVAR. The changes in aortic length reached statistical significance after 12 months (Fig 3).

▶ The widespread use of thoracic endovascular aortic repair (TEVAR) has led to questions of how the aorta remodels after repair. Several studies have been done focusing on the changes in aortic diameter, but information regarding the longitudinal changes of the aorta post-TEVAR is still lacking. This study was a retrospective, single-center review of 53 patients who underwent

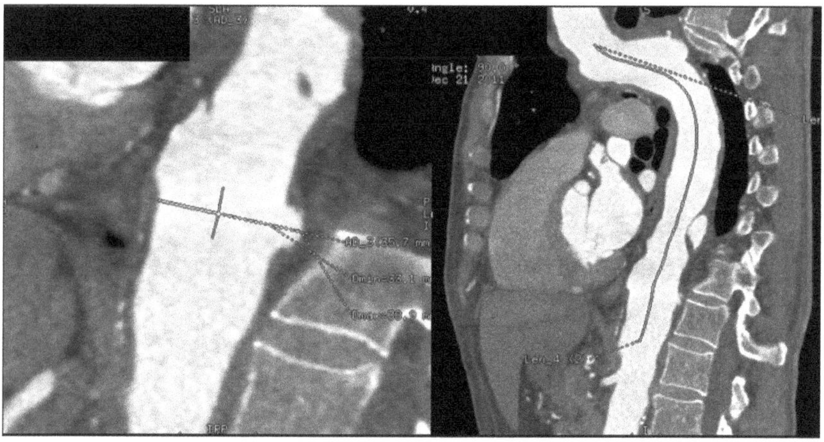

FIGURE 3.—An example of the method of selecting the center line of the aorta (right) and assessing the diameter by using the reconstruction workstation, with the diameter measured perpendicular to the center line of the aorta (left). (Reprinted from Naguib NNN, Zima B, Nour-Eldin N-EA, et al. Long-term changes in aortic length after thoracic endovascular aortic repair. *J Vasc Interv Radiol.* 2016;27:181-187, with permission from SIR.)

TEVAR from October 2002 through May 2010. Nineteen patients had aortic aneurysm, 25 patients had type B dissection, and 9 patients had other pathologic conditions.

Measurements of the aorta were taken before and after stent implantation according to a strict protocol. Diameters were taken at defined points and centerline measurement was performed to determine length (see Fig 3). After 24 months, there was a 9.3% increase in length in the aortic aneurysm group and a 10.5% increase in the dissection group. They observed that the change started to occur around 12 months after implantation. They found no correlation with the initial length of the stented region or with the type of stent used.

This study demonstrates a significant change in aortic length after TEVAR. This is an important component of studying the change in aortic morphology that occurs after TEVAR. Further studies should use these data in conjunction with more complete data on aortic diameter as well as tortuosity to develop a model for expected changes post-TEVAR. In addition, prospective studies may perhaps be able to use these data in planning adjuvant stenting procedures and reinterventions.

M. Arnold, MD

Neuroprotective Strategies Can Prevent Permanent Paraplegia in the Majority of Patients Who Develop Spinal Cord Ischaemia After Endovascular Repair of Thoracoabdominal Aortic Aneurysms

Rossi SH, Patel A, Saha P, et al (St Thomas' Hosp, London, UK)
Eur J Vasc Endovasc Surg 50:599-607, 2015

Objectives.—Spinal cord ischaemia (SCI) following endovascular thoracoabdominal aortic aneurysm (TAAA) repair is a devastating and unpredictable complication. This study describes a single unit's experience of SCI in patients who have had endovascular TAAA repair.

Methods.—A prospectively maintained database of patients having endovascular TAAA repair using branched and fenestrated stent grafts between 2008 and 2014 at a single high volume centre was reviewed. Patients who developed neurological symptoms and signs related to SCI were identified and factors associated with onset and recovery of neurology were analysed.

Results.—Sixty-nine patients (median age 73 years, 52 male; Crawford classification type I [$n = 4$], type II [$n = 11$], type III [$n = 33$], type IV [$n = 14$], type V [$n = 7$]) underwent endovascular TAAA repair. Twelve patients developed neurological symptoms/signs related to SCI but this was successfully reversed in eight patients, leaving four (5.8%) with permanent paraplegia. The median length of aorta covered was not significantly different in the 12 patients who developed SCI compared with the cohort that did not. Eleven of the patients who developed SCI had an intraoperative mean arterial pressure (MAP) below 80 mm Hg. Cutaneous atheroemboli were noted in half of the patients in the SCI group compared with 11% of the non-SCI group ($p < .05$). Strategies used to reverse SCI included raising MAP, cerebrospinal fluid drainage, angioplasty of stenosed internal iliac arteries, and restoring perfusion to the aneurysm sac.

Conclusions.—This series highlights some of the risk factors associated with the development of SCI after endovascular repair of TAAAs. It also illustrates the importance of a dedicated institutional protocol aimed at ensuring the early diagnosis of SCI and prompt intervention to reverse permanent paraplegia in the majority of cases.

▶ The authors present a report of endovascular repair of thoracoabdominal aortic aneurysm (TAAA) and spinal cord injury. Their report mirrors other single-center experiences with an almost 20% rate of paraplegia-related events. In this series, multiple events were reversible, leaving a final paraplegia rate of 6%, which is lower than many reported series. The authors present a nice algorithm that is similar to previous publications with regard to treatment of spinal cord ischemia following surgery. Of note the presence of a spinal drain did not confer protection and was used selectively. In this series, the institution seems experienced and comfortable performing these types of complex endovascular repairs, which allows for spinal ischemia to be identified early. This type of system is imperative if complex aortic procedures are being performed, and this experience argues for such procedures to be referred to high-volume centers of excellence. Although this report does not indicate that length of aortic coverage increased the risk of paraplegia, this is likely secondary to low overall numbers, and the authors believe that longer aortic coverage portends higher risk. This has been established with larger series and continues to be a prevailing belief that should always been considered for endovascular TAAA repair. This series extends the current literature that high-volume endovascular centers can achieve lower rates of spinal ischemic events compared with open repair. Additionally, it is worth noting that current series of endovascular TAAA repair often include patients deemed too high risk for open surgery. While technology evolves to meet the anatomic needs, endovascular repair continues to be tolerated by sicker patients with less physiologic burden compared with open surgery.

B. Propper, MD, FACS

Outcomes of Thoracic Endovascular Aortic Repair and Subclavian Revascularization Techniques

Zamor KC, Eskandari MK, Rodriguez HE, et al (Northwestern Univ Feinberg School of Medicine, Chicago, IL; et al)

J Am Coll Surg 221:93-100, 2015

Background.—Practice guidelines for management of the left subclavian artery (LSA) during thoracic endovascular aortic repair (TEVAR) are based on low-quality evidence, and there is limited literature that addresses optimal revascularization techniques. The purpose of this study was to compare outcomes of LSA coverage during TEVAR and revascularization techniques.

Study Design.—We performed a single-center retrospective cohort study from 2001 to 2013. Patients were categorized by LSA revascularization and by revascularization technique, carotid-subclavian bypass (CSB), or subclavian-carotid transposition (SCT). Thirty-day and mid-term stroke, spinal cord ischemia, vocal cord paralysis, upper extremity ischemia, primary patency of revascularization, and mortality were compared.

Results.—Eighty patients underwent TEVAR with LSA coverage, 25% (n = 20) were unrevascularized and the remaining patients underwent CSB (n = 22 [27.5%]) or SCT (n = 38 [47.5%]). Mean followup time was 24.9 months. Comparisons between unrevascularized and revascularized patients were significant for a higher rate of 30-day stroke (25% vs 2%; $p = 0.003$) and upper extremity ischemia (15% vs 0%; $p = 0.014$). However, there was no difference in 30-day or mid-term rates of spinal cord ischemia, vocal cord paralysis, or mortality. There were no statistically significant differences in 30-day or midterm outcomes for CSB vs SCT. Primary patency of revascularizations was 100%. Survival analysis comparing unrevascularized vs revascularized LSA was statistically significant for freedom from stroke and upper extremity ischemia ($p = 0.02$ and $p = 0.003$, respectively). After adjustment for advanced age, urgency, and coronary artery disease, LSA revascularization was associated with lower rates of perioperative adverse events (odds ratio = 0.23; $p = 0.034$).

Conclusions.—During TEVAR, LSA coverage without revascularization is associated with an increased risk of stroke and upper extremity ischemia. When LSA coverage is required during TEVAR, CSB and SCT are equally acceptable options.

▶ In 2010, the Society for Vascular Surgery published recommendations to perform a left subclavian revascularization before thoracic endovascular repair and for emergency surgeries, to consider revascularization after thoracic endovascular aortic repair (TEVAR). The author group of this article has long advocated left subclavian revascularization and published an article in the past suggesting posterior circulation events were more common when the left subclavian was covered and not revascularized. The present work seeks to evaluate the outcomes of stroke, spinal cord injury, mortality, and graft patency.

Over 12 years, 80 patients required left subclavian coverage (35% of all institutional TEVAR) and 25% of these were not revascularized, most often because of need for urgent or emergent intervention. Although strokes were appreciated in anterior and posterior circulations without significant differences, the severity of the strokes was worse in those without revascularization. Additionally stroke was far more prevalent in the unrevascularized patients (25% vs 1.6%, $P < .003$). Spinal cord injury was not affected by either treatment effect. Ultimately, the authors lend credible evidence that the safest posture is left subclavian revascularization before any elective TEVAR. I further expect this posture will evolve to include endovascualr techniques to accomplish the same left subclavian revascularization, such as chimney or in situ fenestration techniques.

J. H. Black III, MD, FACS

Outcomes of total percutaneous endovascular aortic repair for thoracic, fenestrated, and branched endografts

de Souza LR, Oderich GS, Banga PV, et al (Mayo Clinic, Rochester, MN)
J Vasc Surg 62:1442-1449, 2015

Objective.—Percutaneous endovascular aortic repair (PEVAR) has been increasingly used to treat infrarenal abdominal aortic aneurysms, but few studies have evaluated the results in complex aortic aneurysms. We reviewed the technical success and clinical outcomes of PEVAR using large-diameter sheaths for the treatment of complex aortic aneurysms with thoracic, fenestrated, and branched stent grafts.

Methods.—The clinical data of patients who underwent total PEVAR for descending thoracic aneurysm, thoracoabdominal aortic aneurysm, pararenal, and aortoiliac aneurysms using thoracic, fenestrated, and branched stent grafts between 2009 and 2014 were reviewed. Repairs with fenestrated-branched stent grafts were performed using commercially available or investigational devices under a physician-sponsored

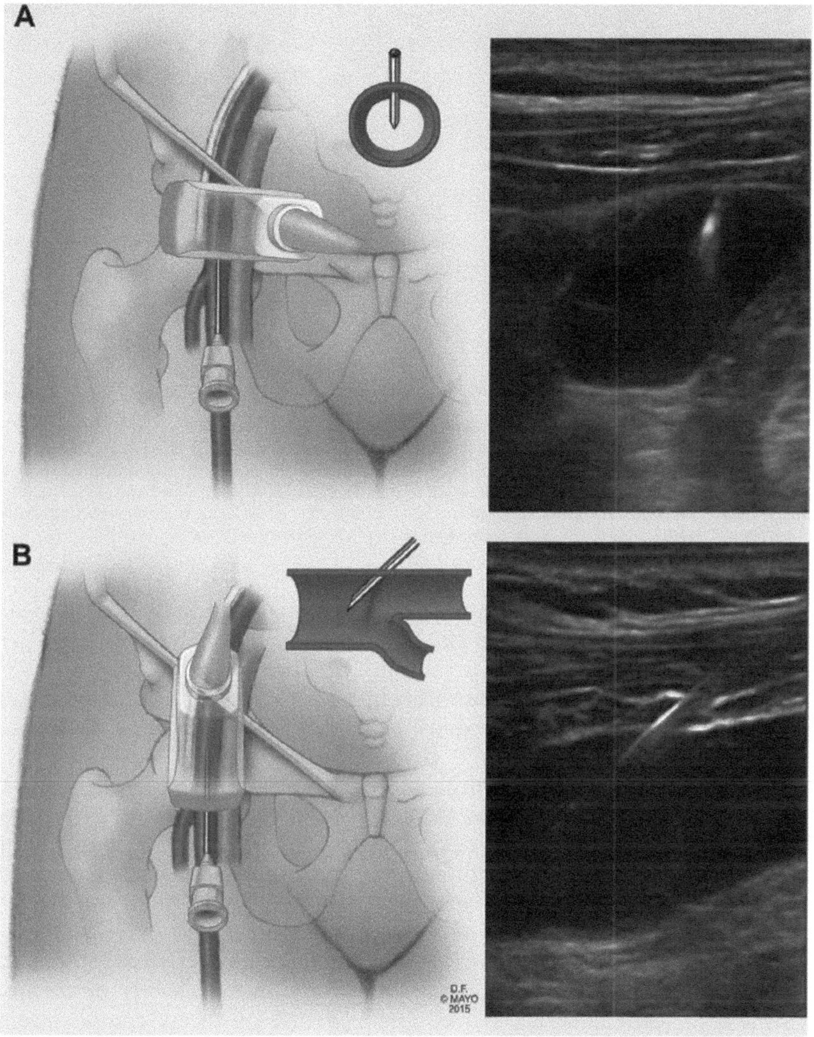

FIGURE 1.—The ultrasound guidance secures a puncture proximal to the femoral bifurcation and in the anterior wall of the artery. Whether to perform the puncture using a (**A**) transverse or a (**B**) longitudinal view is the surgeon's preference. (Reprinted by permission of the Mayo Foundation for Medical Education and Research. All rights reserved.) (Reprinted from de Souza LR, Oderich GS, Banga PV, et al. Outcomes of total percutaneous endovascular aortic repair for thoracic, fenestrated, and branched endografts. *J Vasc Surg*. 2015;62:1442-1449, with permission from the Society for Vascular Surgery.)

investigational device protocols. Percutaneous closure was performed using ultrasound guidance and two Perclose devices (Abbott Vascular, Santa Clara Calif) per femoral puncture site. End points were technical success, access-related complications, morbidity, and mortality.

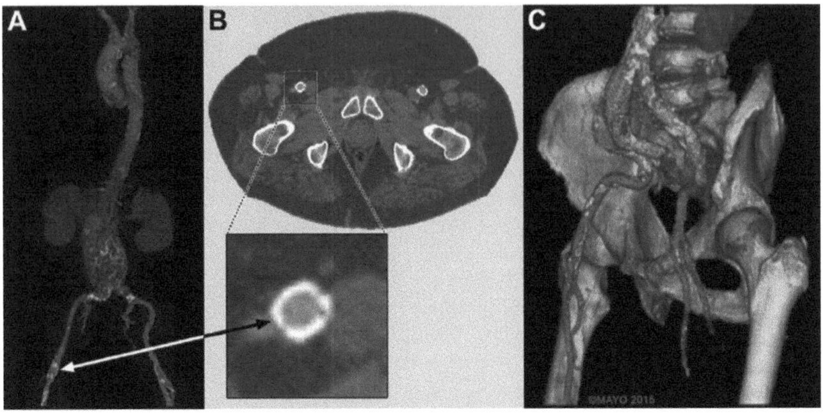

FIGURE 2.—Preoperative imaging evaluation and adequate patient selection are necessary to obtain satisfactory results. **A** and **B**, Areas with severe and circumferential calcification are avoided and may be a contraindication to the total percutaneous procedure. **C**, A high femoral artery bifurcation requires additional care to avoid distal punctures. (Reprinted from de Souza LR, Oderich GS, Banga PV, et al. Outcomes of total percutaneous endovascular aortic repair for thoracic, fenestrated, and branched endografts. *J Vasc Surg*. 2015;62:1442-1449, with permission from the Society for Vascular Surgery.)

Results.—There were 102 patients, 77 male and 25 female, with a mean age of 75 ± 8 years. Aneurysm extent was pararenal in 48 patients (47%), thoracoabdominal aortic aneurysm in 27 (26%), descending thoracic aneurysm in 19 (19%), and aortoiliac in 8 (8%). Fenestrated or branched endografts, or both, were placed in 72 patients (71%). Total percutaneous closure was performed in 170 femoral arteries using ≥20F-diameter sheaths in 163 (96%). Technical success was obtained in 161 femoral arteries (95%). There were no factors associated with technical failure. Access-related complications occurred in five patients (5%), including femoral artery thrombosis in three (3%), and retroperitoneal hematoma or pseudoaneurysm in one patient each (1%). There were no 30-day deaths. Freedom from access-related complications was 97% ± 1% at 30 days and 1 year. No access-related complications occurred >30 days.

Conclusions.—Total percutaneous technique can be safely performed with a high technical success rate and low rate of access complications in patients with thoracic and complex aortic disease requiring large-diameter sheaths. The rate of accessrelated complications (5%) is similar to that reported for PEVAR of infrarenal abdominal aortic aneurysms using smaller-profile devices (Figs 1-4, Table 1).

▶ Percutaneous endovascular aneurysm repair (PEVAR) has been available and described since 1999. The technique is now not considered radical and is likely mainstream for most vascular surgeons. This study further validates the work of those before them including a multi-institutional randomized trial confirming the results (Table 1).[1] The ability to maintain excellent results in this study with the use of some larger devices associated with thoracic, fenestrated, and branched cases is not surprising because many of the percutaneous

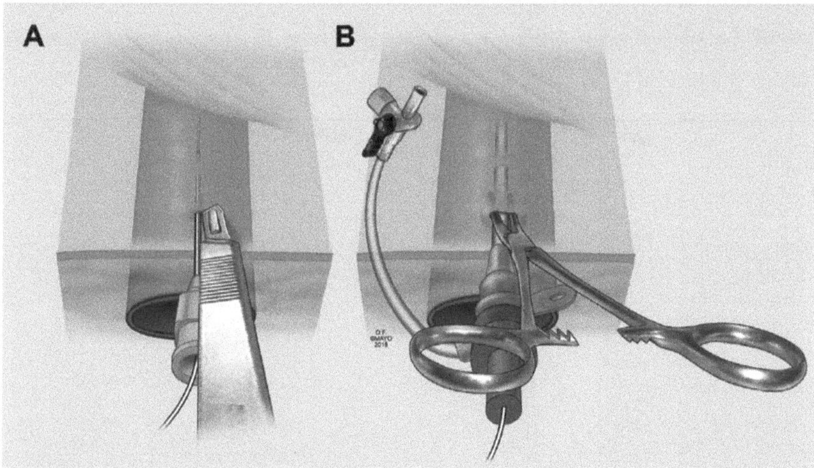

FIGURE 3.—**A**, A small oblique incision is made. **B**, The subcutaneous tissue is dilated circumferentially to facilitate placement of the percutaneous vascular closure devices (PVCDs) and to avoid the inclusion of subcutaneous tissue in the suture. (Reprinted by permission of the Mayo Foundation for Medical Education and Research. All rights reserved.) (Reprinted from de Souza LR, Oderich GS, Banga PV, et al. Outcomes of total percutaneous endovascular aortic repair for thoracic, fenestrated, and branched endografts. *J Vasc Surg*. 2015;62:1442-1449, with permission from the Society for Vascular Surgery.)

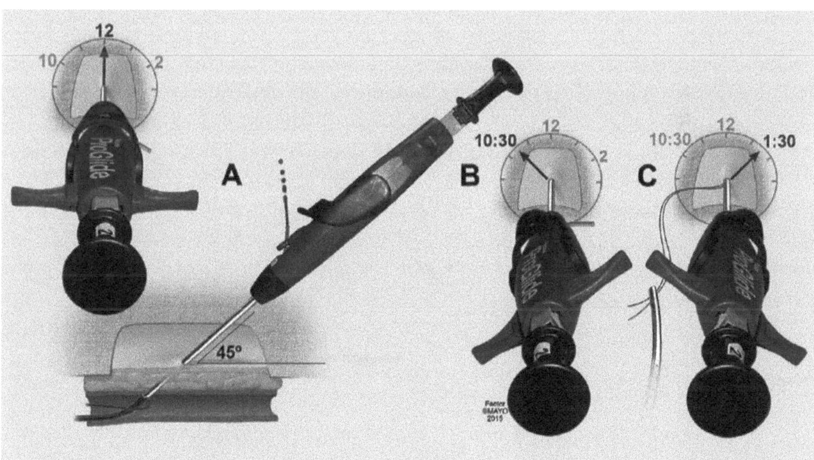

FIGURE 4.—**A**, It is important that both of the devices be introduced at the 12:00 o'clock position and at a ~45° angle from the skin. **B**, After confirmation that the device is inside the vessel, the first one should be rotated to the 10:30 o'clock position before the following steps for its complete delivery. **C**, The second device is introduced in the same fashion as the first one but is rotated to the 1:30 o'clock position. (Reprinted by permission of the Mayo Foundation for Medical Education and Research. All rights reserved.) (Reprinted by permission of the Mayo Foundation for Medical Education and Research. All rights reserved.) (Reprinted from de Souza LR, Oderich GS, Banga PV, et al. Outcomes of total percutaneous endovascular aortic repair for thoracic, fenestrated, and branched endografts. *J Vasc Surg*. 2015;62:1442-1449, with permission from the Society for Vascular Surgery.)

TABLE 1.—Clinical Characteristics in 102 Patients Treated by Thoracic, Fenestrated, and Branched Stent Grafts Using Percutaneous Closure

Variable	Mean ± SD or No. (%)
Age, years	75.1 ± 8.3
Gender	
Male	77 (75)
Female	25 (25)
Cardiovascular risk factors	
Hypertension	89 (87)
Smoking	84 (82)
Hyperlipidemia	78 (76)
Coronary artery disease	59 (58)
Chronic kidney disease	44 (43)
Peripheral arterial disease	21 (21)
Diabetes	14 (14)
BMI, kg/m^2	29.3 ± 5.5
Overweight (25-30 kg/m^2)	39 (38)
Obesity (>30 kg/m^2)	43 (42)
SVS clinical score	9.48 ± 4.63
CFA variables	
More than minimal calcification[a]	62 (36)
Previous exposure[a]	19 (11)
Diameter	10.1 ± 1.9

BMI, Body mass index; *CFA*, common femoral artery; *SD*, standard deviation; *SVS*, Society for Vascular Surgery.
[a]Expressed as number (% by vessel).
(Reprinted from de Souza LR, Oderich GS, Banga PV, et al. Outcomes of total percutaneous endovascular aortic repair for thoracic, fenestrated, and branched endografts. *J Vasc Surg*. 2015;62:1442-1449, with permission from the Society for Vascular Surgery.)

closures that were initially performed were on larger devices before more modern lower profile devices were available. The important aspects of technical success center on proper preoperative selection of patients and avoidance of circumferential calcification (Fig 2) and using ultrasound guidance (Fig 1). Preparation of the access site and accurate deployment are the key intraprocedural aspects of success (Figs 3 and 4). With all of these steps accounted for, a failure of the closure device can still occur, and most experienced operators are able to handle this issue rather easily. It is time to accept PEVAR and understand it is not the device that fails but usually the operator failing to select the proper patient.

N. Singh, MD, FACS

Reference

1. Nelson PR, Kracjer Z, Kansal N, et al. A multicenter, randomized, controlled trial of totally percutaneous access versus open femoral exposure for endovascular aortic aneurysm repair (the PEVAR trial). *J Vasc Surg*. 2014;59:1181-1193.

Results of the Valiant Mona LSA early feasibility study for descending thoracic aneurysms

Roselli EE, on behalf of the Valiant Mona LSA Trial Investigators (Cleveland Clinic, OH; et al)

J Vasc Surg 62:1465-1472, 2015

Objective.—Stent graft coverage of the left subclavian artery (LSA) may be required to achieve an adequate landing zone in up to 40% of descending thoracic aneurysms (DTAs). The Valiant Mona LSA Thoracic Stent Graft System (Medtronic, Santa Rosa, Calif) consists of a main stent graft and a branch stent graft designed to maintain LSA patency while diverting circulation through the encroaching aneurysm. Participating in the United States Food and Drug Administration's new Innovation Pathway, this first-in-human, early feasibility study evaluates early clinical experience of the Valiant Mona LSA Stent Graft System in patients with DTAs where the proximal landing zone necessitates LSA coverage.

Methods.—This premarket, nonrandomized, single-arm prospective study recruited nine patients (age 72.9 ± 7.6 years). Primary end points were aneurysm-related mortality, stroke, paraplegia, left arm/hand ischemia, and treatment success. Neurologic events were assessed by imaging and by independent neurologists. Inclusion criteria required patients with a DTA or penetrating aortic ulcer to have a distance of ≥10 mm between the left common carotid artery and the LSA. Mean aneurysm diameter was 53.7 ± 10.0 mm. The indication for repair was for saccular DTA in five patients or fusiform DTA in four. Seven patients were at American Society of Anesthesiologists Physical Status Classification III/IV.

Results.—All nine patients received one main stent graft (diameter 28 to 42 mm) and one branch stent graft (diameter 10 to 14 mm). To extend device coverage distally, a commercial Valiant Captivia device was implanted in seven patients. No uncorrected endoleaks were observed at the end of the implant procedure. Four endoleaks developed before discharge in four of eight evaluable patients. Two were identified as type II and two were of undetermined type. No endoleak resulted in a secondary intervention. Technical success, defined by the clinical investigational plan, was achieved in all nine patients intraoperatively, and treatment success was achieved in all eight evaluable patients at 1 month. There were no major, disabling strokes. Four minor nondisabling strokes were reported in three patients ≤30 days (days 1, 1, 5, and 24). To date, there have been no reports of death, left arm ischemia, paraplegia, rupture, conversion to open surgery, or secondary endovascular procedure. No patients required surgical LSA revascularization.

Conclusions.—The Valiant Mona LSA system demonstrates technical and treatment success, relative safety, and early durability in its initial

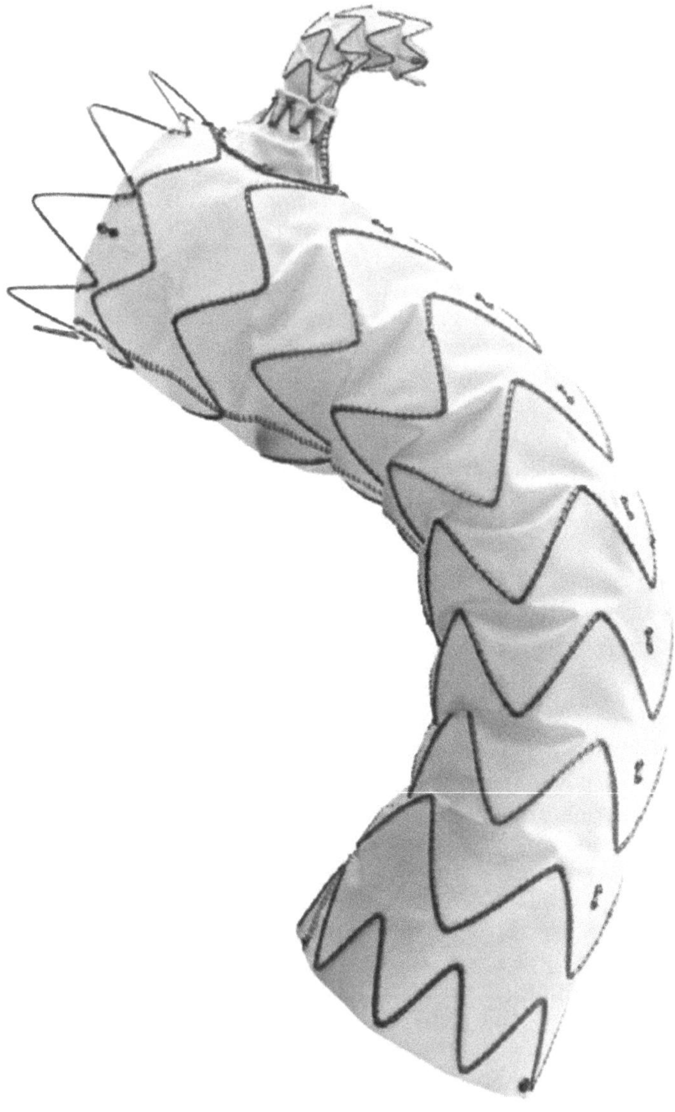

FIGURE 1.—The Valiant Mona LSA stent graft (Medtronic Inc, Santa Rosa, Calif). The main stent graft (MSG) is shown mated with the branch stent graft (BSG). (Reprinted from Roselli EE, on behalf of the Valiant Mona LSA Trial Investigators. Results of the Valiant Mona LSA early feasibility study for descending thoracic aneurysms. *J Vasc Surg*. 2015;62:1465-1472, with permission from the Society for Vascular Surgery.)

use in DTA patients. Midterm results are expected as patients are monitored at regular intervals to 5 years (Fig 1).

▶ The question of revascularizing the left subclavian artery (LSA) at the time of endovascular grafting of thoracic aneurysms (TEVAR) has been debated for decades. Recently a review from the Society of Thoracic Surgeons[1] showed an increased stroke risk by LSA coverage (7.4% vs 4.0%) and a decrease in this risk by revascularization of the LSA (5.6% vs 3.1%). As such, the Society of Vascular Surgery recommends revascularization in all elective TEVARs. Medtronic has attempted to eliminate the need for this second procedure by introducing a single-branched graft (Fig 1) that maintains the patency of the LSA during TEVAR. The primary end points for this premarket, nonrandomized single-arm prospective study were aneurysm-related mortality, stroke, paraplegia, left arm/hand ischemia and treatment success. These end points were successfully met, except for 3 minor nondisabling strokes and 1 major stroke at 30 days. The investigators propose several possible reasons for stroke, particularly specific techniques during deployment such as snaring near LSA origin, common carotid wire access, and multiple manipulations within the arch. In an effort to decrease stroke rate, they have made changes to their procedural adjustments. All stent grafts with branches were implanted successfully. Overall, the Valiant Mona LSA represents a novel way to obviate the need for separate LSA revascularization in patients with descending thoracic aneurysms.

K. C. Orion, MD

Reference

1. Waterford SD, Chou D, Bombien R, Uzun I, Shah A, Khoynezhad A. Left subclavian arterial coverage and stroke during thoracic aortic endografting: a systematic review. *Ann Thoracic Surgery*. 2016;101:381-389.

Risk Factor Analysis of Bird Beak Occurrence after Thoracic Endovascular Aortic Repair

Boufi M, Guivier-Curien C, Deplano V, et al (Aix-Marseille Université, Marseille, France; et al)

Eur J Vasc Endovasc Surg 50:37-43, 2015

Objectives.—The aim was to analyze the role played by anatomy and stent graft in the incidence of incomplete apposition to aortic arch.

Methods.—Between 2007 and 2014 data including available and suitable computed tomographic angiography (CTA) imaging of patients who had undergone thoracic endovascular aortic repair were reviewed. The study included 80 patients (65 men, 54 ± 21 years) treated for traumatic aortic rupture ($n = 27$), thoracic aortic aneurysm ($n = 15$), type B aortic dissection ($n = 24$), penetrating aortic ulcer ($n = 5$), intramural hematoma ($n = 2$), aorto-oesophageal fistula ($n = 2$), and aortic mural thrombus ($n = 5$). Pre- and post-operative CTA images were analyzed to characterize bird beak in terms of length and angle, and to calculate aortic angulation within a 30 mm range at the proximal deployment zone.

Results.—Bird beak configuration was detected in 46 patients (57%): mean stent protrusion length was 16 mm (range: 8—29 mm) and mean bird beak angle was 20° (range: 7—40°). The bird beak effect was significantly more frequent after traumatic aortic rupture treatment ($p = .05$) and in landing zone 2 ($p = .01$). No influence of either stent graft type or generation, or degree of oversizing was observed ($p = .29$, $p = .28$, $p = .81$ respectively). However, the mean aortic angle of patients with bird beak was higher in the Pro-form group than that in the Zenith TX2 group (62° vs. 48°, $p = .13$). Multivariate analysis identified the aortic angle of the deployment zone as the unique independent risk factor of malapposition (HR = 1.05, 95% CI 1–1.10, $p = .005$). The cutoff value of 51° was found to be predictive of bird beak occurrence with a sensitivity of 58% and a specificity of 85%.

Conclusions.—Assessment of proximal landing zone morphology to avoid deployment zones generating an aortic angle of over 50° can be recommended to improve aortic curvature apposition with the current available devices (Fig 1).

▶ This publication highlights the high incidence of bird beaking (BB) after thoracic endovascular aneurysm repair (TEVAR). Of note, this study found that 57% of implanted devices had evidence of BB when examined under set criteria. This number is higher than one would expect at first and truly highlights an area that technology changes are needed. One important note is that the time frame from 2007 to 2014 saw changes to many of the current thoracic devices with a major emphasis focused on BB and conformability. These data show that device deployment in young trauma patients is most likely to yield BB because the aorta is highly angulated and narrow. With age, the aorta elongates, and shifting of the supra-aortic trunk can open the acute aortic angle seen in young patients. Fig 1 nicely demonstrates that device sizing must take into account the estimated deployment angle if full wall apposition is to be achieved. No device was superior using the data from this study, but implant numbers are too low to arrive at a real conclusion for any device. When we evaluate the engineering of TEVAR, BB near the SCA orifice makes sense. Devices created with Z stent configuration are not meant to bend across the Z; rather, divisions between the stents are created for conformability. Couple this with changes in anatomy after stiff wire placement, and precise measurements to limit BB are challenging. The "stack of coins" configuration tends to offer more conformability, but radial force is sacrificed. The article highlights the need for implanters to be aware of the challenges created by acute angulation coupled with the extent needed for coverage. Device selection should be tailored to anatomic constraints versus the "1 device fits all" philosophy. The authors discuss some novel techniques for treatment, including endo-stapler. Caution should be noted as placement of endotacks are challenging in angulated aortic anatomy, and long-term data do not exist regarding durability of the tacks/staples under 3-dimensional vector force (not seen in the infrarenal aorta) against the staple/tack (the flow will be trying to pull the leading edge of the device, causing a pulling force on the tack/staple). Other theoretic complications include inducing aortic dissection with tack malpositioning as most current devices rely on wall-wall apposition before tack placement. This article

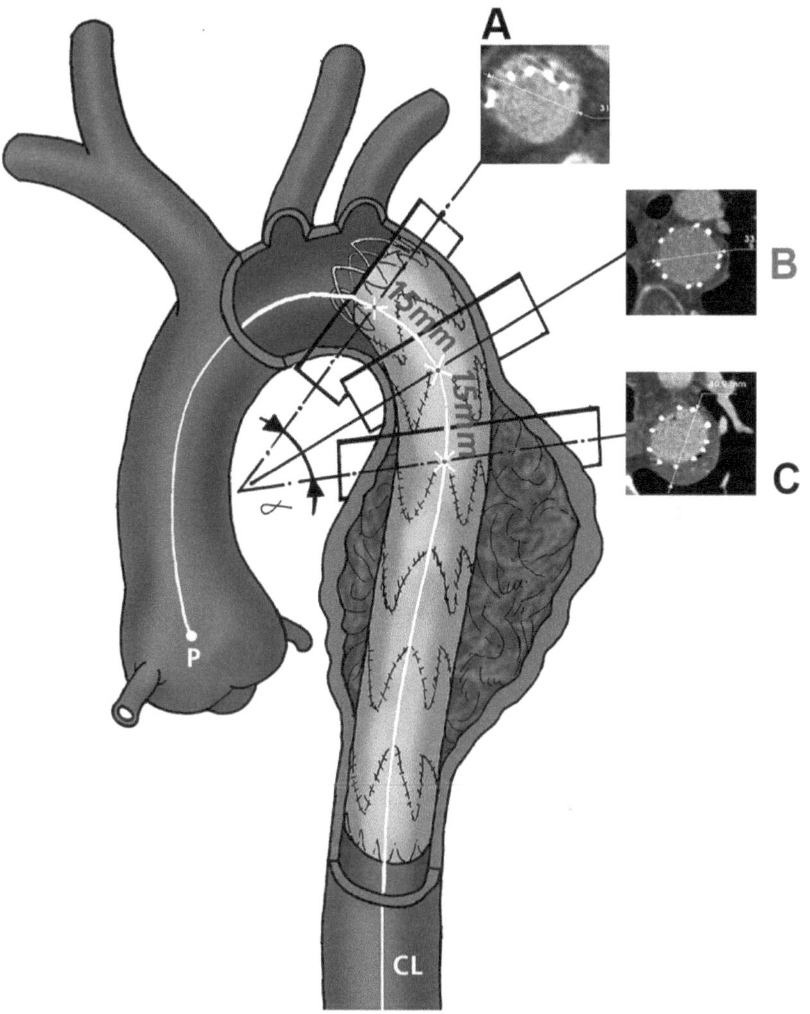

FIGURE 1.—Schematic representation of aortic angle a calculation within α 30-mm range at the proximal deployment zone. (A) Cross-section view of the aorta located 15 mm along the centerline above plane B. (B) Cross-section view showing the stent totally apposed to the wall. (C) Cross-section view of the aorta located 15 mm along centerline below plane B. (Reprinted from Boufi M, Guivier-Curien C, Deplano V, et al. Risk factor analysis of bird beak occurrence after thoracic endovascular aortic repair. *Eur J Vasc Endovasc Surg*. 2015;50:37-43, with permission from European Society for Vascular Surgery.)

is a nice review of the anatomic challenges seen with thoracic repairs and highlights an area in which small engineering changes may offer great benefit.

B. Propper, MD, FACS

Stent graft types for endovascular repair of thoracic aortic aneurysms

Rolph R, Duffy JM, Waltham M (Guys and St Thomas' NHS Foundation Trust, London, UK; Univ of Oxford, UK)

Cochrane Database Syst Rev 9:CD008448, 2015

Background.—The UK prevalence of thoracic aneurysm is estimated at 10.4 per 100,000 person-years. Progressive and unpredictable enlargement can lead to rupture. Endovascular repair of thoracic aortic aneurysms involves a stent graft system being introduced via the femoral artery and manipulated within the aorta under radiological guidance. Following endograft deployment, a seal is formed at the proximal and distal landing zones to exclude the aneurysm sac from the circulation. With the increasing popularity of endovascular repair there has been an increase in the number of commercially available stent graft designs on the market. This is an update of the review first published in 2013.

Objectives.—This review aimed to assess the different stent graft types for endovascular repair of thoracic aortic aneurysms.

Search Methods.—The Cochrane Vascular Group Trials Search Co-ordinator (TSC) searched the Specialised Register (last searched February 2015) and the Cochrane Register of Studies CENTRAL (2015, Issue 1). Trial databases were searched by the TSC for details of ongoing and unpublished studies.

Selection Criteria.—All published and unpublished randomised controlled trials (RCTs) of stent graft types in the repair of thoracic aortic aneurysms were sought without language restriction.

Data Collection and Analysis.—Data collection and analysis was conducted in accordance with the *Cochrane Handbook for Systematic Reviews of Interventions.*

Main Results.—No studies were identified that met the inclusion criteria. It was not possible to assess the quality of the evidence in the absence of studies eligible for inclusion in the review.

Authors' Conclusions.—Unfortunately, no data exist regarding direct comparisons of the performance of different stent graft types. High quality RCTs evaluating stent graft types in thoracic endovascular aneurysm repair are required (Fig 1).

▶ With advancements in endovascular techniques, repair of thoracic aortic aneurysms has shifted away from open repair toward thoracic endovascular aneurysm repair (TEVAR). Although there are no randomized controlled trials (RCTs) comparing open repair with TEVAR, advocates of TEVAR site reduced perioperative morbidity and mortality.[1] In addition, the number of devices available to surgeons for repair of TAA has continued to increase. These devices differ in multiple ways, including their profile, deployment, fixation method, and complication. The Cochrane group sought to examine all RCTs comparing these devices. Despite screening 645 abstracts (Fig 1), no studies were eligible for inclusion in the Cochrane analysis because to date there are no RCTs comparing TEVAR devices. Currently, surgical decision making is made based on

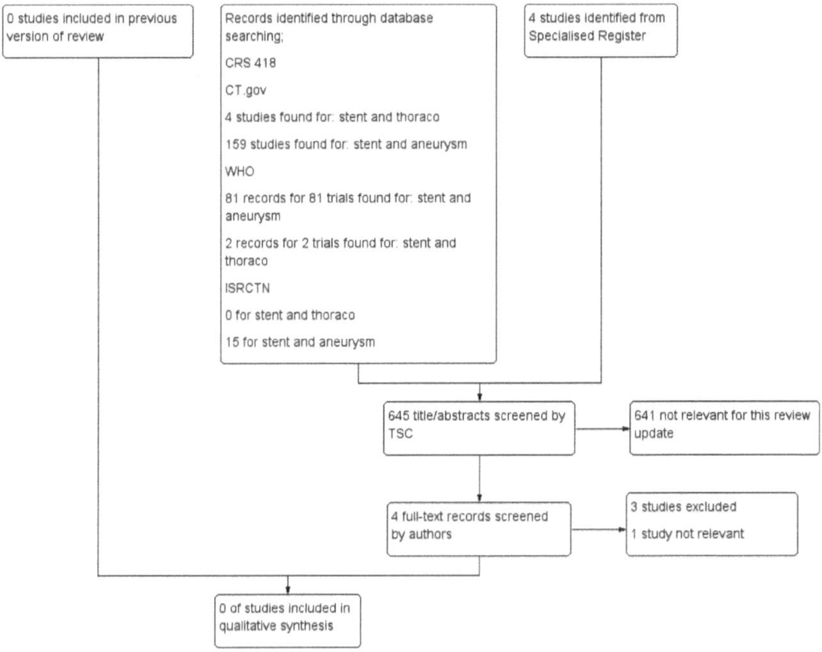

FIGURE 1.—Study flow diagram. (Reprinted from Rolph R, Duffy JM, Waltham M. Stent graft types for endovascular repair of thoracic aortic aneurysms. *Cochrane Database Syst Rev.* 2015;9:CD008448, The Cochrane Collaboration. Published by JohnWiley & Sons, Ltd.)

individual surgeon and institution experience and biases. This article suggests that the devices are largely interchangeable, allowing surgeons to select the best device for their patient.

M. Arnold, MD

Reference

1. Abraha.

Midterm Results of Type B Intramural Hematoma Endovascular Treatment

Felisaz A, Dufranc J, Heyndrickx M, et al (CHU Côte de Nacre, Caen, France)
Ann Vasc Surg 29:898-904, 2015

Background.—Recently, intramural hematoma (IMH) has been characterized as a rare variant of aortic dissection, falling within the acute aortic syndromes (AAS). Although aortic endovascular treatment seems to provide good results, no consensus has been established regarding the optimal management of IMH affecting the descending thoracic aorta (IMH B). The aim of this study was to assess long-term clinical and morphological results of IMH B treated with a stent graft.

Methods.—Between 2002 and 2013, 15 of the 423 (3.5%) consecutive patients with AAS were found to have IMH B. During follow-up, complications related to IMH B were observed in 10 patients, including 5 during the acute period (<14 days). Surgical indications were ulcerations, refractory pain, aneurysm evolution, aortic rupture, and pleural effusion. An endovascular approach was taken for all forms with suitable anatomy.

Results.—Technical success rate was 100%, with complete exclusion of lesions of the descending thoracic aorta in all cases treated with a stent graft. No neurological complications or deaths occurred within the first 30 postoperative days, nor at the end of the mean follow-up of 46 months (1–137 months). After the aortic stent graft, partial or complete regression of the hematoma was observed in all cases.

Conclusions.—IMH B is most often a progressive disease requiring long-term monitoring. In case of complications, stent-graft treatment of the descending thoracic aorta can be performed successfully in most cases. This procedure appears to be a safe technique that provides very good long-term results, with favorable remodeling of the aorta.

▶ Intramural hematoma (IMH) is a recognized variant of aortic dissection, and among 423 consecutive patients in the article by Felisaz et al, the rate of IMH was 3.5%. Although medical therapy is considered primary therapy, the authors provide the results of a more aggressive paradigm. The threshold for intervention are diameter > 50 mm at presentation, rapid enlargement, appearance of dissection, or appearance of ULP (ulcer like projections). The concept of ULP is a reinvention of the more common nomenclature of penetrating aortic ulcer (PAU). The association of IMH and PAU was well studied in a series by Ganaha et al,[1] and the current authors' experience reinforces the association of the concomitant pathology with adverse outcomes. The discussion is an excellent synopsis of the current management controversies in IMH and is informative for the readership.

J. H. Black III, MD, FACS

Reference

1. Ganaha F, Miller DC, Sugimoto K, et al. Prognosis of aortic intramural hematoma with and without penetrating atherosclerotic ulcer: a clinical and radiological analysis. *Circulation.* 2002;106:342-348.

Aneurysmal degeneration of the thoracoabdominal aorta after medical management of type B aortic dissections

Durham CA, Aranson NJ, Ergul EA, et al (Massachusetts General Hosp, Boston)

J Vasc Surg 62:900-906, 2015

Background.—Patients with uncomplicated type B aortic dissections who are managed medically are at risk of aortic aneurysmal degeneration over time. However, the effect of improvement in antihypertensive medications and stricter blood pressure control is unknown. The goal of this study was to determine the rate of aneurysmal degeneration in a contemporary cohort of patients with medically treated type B dissection.

Methods.—Included were all patients with acute uncomplicated type B aortic dissection who were initially managed medically between March 1999 and March 2011 and had follow-up axial imaging studies. Maximum aortic growth was calculated by comparing the initial imaging study to the most current scan or imaging obtained just before any aortic related intervention. An increase of ≥5 mm was the threshold considered as aortic growth. Predictors of aortic aneurysmal degeneration were determined using Cox proportional hazards models.

Results.—We identified 200 patients (61% men) with medically managed acute type B dissections receiving multiple imaging studies. Patients were an average age of 63.4 years, and 75.5% had a history of hypertension. Mean follow-up was 5.3 years (range, 0.1-14.7 years). Mean time between the initial and final imaging studies was 3.2 years (range, 0.1-12.9 years). At 5 years, only 51% were free from aortic growth. Fifty-six patients (28%) required operative intervention (50 open, 6 endovascular repair) for aneurysmal degeneration, and the actuarial 5-year freedom from intervention was 76%. After excluding five patients (2.5%) with early rapid degeneration requiring intervention within the first 2 weeks, the mean rate of aortic growth was 12.3 mm/y for the total aortic diameter, 3.8 mm/y for the true lumen diameter, and 8.6 mm/y for the false lumen diameter. Only aortic diameter at index presentation >3.5 cm was a risk factor for future growth (odds ratio, 2.54; 95% confidence interval, 1.34-4.81; $P < .01$). Complete thrombosis of the false lumen was protective against growth (odds ratio, 0.19; 95% confidence interval, 0.11-0.42; $P < .01$).

Conclusions.—Although medical management of uncomplicated acute, type B aortic dissections has been the standard of care, at 5 years, a significant number of patients will require operative intervention for aneurysmal degeneration. Further studies of early intervention (eg, thoracic endovascular aortic repair) for type B aortic dissection to prevent late aneurysm formation are needed (Table 2).

▶ The management of type B aortic dissection (TBAD) had traditionally been an easy one. If the entry tear was distal to the left subclavian artery, patients

TABLE 2.—Outcome of 200 Patients Presenting with Acute Type B Aortic Dissection Who were Initially Managed Medically

Variables	Outcome
Rapid degeneration <14 days, No. (%)	5 (2.5)
Maximum diameter growth, mm	7.2
True lumen growth, mm	0.2
False lumen growth, mm	7.0
Aortic growth rate,[a] mm/y	12.3
True lumen,[a] mm/y	3.8
False lumen,[a] mm/y	8.6
Completely thrombosed false lumen at first follow-up CT, No. (%)	50 (25.0)
Time between initial and final CT, mean ± SD years	3.2 ± 3.1
Follow-up, mean ± SD years	5.3 ± 3.4
Operative intervention, No. (%)	56 (28.0)
Open	50 (89.3)
Endovascular	6 (10.7)
30-day operative mortality	4 (7.1)

CT, Computed tomography; *SD*, standard deviation.
[a]Excluding 5 patients with rapid expansion.
Reprinted from Durham CA, Aranson NJ, Ergul EA, et al. Aneurysmal degeneration of the thoracoabdominal aorta after medical management of type B aortic dissections. *J Vasc Surg*. 2015;62:900-906, with permission from the Society for Vascular Surgery.

were managed with tightly controlled impulse pressure, heart rate, aspirin, and statins. As the advent of thoracic endografting (TEVAR) becomes more popular, we began to wonder whether simply placing an endograft in uncomplicated dissections would improve patient outcomes. The INSTEAD trial, as reported by Nienaber et al,[1] was a landmark trial that provided for the first time Level 1 evidence to assist us in this decision making. It demonstrated that TEVAR placement failed to improve the rates of 2- year survival and adverse events compared with medical therapy. Most were satisfied again that for uncomplicated TBAD, medical management was still the gold standard of care. The authors herein attempted to answer the question of what exactly happens to aortic remodeling in patients who are treated nonoperatively. They retrospectively examined a large number of patients with acute TBAD who had imaging studies available at time of diagnosis as well as in follow-up. They neatly excluded patients with type A dissections, complicated TBAD and malperfusion necessitating surgical intervention, and 2 patients with rapid degeneration within the first 14 days. Durham and colleagues found a bimodal distribution of patients: those who continued to degenerate their aortas within the first 5-year period and those who did not. The rate of aortic growth was 12.3 mm per year with the false lumen accounting for the majority of this; 8.6 mm/year as shown in Table 2. After multivariate analysis, only initial aortic diameter of > 35 mm was predictive of aortic growth. Complete thrombosis of the false lumen was protective. Their findings suggest that there is a subset of TBAD patients who will continue to degenerate their aorta over time despite best medical therapy and that perhaps we should consider elective TEVAR in these patients in the subacute phase. These sentiments were reinforced when INSTEAD XL[2] trial was published, showing that after 2 years, the addition of TEVAR combined with optimal medical treatment improved survival and disease progression. This is thought to occur because of successful complete thrombosis of the false lumen. Once again we find ourselves reevaluating the best approach to uncomplicated TBAD. Today, surgeons consider early surgical intervention for TBADs initially presenting with a size of > 35 mm, and the indications may expand with future academic evaluations of our outcomes.

K. C. Orion, MD

References

1. Nienaber CA, Rousseau H, Eggebrecht H, et al. Randomized comparison of strategies for type B aortic dissection: the Investigation of STEnt grafts in Aortic Dissection (INSTEAD) trial. *Circulation.* 2009;120:2519-2528.
2. Nienaber CA, Kische S, Rousseau H, et al. Endovascular repair of type B aortic dissection: long-term results of the randomized investigation of stent grafts in aortic dissection trial. *Circ Cardiovasc Interv.* 2013;6:407-416.

Aneurysmal degeneration of the thoracoabdominal aorta after medical management of type B aortic dissections

Durham CA, Aranson NJ, Ergul EA, et al, (Massachusetts General Hosp, Boston)

J Vasc Surg 62:900-906, 2015

Background.—Patients with uncomplicated type B aortic dissections who are managed medically are at risk of aortic aneurysmal degeneration over time. However, the effect of improvement in antihypertensive medications and stricter blood pressure control is unknown. The goal of this study was to determine the rate of aneurysmal degeneration in a contemporary cohort of patients with medically treated type B dissection.

Methods.—Included were all patients with acute uncomplicated type B aortic dissection who were initially managed medically between March 1999 and March 2011 and had follow-up axial imaging studies. Maximum aortic growth was calculated by comparing the initial imaging study to the most current scan or imaging obtained just before any aortic-related intervention. An increase of ≥5 mm was the threshold considered as aortic growth. Predictors of aortic aneurysmal degeneration were determined using Cox proportional hazards models.

Results.—We identified 200 patients (61% men) with medically managed acute type B dissections receiving multiple imaging studies. Patients were an average age of 63.4 years, and 75.5% had a history of hypertension. Mean follow-up was 5.3 years (range, 0.1-14.7 years). Mean time between the initial and final imaging studies was 3.2 years (range,

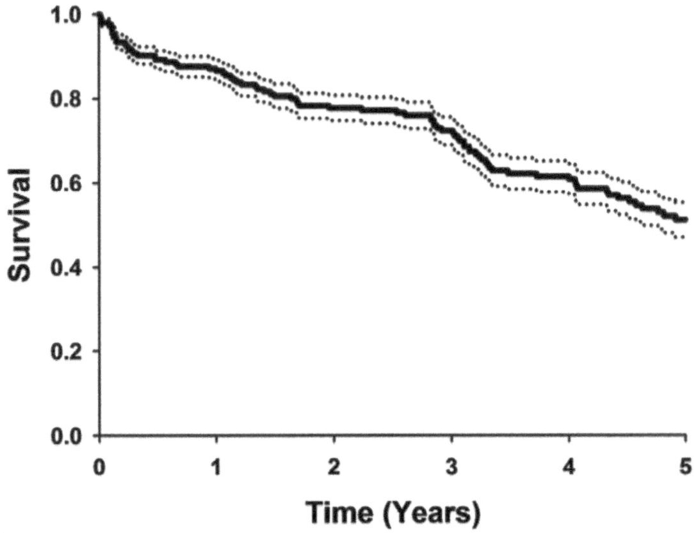

At risk:	200	161	134	117	85	54
Survival (%):	100.0	86.6	77.8	72.3	60.8	51.1
SE (%):	0.0	2.5	3.0	3.3	3.7	4.1

FIGURE 1.—Kaplan-Meier curve shows freedom from aortic growth in 200 patients with uncomplicated, acute type B dissection. (Reprinted from Durham CA, Aranson NJ, Ergul EA, et al. Aneurysmal degeneration of the thoracoabdominal aorta after medical management of type B aortic dissections. *J Vasc Surg*. 2015;62:900-906, with permission from the Society for Vascular Surgery.)

0.1-12.9 years). At 5 years, only 51% were free from aortic growth. Fifty-six patients (28%) required operative intervention (50 open, 6 endovascular repair) for aneurysmal degeneration, and the actuarial 5-year freedom from intervention was 76%. After excluding five patients (2.5%) with early rapid degeneration requiring intervention within the first 2 weeks, the mean rate of aortic growth was 12.3 mm/y for the total aortic diameter, 3.8 mm/y for the true lumen diameter, and 8.6 mm/y for the false lumen diameter. Only aortic diameter at index presentation >3.5 cm was a risk factor for future growth (odds ratio, 2.54; 95% confidence interval, 1.34-4.81; $P < .01$). Complete thrombosis of the false lumen was protective against growth (odds ratio, 0.19; 95% confidence interval, 0.11-0.42; $P < .01$).

Conclusions.—Although medical management of uncomplicated acute, type B aortic dissections has been the standard of care, at 5 years, a significant number of patients will require operative intervention for aneurysmal degeneration. Further studies of early intervention (eg, thoracic endovascular aortic repair) for type B aortic dissection to prevent late aneurysm formation are needed (Fig 1, Tables 2 and 3).

▶ This is an important retrospective natural history study on the longer term outcomes of 200 patients with medically managed type B aortic dissections

TABLE 2.—Outcome of 200 Patients Presenting with Acute Type B Aortic Dissection Who were Initially Managed Medically

Variables	Outcome
Rapid degeneration <14 days, No. (%)	5 (2.5)
Maximum diameter growth, mm	7.2
True lumen growth, mm	0.2
False lumen growth, mm	7.0
Aortic growth rate,[a] mm/y	12.3
True lumen,[a] mm/y	3.8
False lumen,[a] mm/y	8.6
Completely thrombosed false lumen at first follow-up CT, No. (%)	50 (25.0)
Time between initial and final CT, mean ± SD years	3.2 ± 3.1
Follow-up, mean ± SD years	5.3 ± 3.4
Operative intervention, No. (%)	56 (28.0)
Open	50 (89.3)
Endovascular	6 (10.7)
30-day operative mortality	4 (7.1)

CT, Computed tomography; *SD*, standard deviation.
[a]Excluding 5 patients with rapid expansion.
Reprinted from Durham CA, Aranson NJ, Ergul EA, et al. Aneurysmal degeneration of the thoracoabdominal aorta after medical management of type B aortic dissections. *J Vasc Surg*. 2015;62:900-906, with permission from the Society for Vascular Surgery.

(TBAD) between 1999 and 2011. The patients were identified using *International Classification of Disease*, 9th revision, coding acute TBAD. The study adds to the body of contemporary literature by helping us understand the natural history of medically managed TBAD and ultimately adds to our efforts to appropriately select TBAD patients who would benefit from preemptive thoracic endovascular aneurysm repair (TEVAR) to prevent future aneurysmal degeneration of the dissected aorta. The study focused on 3 primary outcomes: freedom from aortic growth (defined as an increase of > 5 mm in the maximal aortic diameter on subsequent imaging compared with the initial imaging study, assuming linear growth of the dissected aorta), freedom from intervention for aneurysmal degeneration, and rate of aortic growth. Table 2 summarizes the outcomes. The study showed a mean rate of aortic growth of 12.3 mm per year with a mean time between the initial and final imaging studies of 3.2 years (range 0.1–12.9 years). Freedom from aortic growth is illustrated nicely using a Kaplan-Meier curve in Fig 1. During a median follow-up of 4.8 years, 46.5% exhibited growth of the maximum aortic diameter by at least 5 mm and 28.0% required operative intervention for aneurysmal degeneration. Two clinical factors stood out in a multivariate model (Table 3) as related to aneurysmal degeneration: an aortic diameter at index presentation greater than 3.5 cm as a risk factor while complete false lumen thrombosis as a protective factor. Data

TABLE 3.—Univariate analysis of demographic, comorbid, and aortic characteristics of 200 patients with acute Type B aortic dissection, stratified by those with and without aortic growth

Variables	No Growth (n = 107)	Growth (n = 93)	P^a
Demographic			
Age, mean ± SD years	64.6 ± 14.3	62.0 ± 16.1	.22
Male, %	55.1	67.7	.07
Caucasian, %	85.1	77.4	.17
Comorbidities, %			
Hypertension	73.6	79.4	.34
Coronary artery disease	40.2	46.2	.39
Cerebrovascular disease	25.2	10.8	.02
Chronic obstructive pulmonary disease	16.8	19.3	.64
Diabetes mellitus	16.8	18.3	.79
End-stage renal disease	8.4	2.2	.06
Marfan disease	3.7	5.4	.58
Aortic anatomy			
Initial aortic diameter, mean ± SD mm	35.8 ± 9.9	38.9 ± 8.0	.03
Initial aortic diameter >35 mm, %	43.9	68.9	<.01
Completely thrombosed false lumen, %	37.4	10.8	<.01

SD, Standard deviation.
[a]$P < .05$ is statistically significant.
Reprinted from Durham CA, Aranson NJ, Ergul EA, et al. Aneurysmal degeneration of the thoracoabdominal aorta after medical management of type B aortic dissections. *J Vasc Surg*. 2015;62:900-906, with permission from the Society for Vascular Surgery.

from this study could serve as preliminary data for future prospective studies assessing the role of TEVAR in the altering the natural history of TBAD.[1,2]

S. Shalhub, MD, MPH, FACS

References

1. Van Bogerijen GH, Tolenaar JL, Rampoldi V, et al. Predictors of aortic growth in uncomplicated type B aortic dissection. *J Vasc Surg*. 2014;59:1134-1143.
2. Tsai TT, Fattori R, Trimarchi S, et al. Long-term survival in patients presenting with typeB acute aortic dissection: insights from the International Registry of Acute Aortic Dissection. *Circulation*. 2006;114:2226-2231.

Aortic dissection with acute malperfusion syndrome: Endovascular fenestration via the funnel technique

Vendrell A, Frandon J, Rodiere M, et al (Centre Hospitalier Universitaire de Grenoble, France; et al)

J Thorac Cardiovasc Surg 150:108-115, 2015

Objective.—To analyze the short- and long-term results of an original aortic fenestration method using the funnel technique during aortic dissection complicated by malperfusion syndrome.

Methods.—The funnel technique consists of deployment of an uncovered aortic stent graft placed from the false to the right lumen through

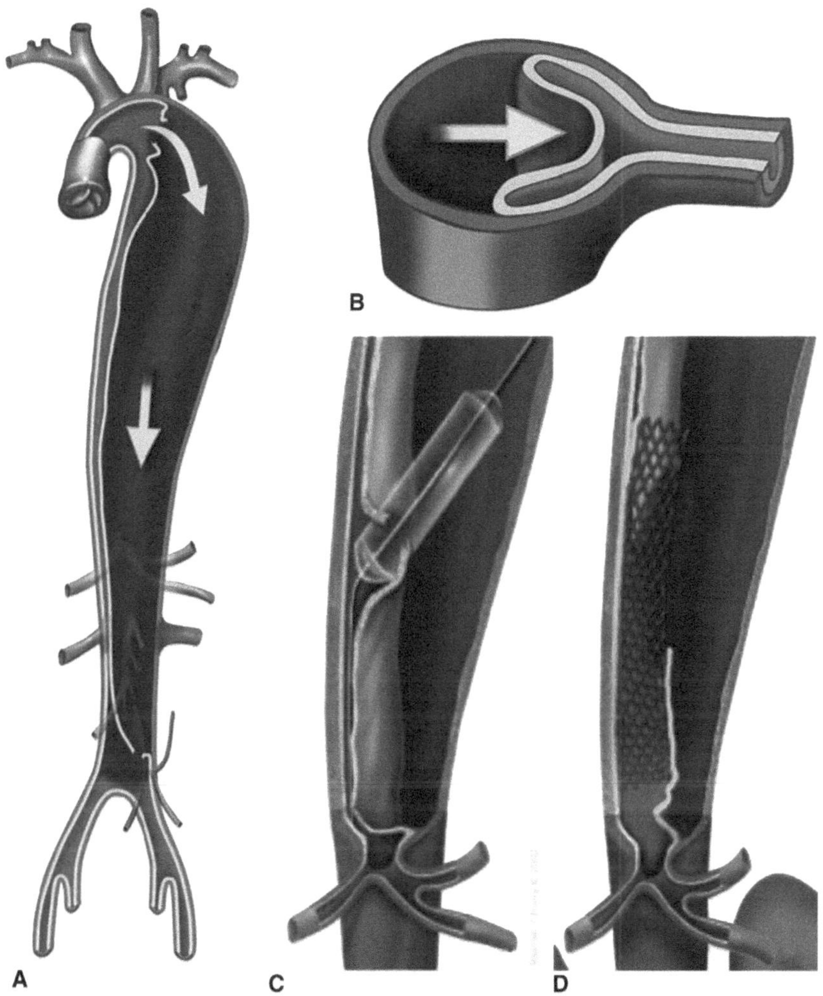

FIGURE 2.—Illustration of the funnel technique: A and B, shows the dynamic compression. The true lumen is collapsed by the large false lumen. C and D, Aortic fenestration with balloon angioplasty of the fenestration opening and deployment of the stent graft across the false and the true lumen. (Reprinted from Vendrell A, Frandon J, Rodiere M, et al. Aortic dissection with acute malperfusion syndrome: endovascular fenestration via the funnel technique. *J Thorac Cardiovasc Surg*. 2015;150:108-115, with permission from The American Association for Thoracic Surgery.)

an intimal flap aortic fenestration made by balloon angioplasty. Twenty-eight patients presenting with an aortic dissection (type A, n = 19; type B, n = 9) were treated for malperfusion syndrome owing to dynamic compression (16 renal, 17 bowel, and 13 lower limb ischemia) using the aforementioned technique, and had follow-up evaluation at short term (30 days) and long term (mean: 55 ± 40 months). Eight patients had severe ischemia on arrival (6 bowel, 7 renal, 3 lower limb).

Results.—Technical success was achieved in 27 of 28 patients (96%), and ischemic symptoms had disappeared in 25 of 28 patients (89%) at short-term follow up. Five patients presented postprocedure complications: 4 minor and 1 major with arterial thrombosis which caused technical failure (3.6%). The 30-day mortality rate was 7% (n = 2), related to bowel ischemia complications. At long-term follow up, 21 patients had a stable thoracic aortic diameter (91%).

Conclusions.—The funnel technique, in cases of malperfusion syndrome after aortic dissection, safely improves short- and long-term clinical outcome, and could represent an interesting alternative in the management of patients. The hemodynamic efficiency of this technique may account for a lower mortality in our series (Fig 2).

▶ Methods to resolve malperfusion syndrome in the setting of acute aortic dissection are inherently hazardous. As surgeons' comfort with thoracic endovascular aneurysm repair (TEVAR) has inreased, it has become the key modality to address dynamic aortic obstruction from the intimal flap at the reno-visceral segment. Of course, TEVAR may not be feasible with a type A dissection in which the arch dissection obliterates the fixation zone. In these cases, as well as select type B dissection cases, the authors offer a strategy that may supplant typical fenestration strategies that most surgeons and interventionalists deem too risky.

The funnel technique employs a balloon septostomy and then an indwelling large diameter Wallstent (24 mm) across the true and false lumen. The stent serves the purpose of promoting equalization of the pressure gradients that drive the mobility of the dissection flap through the cardiac cycle. I further suspect the resolution of the visceral ischemia is related to the large stent preventing the flap from getting anywhere near the reno-visceral branch origins. Long-term follow-up of the technique described is an added bonus, as the long-term results of most fenestration reports is lacking; the additional benefit to reduce aortic growth to 1.46 mm per annum suggests a true relief of pressure in the false lumen with the funnel technique.

J. H. Black III, MD, FACS

Endovascular Management of Rupture in Acute Type B Aortic Dissections

Faure EM, Canaud L, Marty-Ané C, et al (Arnaud de Villeneuve Univ Hosp, Montpellier, France; et al)

Eur J Vasc Endovasc Surg 49:655-660, 2015

Objective.—Reports of thoracic endovascular aortic repair (TEVAR) for complicated acute type B aortic dissection (ABAD) bring together a large range of clinical presentations. With a 30 day mortality of 50% when managed with open surgery, rupture is the most devastating complication of ABAD. This study investigated the outcome of TEVAR for ABAD complicated by rupture (r-ABAD) to assess the results of this particularly critical subgroup.

Methods.—A review of consecutive TEVAR for r-ABAD in two tertiary referral centers was performed using a prospectively maintained database.

Results.—Between 2000 and 2013, 24 patients (mean age 71 years; 14 males) underwent TEVAR for r-ABAD. Sixteen (67%) were in shock (Systolic blood pressure <80 mm Hg) before surgery. Seven patients had coverage of the left subclavian artery, of whom four had partial arch debranching procedures via cervical access concomitant with TEVAR. Median length of aortic coverage was 150 mm, median proximal oversizing was 13.3% (range 6.2—33.3%). Technical success was achieved in 100%. There were four in hospital deaths (16%). Two patients (8%) had paraplegia, but neither stroke nor renal insufficiency requiring dialysis occurred. During a mean follow up of 28 months, there was one aortic dissection related death and eight patients (40% of the surviving patients) required re-intervention. All re-interventions were managed endovascularly. At last follow up CT scan, eight patients (40%) had complete remodeling of the aortic wall.

Conclusion.—With 16% in hospital mortality and 8% early major complications, this study confirms the feasibility of TEVAR for r-ABAD with a lower peri-operative morbidity and mortality rate compared with open surgery. Given the high rate of re-intervention, close follow up is required in surviving patients.

▶ The authors of this study report on the success of treatment for ruptured type B dissections at 2 tertiary referral centers in Europe. The authors highlight that the term "complicated" when referring to type B dissection encompasses a large subset of conditions, and they chose to focus on rupture. One could also argue that rupture also presents in a variety of fashions including immediate hemodynamic compromise to contained rupture, and the full spectrum between. The data reported ultimately show 5 dissection-related deaths and 2 patients with paraplegia yielding clinical success in more than two-thirds of the patients treated. They conclude that thoracic endovascular aortic repair (TEVAR) can be used to treat rupture successfully. I am not sure that this was still a topic of significant debate. In fact, I would argue that patients with type B dissection and rupture should be primarily offered an endovascular solution as open surgery carries prohibitive risk. Although the etiology of blunt traumatic injury is different, the evolution in treatment can be applied to type B dissection with rupture. What is lacking in this article is the data from all of the other patients treated with type B dissection that did not rupture. It would be interesting to compare the operative results for those treated for rupture against those treated for other "complicating" factors. Additionally it would be interesting to compare the follow-up data for the rupture cohort against those with other surgical indication. Based on the high reintervention rate following TEVAR, I do agree with the conclusion that patients with TEVAR for rupture should be surveyed closely.

B. Propper, MD, FACS

Hospital survival of aortic dissection in children

Hua H-U, Tashiro J, Allen CJ, et al (Univ of Miami, FL)

J Surg Res 196:399-403, 2015

Background.—Thoracic aortic dissection (AD) is a rare occurrence in childhood and mostly associated with connective tissue disorders or congenital abnormalities. We examined the characteristics associated with AD and predictors of survival.

Methods.—The Kids' Inpatient Database (1997–2009) was used to identify thoracic ADs occurring in patients <20-y-old. Clinical characteristics, as well as determinants of survival, were analyzed using standard statistical methods.

Results.—One hundred sixty-eight cases of thoracic AD were identified during the study period. Overall survival was 83%. Average length of stay was 15.9 ± 16.9 d, with charges 181,867.92 ± $211,985.00. Thoracic dissection tended to affect adolescents aged 15–19 y (67%), males (76%), and Caucasians (56%) most frequently. Most patients were privately insured (64%) and treated at urban teaching centers (86%). Commonly associated diagnoses were hypertension (18%), Marfan syndrome (15%), and aortic valve disorders (8%). When repair was performed, open repair was more frequent (88%) than endovascular repair (6%). Hemorrhage was the most common complication (19%). Multiple determinants of survival were found. Girls (mortality odds ratio: 0.21 [0.05–0.91]) fared better than boys, $P = 0.023$. Patients with Medicaid (2.84 [1.21–6.69]) had higher mortality *versus* privately insured, $P = 0.014$. Income, race, and hospital characteristics, and type of repair were not significant predictors, even on sub-analyses of surgical and nonsurgical groups separately.

Conclusions.—Dissection of the thoracic aorta is a rare but significant condition affecting the pediatric population. Most repairs are performed using open technique. Payer status and gender are predictors of survival in these cases (Fig 1).

▶ Acute aortic dissection (AD) is predominantly known as a disease of old men; however, it does rarely occur in children. The International Registry of Acute Aortic Dissections is a consortium of research centers in 11 countries to study the management and outcomes of AD but that do not include pediatric patients. To date, there have been no large, population-based analyses of pediatric AD patients. The authors here skillfully utilize the Kids' Inpatient Database (KID) to identify and review AD in pediatric patients. They found that pediatric AD is still carries high mortality despite children presumably having fewer comorbidities, which often play a role in morbidity and mortality in adult patients. The overall in-hospital mortality was 17% in patients < 20 years of age, with male sex and Medicaid payer status having the worse predictors of survival. In contradistinction to previous studies, they did not

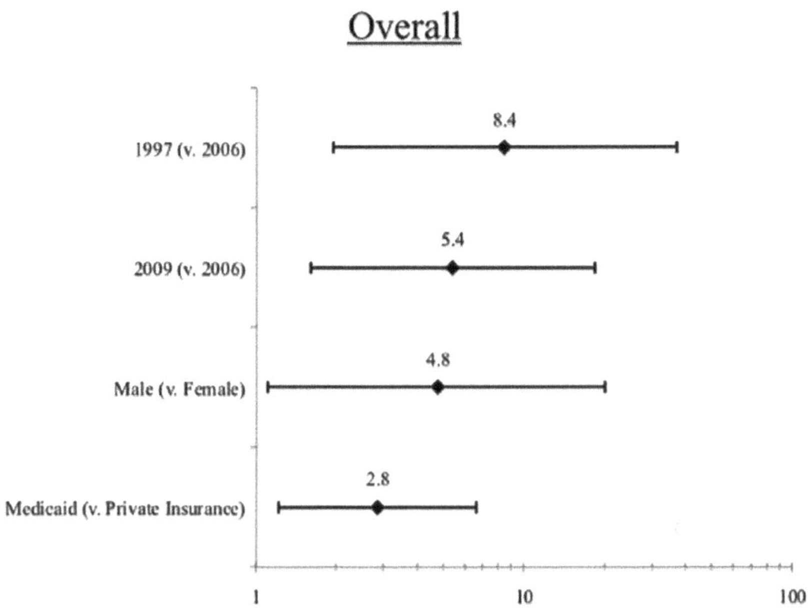

FIGURE 1.—Factors associated with in-hospital mortality in pediatric patients presenting with AD in the KID, 1997–2009. Bivariate analyses were performed with chi-square or Fisher exact test, as appropriate. Mortality odds ratios are depicted as diamonds, with values indicated previously. Error bars represent 95% confidence intervals. (Reprinted from Hua H-U, Tashiro J, Allen CJ, et al. Hospital survival of aortic dissection in children. *J Surg Res*. 2015;196:399-403, with permission from Elsevier.)

find a strong association of trauma with AD in this young age group. This may be because of the limitations of the coding within the KID database. Not surprisingly, many of the patients had connective tissue disease or congenital heart and aortic anomalies. However, the most common predisposing factor was actually hypertension, which leads to a lengthy discussion about why more American children have high blood pressure. Repair type and complications—namely, bleeding—did not affect survival outcomes in this study. Pediatric patients with connective tissue disease who require surgical intervention underwent open repair more often than an endovascular approach. This is unaccountably because patients with Marfan', Loeys-Dietz, and Ehler-Danlos will continue to experience degeneration of their aortas, making endografts highly likely to fail in the future.

K. C. Orion, MD

Impact of alterations in target vessel curvature on branch durability after endovascular repair of thoracoabdominal aortic aneurysms

Sylvan J, Brier C, Wolski K, et al (Cleveland Clinic Lerner College of Medicine-CWRU, OH)

J Vasc Surg 63:634-641, 2016

Objective.—The aim of this study was to evaluate curvature and its effect on the durability of visceral and renal branches in patients undergoing endovascular repair of thoracoabdominal aortic aneurysms (TAAAs) with fenestrated/branched endovascular aneurysm repair (F/B-EVAR).

Methods.—Quantitative branch vessel curvature assessment on branches arising from reinforced fenestrations was performed for 168 patients undergoing F/B-EVAR for type II and type III TAAAs. Preoperative and postoperative centerline coordinates were obtained using iNtuition (TeraRecon, Foster City, Calif) and exported into MATLAB (The MathWorks, Inc, Natick, Mass) based on thin-slice computed tomography imaging. Spline interpolation was applied to the centerline coordinates and resampled at 100 equally spaced points, and curvature calculations (κ, mm^{-1}) were applied. Global and maximal curvatures for each of the target vessels were measured and categorized by severity. Categories for curvature were 0 to 0.05 mm^{-1} (low), 0.05 to 0.1 mm^{-1} (medium), 0.1 to 0.15 mm^{-1} (high), and >0.15 mm^{-1} (extreme) for global curvature and 0 to 0.2 mm^{-1}, 0.2 to 0.4 mm^{-1}, 0.4 to 0.6 mm^{-1}, and >0.6 mm^{-1}, respectively, for maximum curvature. Curvature variances were assessed for an association with vessel patency and need for reintervention.

Results.—There were 558 vessels that underwent analysis based on repairs involving 650 vessels, whereby 92 vessels were excluded as they were treated with an external helical branch (58 celiac arteries and 34 superior mesenteric arteries). There was a significant difference found before and after F/B-EVAR for the global celiac artery curvature (median difference, −0.01; $P < .001$), global left renal artery curvature (median, −0.01; $P = .014$), maximum left renal artery curvature (median, 0.05; $P < .001$), and maximum right renal artery curvature (median, 0.03; $P = .009$). Maximum artery curvature was found to have shifted distally in all vessels postoperatively; 37 adverse events (AEs) were observed in 30 patients (6 branched occlusions and 31 reinterventions [24 type III endoleaks, 5 vessel stenoses, and 2 vessel occlusions]). The majority of AEs (>70%) occurred within the range of low to medium curvature. Univariate analysis found gender to be a dependent variable associated with high (maximum) preoperative curvature (odds ratio, 0.395; $P = .02$). The use of self-expanding stents (vs balloon-expandable stents alone) in vessels with high preoperative curvature (>0.6 mm^{-1}) was significant in the right renal artery ($P = .044$).

TABLE 5.—Number of Adverse Events (AEs) that Occur in a Low, Medium, High, and Outlier Range of Curvatures

Range (mm^{-1})	Preoperative Global Curvature, No. (%)	Postoperative Global Curvature, No. (%)
Low (0-0.05)	15 (40.5)	15 (40.5)
Medium (0.05-0.1)	14 (37.8)	18 (48.6)
High (0.1-0.15)	7 (18.9)	4 (10.8)
Extreme (>0.15)	1 (2.7)	0 (0)
	Preoperative Maximum Curvature, No. (%)	Postoperative Maximum Curvature, No. (%)
Low (0-0.2)	14 (37.8)	8 (21.6)
Medium (0.2-0.4)	14 (37.8)	19 (51.4)
High (0.4-0.6)	6 (16.2)	4 (10.8)
Extreme (>0.6)	3 (8.1)	6 (16.2)

Reprinted from Sylvan J, Brier C, Wolski K, et al. Impact of alterations in target vessel curvature on branch durability after endovascular repair of thoracoabdominal aortic aneurysms. *J Vasc Surg*. 2016;63:634-641, with permission from the Society for Vascular Surgery.

Conclusions.—This study did not show a significant relationship between the severity of artery curvature or changes in curvature and AEs found for visceral or renal branches after F/B-EVAR for extensive TAAA. Surprisingly, the majority of AEs occurred in low- and medium-curved vessels. This study is limited in that it does not take into account other factors that may affect AEs, like motion, which would be valuable in future studies (Table 5).

▶ Branch vessel stenosis and occlusions, although rare after endovascular repair of thoracoabdominal aneurysms (TAA), are one the more feared complications. In fact, many would argue that only if we can maintain the patency of these branches should we continue to push the endovascular technology further in complex thoracoabdominal aneurysms. The authors from the Cleveland Clinic sought to determine whether target vessel curvature may contribute to branch durability after fenestrated/branched endovascular aneurysm repair (F/B-EVAR). They provide a truly extensive experience of these surgeries, reviewing 168 cases over a mere 3-year period. This provided 558 target vessels, which included only those stented with a reinforced fenestration and balloon-expandable stent (BES). Vessels treated with helical directional branches or bridged with self-expanding stents (SES) were excluded. The authors then analyzed preoperative thin-sliced CT scans, and centerlines were used to determine curvature. Maximum curvature was defined as the region along the curve where the greatest amount of deviation from a straight line occurs, and global curvature is the average curvature along the entire length of the vessel taken at 100 points. Maximum and global curvatures were determined preoperatively and postoperatively. The authors predicted that greater curvature, either pre- or postoperatively, would be associated with branch vessel failure and need for reintervention. Instead, they found that the majority of adverse events (> 70%) occurred within the range of low to medium curvature, as seen in

Table 5. Also, factors that were predictive of renal branch occlusion were the use of cranially directed branches and long mean renal artery length. Aortic angulation relative to the renal artery did not appear to be a factor in renal artery branch patency. Interestingly, it was observed that the global curvature of vessels remained unchanged postoperatively in the superior mesenteric artery and right renal artery and decreased in the celiac artery and left renal artery after placement of a stiff BES. However, the degree of maximum curvature was increased; in other words, the placement of a stiff stent within a curved vessel simply advances the vessel curvature to a single location at the end of the stent-artery interface. This observation is remarkable and has, in practice, been foreseen by vascular surgeons as many will place an SES distally to ease the transition of the stiff BES to a tortuous, more compliant target vessel. What this study confirms is that although tremendous effort is being placed into aortic endograft development, an even greater amount of energy needs to evaluate and improve the stents we use to maintain the visceral and renal branches. Only then will F/B-EVAR surpass open TAA repair.

K. C. Orion, MD

Modified Petticoat Technique with Pre-placement of a Distal Bare Stent Improves Early Aortic Remodeling after Complicated Acute Stanford Type B Aortic Dissection

He H, Yao K, Nie WP, et al (The Third Xiangya Hosp of Central South Univ, Changsha, China; et al)

Eur J Vasc Endovasc Surg 50:450-459, 2015

Objective.—This study evaluates the safety and efficacy of pre-placement of a distal bare stent as an adjunct to thoracic endovascular aortic repair (TEVAR) in the setting of complicated acute Stanford type B aortic dissection (cTBAD).

Methods.—The records of all patients diagnosed with cTBAD at the institution between 2010 and 2013 were reviewed. Indications for the pre-placement of a distal bare stent included symptomatic malperfusion and/or radiological evidence of true lumen collapse. Computed tomography angiography was performed post-operatively to assess aortic remodeling.

Results.—148 patients were treated for cTBAD: 113 patients (76.4%) were treated with standard TEVAR and 35 (23.6%) were treated by combined proximal TEVAR with pre-placement of an adjunctive distal bare stent. Primary technical success was 95.9%. The 30 day mortality rate was 4.1% and was not different between groups. The 30 day morbidity included transient renal failure (10.1%), endoleak (7.4%), and paraplegia (2.7%), and was not different between groups. The mean follow up was 10 months (range 2–12 months). No late stent complications were observed; patients with an adjunctive bare stent had less distal re-dissection (0% vs. 15%; $p = .01$) and fewer endovascular re-interventions (5.7% vs. 20.4%; $p = .04$). At 1 year, patients treated with

TEVAR and an adjunctive distal bare stent had increased true lumen volume (166 vs. 110 mL; $p = .022$), decreased false lumen volume (60 vs. 90 mL; $p = .043$), and increased complete false lumen thrombosis in the thoracic (76.5% vs. 29.5%; $p < .001$) and abdominal (20.6% vs. 3.8%; $p = .002$) segments.

Conclusions.—Combined pre-placement of a distal bare stent as an adjunct to proximal TEVAR to treat cTBAD restricts oversizing of the distal stent graft, reducing the potential for distal true lumen collapse and visceral malperfusion, and improving remodeling of the dissected thoracic aorta. Long-term follow up and prospective studies are needed to assess the overall effectiveness of this treatment strategy.

▶ This reports discussed the use of the petticoat technique for repair of acute type B dissection. In general, the premise of this technique involves placing a self-expanding stent in the targeted distal true lumen of the dissection to limit the expansion of the proximal covered device. The authors postulate that this technique would induce true lumen remolding and raise concern about oversizing the thoracic endovascular aortic repair (TEVAR) device. Overall, I feel that this article tries to solve an issue that is secondary to the indication for surgery. A large portion of patients with type B dissection are treated medically with TEVAR used to induce aortic remodeling long term; however, patients requiring emergent surgical intervention for type B dissections are usually the result of visceral malperfusion. In these cases, although aortic remodeling is important, the acute need is to reestablish true lumen and visceral flow. Using TEVAR to "move" the flap can be successful, and if visceral flow is established after TEVAR, then other procedures can be delayed. Those with continued malperfusion represent the highest risk group. In these patients, aortic remodeling is essentially ignored at the initial setting, and all focus is on restoring true lumen and visceral flow. The patient sample presented comprises a large group of patients with refractory pain. This subset may represent the group that benefits from aggressive true lumen remodeling. The stent used for this study (Sinus XL) does not appear to be available in the United States but is a large self-expanding nitinol stent. Assuming the distal target of TEVAR is proximal to the celiac, I am unsure how using an uncovered stent is beneficial compared with a smaller-sized TEVAR device. Using sequentially placed distal to proximal TEVAR devices, the same goal can be accomplished, and all fenestrations can be excluded. This technique may confer higher spinal ischemic rates, but this article does not discuss spinal ischemia with regard to the petticoat technique. Use of covered stenting has the advantage if rupture occurs while stenting, as reported in 1 patient in this series. The authors conclude that bare metal stenting is protective for malperfusion. I do not think this article has data to support this, and what is not discussed is the bare metal stent causing flap tear in the paravisceral aorta changing the dynamic nature of the dissection flap. One conclusion that does seem supported is the improvement in continued dissection with stenting. Again, I am not sure that bare metal stenting offers advantage over covered stenting for this outcome.

B. Propper, MD, FACS

Modified Petticoat Technique with Pre-placement of a Distal Bare Stent Improves Early Aortic Remodeling after Complicated Acute Stanford Type B Aortic Dissection

He H, Yao K, Nie WP, et al (The Third Xiangya Hosp of Central South Univ, Changsha, China; et al)

Eur J Vasc Endovasc Surg 50:450-459, 2015

Objective.—This study evaluates the safety and efficacy of pre-placement of a distal bare stent as an adjunct to thoracic endovascular aortic repair (TEVAR) in the setting of complicated acute Stanford type B aortic dissection (cTBAD).

Methods.—The records of all patients diagnosed with cTBAD at the institution between 2010 and 2013 were reviewed. Indications for the pre-placement of a distal bare stent included symptomatic malperfusion and/or radiological evidence of true lumen collapse. Computed tomography angiography was performed postoperatively to assess aortic remodeling.

Results.—148 patients were treated for cTBAD: 113 patients (76.4%) were treated with standard TEVAR and 35 (23.6%) were treated by combined proximal TEVAR with pre-placement of an adjunctive distal bare stent. Primary technical success was 95.9%. The 30 day mortality rate was 4.1% and was not different between groups. The 30 day morbidity included transient renal failure (10.1%), endoleak (7.4%), and paraplegia (2.7%), and was not different between groups. The mean follow up was 10 months (range 2–12 months). No late stent complications were observed; patients with an adjunctive bare stent had less distal re-dissection (0% vs. 15%; $p = .01$) and fewer endovascular re-interventions (5.7% vs. 20.4%; $p = .04$). At 1 year, patients treated with TEVAR and an adjunctive distal bare stent had increased true lumen volume (166 vs. 110 mL; $p = .022$), decreased false lumen volume (60 vs. 90 mL; $p = .043$), and increased complete false lumen thrombosis in the thoracic (76.5% vs. 29.5%; $p < .001$) and abdominal (20.6% vs. 3.8%; $p = .002$) segments.

Conclusions.—Combined pre-placement of a distal bare stent as an adjunct to proximal TEVAR to treat cTBAD restricts oversizing of the distal stent graft, reducing the potential for distal true lumen collapse and visceral malperfusion, and improving remodeling of the dissected thoracic aorta. Long-term follow up and prospective studies are needed to assess the overall effectiveness of this treatment strategy (Fig 1, Tables 3 and 5).

► The management of acute type B aortic dissection (TBAD) continues to evolve. There is a growing interest in addressing the issue of distal endoleak

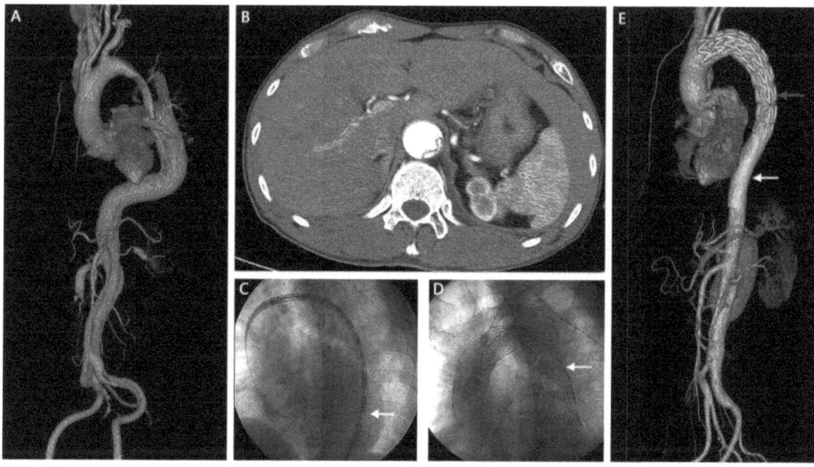

FIGURE 1.—(A,B) Preprocedure computed tomographic scan showing acute type B dissection with false lumen compression of the true lumen. (A) Three dimensional reconstruction. (B) Abdominal aorta showing collapsed true lumen. (C,D) Digital subtraction angiography showing (C) initial release of the distal bare stent (arrow) at the distal landing zone and then (D) subsequent deployment the stent graft (arrow) in the proximal thoracic aorta. (E) Computed tomographic scan 6 months after the procedure showing the position of the covered stent (blue arrow) and distal bare stent (white arrow) with re-expansion of the true lumen and obliteration of the false lumen. (Reprinted from He H, Yao K, Nie WP, et al. Modified petticoat technique with pre-placement of a distal bare stent improves early aortic remodeling after complicated acute stanford type B aortic dissection. *Eur J Vasc Endovasc Surg.* 2015;50:450-459, with permission from European Society for Vascular Surgery.)

TABLE 3.—Patient Outcomes After TEVAR

	TEVAR ($n = 113$)	TEVAR with Bare Stent ($n = 35$)	p
Technical success	108 (95.6%)	34 (97.1%)	.98
30 day mortality	5 (4.4%)	1 (2.8%)	.46
30 day morbidity			
Endoleak	9 (7.9%)	2 (5.7%)	.66
Aortic rupture	5 (4.4%)	1 (2.8%)	.46
Stroke	0 (0%)	0 (0%)	–
Paraplegia	3 (2.7%)	1 (2.8%)	.95
Acute renal failure	10 (8.8%)	5 (14.3%)	.35
>30 day mortality	3 (2.7%)	0 (0%)	.38
>30 day morbidity			
Permanent dialysis	8 (7.1%)	0 (0%)	.11
Late aortic rupture	3 (2.7%)	0 (0%)	.38
SIDR	17 (15%)	0 (0%)	.01[a]
Secondary intervention			
Surgical	4 (3.5%)	0 (0%)	.26
Endovascular	23 (20.4%)	2 (5.7%)	.04[a]

TEVAR = thoracic endovascular aortic repair; SIDR = stent graft induced distal re-dissection.
[a]Significant, <.05.
Reprinted from He H, Yao K, Nie WP, et al. Modified petticoat technique with pre-placement of a distal bare stent improves early aortic remodeling after complicated acute stanford type B aortic dissection. *Eur J Vasc Endovasc Surg.* 2015;50:450-459, with permission from European Society for Vascular Surgery.

TABLE 5.—Qualitative Assessments of the False Lumen After TEVAR

			TEVAR ($n = 113$)	TEVAR with bare stent ($n = 35$)	T test	p
Pre-operative	Thoracic	Patent	53 (50.5%)	16 (47.1%)	0.12	.7291
		Partially thrombosed	52 (49.5%)	18 (52.9%)		
		Completely thrombosed	0 (0%)	0 (0%)		
	Abdominal	Patent	76 (73.8%)	24 (70.6%)	0.145	.9301
		Partially thrombosed	27 (25.7%)	9 (26.5%)		
		Completely thrombosed	2 (1.9%)	1 (2.9%)		
12-month follow up	Thoracic	Patent	0 (0%)	0 (0%)	23.4	<0.001[a]
		Partially thrombosed	74 (70.5%)	8 (23.5%)		
		Completely thrombosed	31 (29.5%)	26 (76.5%)		
	Abdominal	Patent	32 (30.5%)	4 (11.8%)	12.62	.0018[a]
		Partially thrombosed	69 (65.7%)	23 (67.6%)		
		Completely thrombosed	4 (3.8%)	7 (20.6%)		

TEVAR = thoracic endovascular aortic repair.
[a]Significant, <.05.
Reprinted from He H, Yao K, Nie WP, et al. Modified petticoat technique with pre-placement of a distal bare stent improves early aortic remodeling after complicated acute stanford type B aortic dissection. *Eur J Vasc Endovasc Surg.* 2015;50:450-459, with permission from European Society for Vascular Surgery

or stent-induced distal redissection (SIDR) at the distal edge of the stent graft and lack of subsequent aortic remodeling. One potential solution is to deploy a bare stent distal to the stent graft via the Provisional ExTension To Induce COmplete Attachment (Petticoat) technique. The Petticoat technique aims to enhance distal anchoring of the thoracic stent graft and to induce positive aortic remodeling with true lumen expansion and false lumen thrombosis with preservation of the visceral arteries. The authors here present a similar but alternative approach with preplacement of an adjunctive distal bare stent in the distal aorta (Fig 1) to stabilize the dissection flap, restore the normal diameter of the distal aorta, reverse true lumen collapse, and enhance false lumen thrombosis. This is a retrospective study of 35 complicated TBAD cases treated by a combined proximal thoracic endovascular aortic repair (TEVAR) compared with 113 patients treated with standard TEVAR between 2010 and 2013 in China. The mean follow-up was 10 months (range 2–12 months). Table 3 summarizes the patient outcomes. The most notable finding is the absence of SIDR in the TEVAR with distal bare stent group (0% vs 15%; $P < .01$) and subsequently lower secondary interventions (5.7% vs 20.4%; $P < 04$), which most commonly were needed for SIDR occurring in the conventional TEVAR group. At the 1-year follow-up, patients treated with an adjunctive distal bare stent also had increased complete false lumen thrombosis in the thoracic (76.5% vs 29.5%; $P < .001$) and abdominal (20.6% vs 3.8%; $P < .002$) segments (Table 5). Although this approach offers acceptable results, long-term results and future prospective studies assessing the role of TEVAR in the altering the natural history of complicated TBAD are necessary.[1,2]

S. Shalhub, MD, MPH, FACS

References

1. Melissano G, Bertoglio L, Rinaldi E, et al. Volume changes in aortic true and false lumen after the "PETTICOAT" procedure for type B aortic dissection. *J Vasc Surg.* 2012;55:641-651.
2. Lombardi JV, Cambria RP, Nienaber CA, et al. STABLE Investigators. Aortic remodeling after endovascular treatment of complicated type B aortic dissection with the use of a composite device design. *J Vasc Surg.* 2014;596:1544-1554.

The Impact of Pre-Operative Malperfusion on Outcome in Acute Type A Aortic Dissection: Results From the GERAADA Registry

Czerny M, Schoenhoff F, Etz C, et al (Univ Hosp Zurich, Switzerland; Univ Hosp Bern, Switzerland; Heart Ctr Leipzig, Germany; et al)

J Am Coll Cardiol 65:2628-2635, 2015

Background.—Malperfusion adversely affects outcomes in patients with acute type A aortic dissection, but reliable quantitative data are lacking.

Objectives.—The aim of this study was to analyze the impact of various forms of malperfusion on early outcome.

Methods.—A total of 2,137 consecutive patients enrolled in GERAADA (German Registry for Acute Aortic Dissection Type A) who underwent surgery between 2006 and 2010, of whom 717 (33.6%) had any kind of pre-operative malperfusion, were retrospectively analyzed.

Results.—All-cause 30-day mortality was 16.9% and varied substantially according to the number of organ systems affected by malperfusion (none, 12.6%; 1 system, 21.3%; 2 systems, 30.9%; 3 systems, 43.4%; $p < 0.001$). Pre-operative cerebral malperfusion, comatose state, peripheral malperfusion, visceral malperfusion, involvement of supra-aortic branches, coronary malperfusion, and renal malperfusion were all independent predictors of developing any post-operative malperfusion syndrome. When survival was considered, age, peripheral malperfusion, involvement of supraaortic branches, coronary malperfusion, spinal malperfusion, a primary entry in the descending aorta, and pre-operative comatose state were independent predictors, again with increasing significance.

Conclusions.—Malperfusion remains a severe clinical condition with strong potential for adverse outcomes in patients undergoing surgery for acute type A aortic dissection. The GERAADA registry suggests that the impact of the number of organs involved and the type of malperfusion on outcome differs substantially. Introducing an appropriate classification system, such as "complicated" and uncomplicated" acute type A aortic dissection, might help predict individual risk as well as select a surgical strategy that may quickly resolve malperfusion (Table 2).

▶ Malperfusion events drive substantial morbidity and mortality in the episode of Type A aortic dissection. The authors report from the German Registry for

TABLE 2.—Survival per Number of Pre-Operative Malperfused Organ Systems

Malperfused Organ Systems	Total	Survivors	Dead	Percent Dead per Group
None	1,420 (66.4)	1,241 (58.1)	179 (8.4)	12.6
1	494 (23.1)	389 (18.2)	105 (4.9)	21.3
2	139 (6.5)	96 (4.5)	43 (2.0)	30.9
3	53 (2.5)	30 (1.7)	23 (1.1)	43.4

Values are n (%).

Reprinted from Czerny M, Schoenhoff F, Etz C, et al. The impact of pre-operative malperfusion on outcome in acute type A aortic dissection: results from the GERAADA registry. *J Am Coll Cardiol.* 2015;65:2628-2635, with permission from The American College of Cardiology Foundation.

Acute Aortic Dissection Type A 2137 patients in whom 717 (33%) were detected to have any type of preoperative malperfusion. Because malperfusion is so common, it is worthwhile to consider the aortic territories involved and the "weight" of an event in the area; in such an examination, tailoring the operation would have potential benefit. In their rigorous analysis, the authors have provided this insight.

Registry data can create a bias, and aortic dissection surgery is not immune; for example, a hemiarch or total arch repair has a substantially different risk profile, and likely the latter would be required for extensive dissection of the supra-aortic branches by the dissection. In this example, the risk for stroke would rise but may have been proffered anyway by a comatose patient preoperatively. Nonetheless, an odds ratio of 9.4 for postoperative renovisceral malperfusion when it was present preoperatively makes the argument that a corrective surgery in the ascending or arch may be insufficient to reverse the more distal malperfusion event. These patients should be considered for an endovascular procedure before undergoing type A dissection surgery. This is reversal of the paradigm for emergency management of the type A dissection patient, but this article builds a solid argument.

J. H. Black III, MD, FACS

Volumetric analysis of the initial index computed tomography scan can predict the natural history of acute uncomplicated type B dissections

Lavingia KS, Larion S, Ahanchi SS, et al (Eastern Virginia Med School, Norfolk)
J Vasc Surg 62:893-899, 2015

Objective.—Our objective was to characterize the predictive impact of computed tomography (CT) scan volumetric analysis on the natural history of acute uncomplicated type B aortic dissections (ADs).

Methods.—We conducted a retrospective review of patients with acute type B ADs from 2009 to 2014. On an iNtuition workstation (TeraRecon, Foster City, Calif), volume measurements were obtained using the true lumen volume (TLV), false lumen volume (FLV), and total aortic volume from the left subclavian artery to the celiac artery. Growth rate was calculated as the change in maximal diameter between first and last available CT scans during the time interval. The primary outcome of the study was delayed aortic intervention. $P < .05$ was considered statistically significant.

Results.—During a 5-year period, 164 patients had CT scan evidence of acute type B ADs; 11 patients were excluded for lack of subsequent follow-up imaging; 36 patients who underwent urgent repair (<14 days from presentation) were also excluded. We evaluated a total of 117 patients: 85 patients who did not require intervention and 32 who underwent delayed (>14 days) thoracic endovascular aneurysm repair (29) or open repair (3). Mean age was 66 ± 12 years. Mean TLV/FLV ratio on initial CT scan was significantly higher in patients who did not eventually require an operation (1.55 vs 0.82; $P = .02$). The mean growth rate was higher in those eventually requiring operation (2.47 vs 0.42 mm/mo; $P = .003$). Patients were divided into three subgroups on the basis of their initial imaging TLV/FLV ratios (<0.8, 0.8-1.6, and >1.6). There was a significant difference in the growth rates between these three groups (4.6 vs 2.4 vs 0.8 mm/mo; $P < .025$). Area under the receiver operating characteristic curve analysis revealed that a TLV/FLV ratio <0.8 was highly predictive for requiring an intervention (area = 0.8; sensitivity, 69%; specificity, 84%: positive predictive value, 71%; negative predictive value, 81%), with an odds ratio of 12.2 (confidence interval, 5-26; $P < .001$). Conversely, a TLV/FLV ratio of >1.6 was highly predictive for freedom from delayed operation (sensitivity, 91%; specificity, 42%; positive predictive value, 61%; negative predictive value, 86%). After Kaplan-Meier analysis, 1-year and 2-year survival free of aortic interventions was 60% and 42% with a TLV/FLV ratio <0.8 and 92% and 82% with a ratio >1.6 ($P = .001$).

Conclusions.—Initial CT scan volumetric analysis in patients presenting with uncomplicated acute type B ADs is a useful tool to predict growth and need for future intervention (Fig 2, Table 3).

▶ The authors sought to use initial index computed tomography scan volumetric analysis to predict the natural history of acute uncomplicated acute type B aortic dissections (TBAD). This is a retrospective review of 117 patients with TBAD from 2009 to 2014. The patients were identified using *International Classification of Diseases*, 9th Revision, coding for acute TBAD. Volumetric analysis was performed using the summation of area technique on the TeraRecon software from the left subclavian artery to the origin of the celiac artery. Patients who required repair for aneurysmal degeneration or rupture (27.4%, mean time to repair was 23 months, range, 2–61) were compared with those who did not. Table 3 summarizes the aortic diameters and volumetric measurements between the 2 groups. The authors demonstrated a larger false lumen volume (FLV) and a smaller true lumen volume (TLV)/FLV ratio were significantly different between the patient groups on univariate analysis and in a multivariate model. Fig 1 illustrates the Kaplan-Meier analysis for freedom from intervention

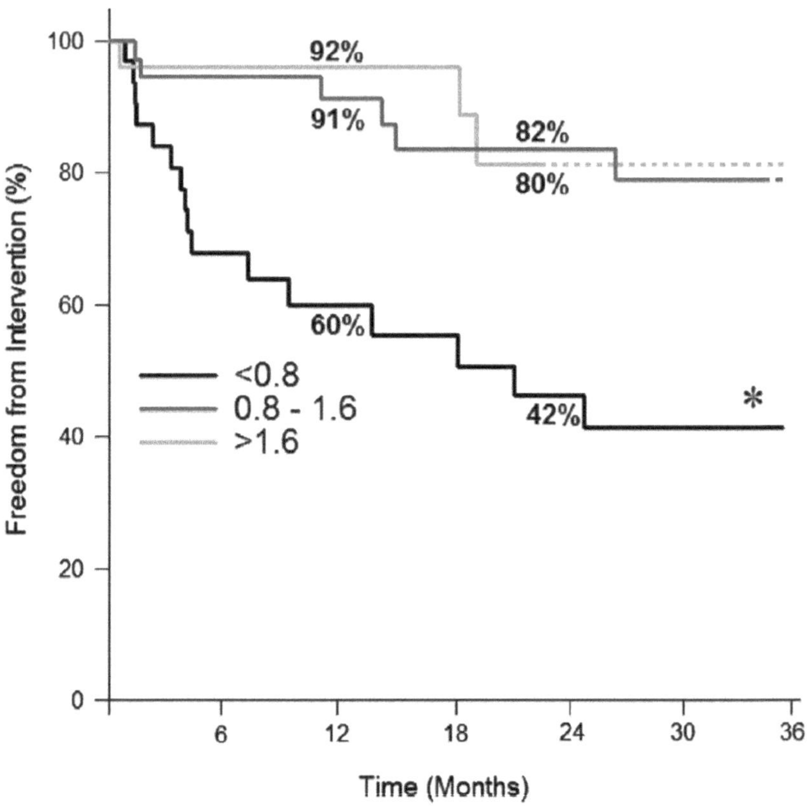

FIGURE 2.—Kaplan-Meier analysis for freedom from intervention (%) stratified between study participants with true lumen to false lumen volume (TLV/FLV) ratios listed. The *dashed line* indicates the time point at which standard error exceeds 10%. *Statistically different from other groups at $P < .001$. (Reprinted from Lavingia KS, Larion S, Ahanchi SS, et al. Volumetric analysis of the initial index computed tomography scan can predict the natural history of acute uncomplicated type B dissections. *J Vasc Surg*. 2015;62:893-899, with permission from the Society for Vascular Surgery.)

TABLE 3.—Mean Vessel Characteristics Between Patients Who Required Intervention and Those Who Did Not

	No Intervention (SD) (n = 85)	Intervention (SD) (n = 32)	*P* Value
Maximum aortic diameter, mm	45.1 (7.4)	48.4 (9.4)	.047
TLV, mm^3	180 (61)	167 (86)	.386
FLV, mm^3	139 (64)	223 (65)	<.001
TLV/FLV	1.557 (0.82)	0.822 (.55)	<.001
Aortic diameter at LSA, mm	27.4 (7.8)	28.9 (14)	.475
Mean growth rate, mm/mo	0.42 (1.9)	2.47 (5.3)	.003

FLV, False lumen volume; *LSA*, left subclavian artery; *SD*, standard deviation; *TLV*, true lumen volume

Reprinted from Lavingia KS, Larion S, Ahanchi SS, et al. Volumetric analysis of the initial index computed tomography scan can predict the natural history of acute uncomplicated type B dissections. *J Vasc Surg*. 2015;62:893-899, with permission from the Society for Vascular Surgery.

stratified by TLV/FLV ratios with a significantly decreased freedom from intervention in patients with TLV/FLV ratio <0.8 compared with >1.6. Data from this study would serve as a preliminary data for future prospective studies to predict the natural history of TBAD.[1]

S. Shalhub, MD, MPH, FACS

Reference

1. Trimarchi S, Jonker FH, van Bogerijen GH, et al. Predicting aortic enlargement in type B aortic dissection. *Ann Cardiothorac Surg*. 2014;3:285-291.

Moderate to Deep Hypothermia in Patients Undergoing Thoracoabdominal Aortic Repair

Fukui T, Takanashi S (Sakakibara Heart Inst, Tokyo, Japan)

Ann Vasc Surg 31:39-45, 2016

Background.—The aim of this study was to determine early and mid-term outcomes after open repair of thoracoabdominal aortic aneurysm, with moderate to deep hypothermia as part of proximal aortic management.

Methods.—Between April 2009 and March 2015, 44 patients underwent thoracoabdominal aortic repair by total cardiopulmonary bypass at our institute. Our strategy was to use deep (<25°C) hypothermic circulatory arrest when open proximal anastomosis is necessary ($n = 18$). Otherwise, proximal anastomosis with an aortic clamp was performed with moderate (25–30°C) hypothermia without circulatory arrest ($n = 26$). Early and mid-term outcomes were assessed in all patients.

Results.—In-hospital mortality was observed in 1 patient (2.3%). Stroke was observed in 2 (4.5%) patients and a spinal cord ischemic injury in 4 (9.1%). Renal failure requiring new hemodialysis was observed in 5 patients (11.4%). There were 9 patients (20.5%) with early major adverse events (in-hospital death, stroke, spinal cord ischemic injury, renal failure requiring new hemodialysis, and prolonged intubation). Multivariable logistic regression analysis demonstrated that a history of abdominal aortic aneurysm repair (odds ratio 17.711, 95% confidence interval 1.274–246.426, $P = 0.032$) was the only independent predictor of early major adverse events. Deep hypothermic circulatory arrest was not an independent predictor of early major adverse events. At 5 years, overall freedom from death was 89.4 ± 6.1%.

Conclusion.—Moderate to deep hypothermia as a constituent of proximal aortic management was safe and effective in patients undergoing open repair of thoracoabdominal aortic aneurysm.

► The authors provide a look at 44 patients undergoing thoracoabdominal bypass surgery over a 6-year period. In general, this breaks down to 7 surgeries per year for thoracoabdominal aortic surgery. The goal of the study was to evaluate hypothermic circulatory arrest using both deep and moderate temperatures. This was a retrospective review, and its cannot be used to make any determination about a particular technique with regard to Crawford extent. The patients in this study were distributed among the various type of thoracoabdominal aortic repair (TAAA) and surgeon preferences directed the approach. Of note, the complication rates from this report mimic other reporting with major adverse complications occurring in more than 20% of patients. This is similar to the 2016 Cosseli et al report on more than 3000 TAAA repairs. The take-home message form this report, like many before, is that TAAA should be performed in centers of excellence by high-volume surgeons given the high rate of periprocedural complications. With regard to hypothermic circulatory arrest (HCA) versus partial cooling and left heart bypass, this remains surgeon preference and largely determined by anatomic constraints. The authors clearly define the advantages of HCA, which include a bloodless field and the ability to access the inside of the aortic arch to remove plaque or debris. At the same time, the authors point out the downside to HCA including prolonged operative times and profound coagulopathy. In general, the use of HCA seems most appropriate for extent I and extent II repairs when the proximal aortic anastomosis presents the most challenge. While reported it is hard to imagine a scenario in which is more advantages for extent III or IV repairs. Although the data presented represent a group 44 patients, the authors do not break down the complication profile by the extent of TAAA. This would have been helpful because benefit to hypothermia is not likely sustained in the extent 4 repairs.

B. Propper, MD, FACS

Open versus Endovascular Repair of Arch and Descending Thoracic Aneurysms: A retrospective Comparison

Shiraev TP, Qasabian R, Tardo D, et al (Royal Prince Alfred Hosp, Camperdown, New South Wales, Australia; The Univ of Notre Dame, Darlinghurst, New South Wales, Australia)

Ann Vasc Surg 31:30-38, 2016

Background.—Thoracic aortic aneurysms (TAAs) contribute significant mortality if left untreated, but surgical repair has historically carried substantial risks.

Methods.—We sought to observe trends and outcomes of open and endovascular thoracic endovascular aneurysm repair thoracic aortic repairs, so conducted a retrospective review of all patients who presented for management of TAAs from 2003 to 2013 at 2 hospitals in Sydney, Australia.

Results.—A total of 179 patients presented with TAAs over the study period, including 5 ruptures. Fifty-two were treated nonoperatively, with 127 surgically repaired. Operative duration was significantly shorter in endovascular than open repair of arch (193 ± 108 vs. 396 ± 98 min, $P = 0.0001$) and descending aneurysms (242 ± 116 vs. 422.5 ± 161 min, $P = 0.003$). There were no differences in mortality or

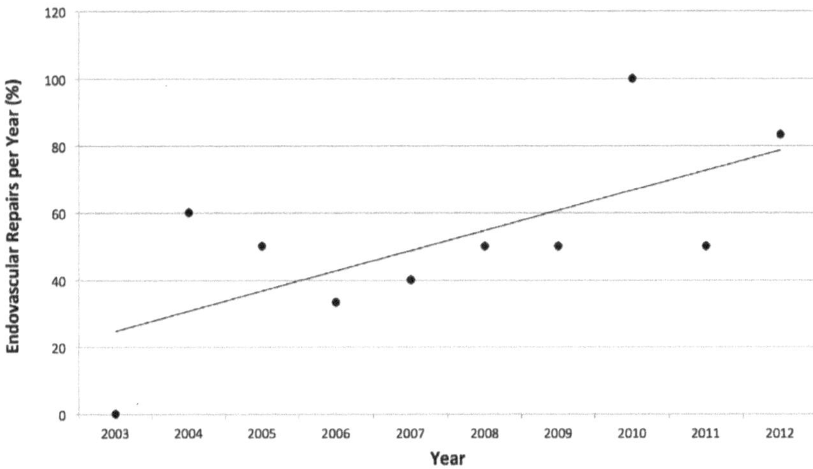

FIGURE 1.—Percentage of patients undergoing endovascular descending aneurysm repair per year over the study period. $R^2 = 0.453$, $\beta = 0.673$, and $P = 0.033$. (Reprinted from Shiraev TP, Qasabian R, Tardo D, et al. Open versus endovascular repair of arch and descending thoracic aneurysms: a retrospective comparison. *Ann Vasc Surg*. 2016;31:30-38, with permission from Elsevier.)

complication rates (including paraplegia), duration of hospital or intensive care unit stay, or transfusion requirements between endovascular and open TAA repairs.

Conclusions.—Apart from reduced surgical duration, this study revealed no benefits of endovascular over open TAA repair. Overall morbidity and mortality were low, even in elderly patients (Fig 1).

▶ Thoracic aortic aneurysms (TAA), although relatively rare in occurrence, have substantial morbidity and mortality. Surgical repair has traditionally been associated with substantial risks. The authors of this study sought to look at contemporary outcomes for patients undergoing TAA repair and compare open repair with thoracic endovascular aneurysm repair (TEVAR). They performed a retrospective analysis of 179 patients diagnosed with TAA seen at 1 of 2 large tertiary referral centers in Sydney, Australia, from 2003 to 2013. All patients with Crawford type 0–III anatomy were included, but they did not include type IV, thoracoabdominal aneurysms.

One hundred twenty-seven patients underwent surgical repair. Sixty-nine patients had open repair of the ascending aorta, 27 patients had arch repair, 20 open repair, and 7 endovascular. Thirty-one patients had repair of the descending aorta, 12 open, and 19 endovascular. Although operative repair of TAA is associated with high perioperative mortality, only 3 of the patients who underwent surgical management died during the study period. Patients over age 75 were almost twice as likely to have an endovascular procedure (83.3 vs 47.4%, $P = .045$). They also found a significant increase in the percentage of descending TAA treated with TEVAR over time (Fig 1). Operative duration was significantly longer in the open repair compared with TEVAR in the arch (396 ± 98 min vs 193 ± 108 min, $P = .0001$) as well as descending aorta (422.5 ± 161 min vs 242 ± 116, $P = .003$). Most importantly, they found no differences in mortality or complication rates, duration of hospital or intensive care unit stay, spinal cord ischemia, or transfusion requirements between the 2 groups.

Although this article illustrates that TAA can safely be performed as both open or TEVAR, it is a retrospective study and thus not a true comparison between the 2 modalities. Patients for each cohort were carefully selected, and therefore the 2 techniques should not be seen as equivocal. In addition, many of the patients included in the TEVAR group underwent hybrid procedures and did not have a purely endovascular approach. A larger, prospective study, perhaps with 3 arms to include open, hybrid, and TEVAR, would give a more robust perspective on differences between the techniques.

M. Arnold, MD

Staged hybrid repair of extensive thoracoabdominal aortic aneurysms secondary to chronic aortic dissection

Jain A, Flohr TF, Johnston WF, et al (Univ of Cincinnati, OH; Univ of Virginia, Charlottesville)

J Vasc Surg 63:62-69, 2016

Objective.—Many patients with aortic dissection develop Crawford extent I or II thoracoabdominal aortic aneurysms (TAAA). Because open repair is associated with a high morbidity and mortality, hybrid approaches to TAAA repair are emerging. In this study, we evaluated the midterm outcomes and aortic remodeling of a hybrid technique that combines proximal thoracic endovascular aneurysm repair (TEVAR), followed by staged distal open thoracoabdominal repair for patients with Crawford extent I or II TAAAs secondary to chronic aortic dissection.

Methods.—We identified 19 patients with Crawford extent I (n = 1) or extent II (n = 18) TAAAs secondary to chronic aortic dissection who underwent a staged hybrid repair from 2007 to 2014 at our institution. Nine patients had previous open ascending aortic surgery for type I aortic dissection. Stage 1 TEVAR was performed via percutaneous (n = 8), femoral cutdown (n = 8), or iliac exposure (n = 3). The left subclavian artery was covered in nine patients and revascularized in eight patients using carotid-subclavian bypass (n = 7) or laser fenestration (n = 1). Stage 2 open repair was performed a median of 18 weeks later with partial cardiopulmonary bypass via left femoral arterial and venous cannulation for visceral and lower body perfusion. The open thoracoabdominal graft was anastomosed proximally in an end to end fashion with the endograft. We then assessed surgical morbidity and mortality, midterm survival, and freedom from reintervention. Aortic remodeling was measured and change in maximum aortic and false lumen diameter at last followup (median, 3 years) from baseline was assessed.

Results.—There were no deaths, strokes, or chronic renal failure in this cohort. After stage 1 TEVAR, three patients required repeat intervention for endoleak (type Ia, n = 1; type Ib, n = 1; type II, n = 1) before open repair. After stage 2 open repair, there was a single delayed permanent paralysis 2 weeks after discharge. At a median 3-year follow-up (range, 6 months-6.2 years), there were no deaths, neurologic events, endoleaks, or TAAA reinterventions. Complete false lumen thrombosis occurred in 100% of the patients, with maximum false lumen diameter decreasing from 34.3 ± 15.3 mm to 13.2 ± 12.0 mm ($P < .01$) and total aortic diameter decreasing from 60.2 ± 9.0 mm to 49.4 ± 9.6 mm ($P < .01$).

Conclusions.—Staged hybrid TAAA repair, using a combination of proximal TEVAR with open distal repair, can be performed using established endovascular skills and technology coupled with traditional open aortic surgical techniques, with low surgical morbidity and mortality. In the midterm, staged hybrid TAAA repair was associated favorable survival, aortic remodeling, and freedom from reintervention.

▶ The authors discuss present a single-center case series of 19 thoracoabdominal aortic aneurysms (TAAA) of which 18 are extent 2 repairs. They propose that thoracic endovascular aneurysm repair (TEVAR) followed by open repair is an acceptable alternative to single-stage repair. The premise of the hybrid approach stems from the high paraplegia rate and mortality associated with open extent reconstructions. The authors propose that staged approach improves these outcomes. Although the study includes only 19 patients, there is 1 reported incident of paraplegia that occurred late for a total rate of 5%. This is below the reported rate of paraplegia reported at large volume TAAA centers. The idea of staged reconstruction hinges on the benefit of aortic and spinal cord ischemic conditioning; moreover, the thought that covering the proximal aorta allows the distal aorta to collateralize flow and conditions the spinal cord for the eventual ischemia. Variations of this theory were proposed in 2006 by Resch et al as they performed alternative hybrid approach for those unfit for open TAAA. Similar to this article, the overall complications rates were high, particularly renal failure. The reported 5% rate of paraplegia in this case is low compared with other open TAAA repair literature. This is the area where future research should focus. It is possible that turning an extent II repair into an extent IV lessens the physiologic burden and hence lessens the chance of spinal ischemia. The renal failure rate presented is no different from other large TAAA reports. Lastly, 2 other areas that require some clarification include cost and loss to follow-up. The cost of staged approach is almost certainly higher, and the gains in complication profile are likely needed to justify the additional cost. In this series all patients returned for stage II procedures, but there will be patients who do not tolerate stage I or do not return for stage II. I view this as a benefit, because those who cannot tolerate TEVAR or return for stage II are not likely to be patients who derive benefit from open complex aortic reconstruction (stage II).

B. Propper, MD, FACS

Staged hybrid repair of extensive thoracoabdominal aortic aneurysms secondary to chronic aortic dissection

Jain A, Flohr TF, Johnston WF, et al (Univ of Cincinnati, OH; Univ of Virginia, Charlottesville)

J Vasc Surg 63:62-69, 2016

Objective.—Many patients with aortic dissection develop Crawford extent I or II thoracoabdominal aortic aneurysms (TAAA). Because open repair is associated with a high morbidity and mortality, hybrid approaches to TAAA repair are emerging. In this study, we evaluated the midterm outcomes and aortic remodeling of a hybrid technique that combines proximal thoracic endovascular aneurysm repair (TEVAR), followed by staged distal open thoracoabdominal repair for patients with Crawford extent I or II TAAAs secondary to chronic aortic dissection.

Methods.—We identified 19 patients with Crawford extent I (n = 1) or extent II (n = 18) TAAAs secondary to chronic aortic dissection who underwent a staged hybrid repair from 2007 to 2014 at our institution. Nine patients had previous open ascending aortic surgery for type I aortic dissection. Stage 1 TEVAR was performed via percutaneous (n = 8), femoral cutdown (n = 8), or iliac exposure (n = 3). The left subclavian artery was covered in nine patients and revascularized in eight patients using carotid-subclavian bypass (n = 7) or laser fenestration (n = 1). Stage 2 open repair was performed a median of 18 weeks later with partial cardiopulmonary bypass via left femoral arterial and venous cannulation for visceral and lower body perfusion. The open thoracoabdominal graft was anastomosed proximally in an end to end fashion with the endograft. We then assessed surgical morbidity and mortality, midterm survival, and freedom from reintervention. Aortic remodeling was measured and change in maximum aortic and false lumen diameter at last followup (median, 3 years) from baseline was assessed.

Results.—There were no deaths, strokes, or chronic renal failure in this cohort. After stage 1 TEVAR, three patients required repeat intervention for endoleak (type Ia, n = 1; type Ib, n = 1; type II, n = 1) before open repair. After stage 2 open repair, there was a single delayed permanent paralysis 2 weeks after discharge. At a median 3-year follow-up (range, 6 months-6.2 years), there were no deaths, neurologic events, endoleaks, or TAAA reinterventions. Complete false lumen thrombosis occurred in 100% of the patients, with maximum false lumen diameter decreasing from 34.3 ± 15.3 mm to 13.2 ± 12.0 mm ($P < .01$) and total aortic diameter decreasing from 60.2 ± 9.0 mm to 49.4 ± 9.6 mm ($P < .01$).

Conclusions.—Staged hybrid TAAA repair, using a combination of proximal TEVAR with open distal repair, can be performed using established endovascular skills and technology coupled with traditional open aortic surgical techniques, with low surgical morbidity and mortality. In the midterm, staged hybrid TAAA repair was associated favorable survival, aortic remodeling, and freedom from reintervention (Tables 3 and 4).

▶ The authors present the largest series of hybrid extent II thoracoabdominal aneurysm (TAAA II) repair in patients with dissection-related aneurysmal degeneration. The staged approach involves a proximal thoracic stent graft (TEVAR) to convert an extent I or II TAAA to an extent III, IV, or V TAAA thus eliminating the need for surgical dissection and clamping around the aortic arch, followed by a staged open distal TAAA repair via a thoraco-retroperitoneal exposure. The goal of this approach is to distribute ischemia to the spinal cord over time, which allows potential collateral vessel development. This is a retrospective review of 19 cases of dissection related TAAA requiring repair (9 type A, 10 type B). The patients underwent a staged hybrid repair for Crawford extent I (n = 1) or extent II (n = 18) TAAA from 2007 to 2014. TEVAR was performed from the left subclavian artery (including coverage if needed) to just above the level of the celiac artery. The authors are proponents of routine revascularization of the left subclavian artery before coverage and routine spinal drainage at the time of TEVAR. The median time interval between the 2 stages was 18 weeks. During the second stage, the distal body and visceral artery perfusion was used

TABLE 3.—Surgical Outcomes of Staged Hybrid Repair of Extensive Thoracoabdominal Aortic Aneurysm (*TAAA*) Secondary to Aortic Dissections (N = 19)

Outcome	No. (%)
Thoracic stent graft (stage 1)	
Death	0 (0)
Stroke	0 (0)
Paraplegia	0 (0)
Acute renal failure	1 (5)
Reintervention for endoleak	
Type Ia endoleak	1 (5)
Type Ib endoleak	1 (5)
Type II endoleak	1 (5)
Atrial fibrillation (new onset)	1 (5)
Pleural effusion	3 (16)
Brachial artery pseudoaneurysm	1 (5)
Open distal TAAA repair (stage 2)	
Death	0 (0)
Stroke	0 (0)
Paraplegia (delayed)[a]	1 (5)
Acute renal failure	5 (26)
PEA arrest (full recovery)	1 (5)
Retrograde dissection (delayed)	1 (5)

PEA, Pulseless electrical activity.
[a]The patient developed paraplegia after discharge during hemodialysis (HD).
Reprinted from Jain A, Flohr TF, Johnston WF, et al. Staged hybrid repair of extensive thoracoabdominal aortic aneurysms secondary to chronic aortic dissection. *J Vasc Surg*. 2016;63:62-69, with permission from the Society for Vascular Surgery.

TABLE 4.—Midterm Outcome (Median, 3 Years)

Outcome	No. (%)
Death	0 (0)
Stroke	0 (0)
Paralysis	1 (5)
Chronic renal failure	0 (0)
Aortic reintervention	
Endoleak	0 (0)
Thoracoabdominal aorta	1 (5)
Ascending aorta	2 (10)
Aortic remodeling	
Complete false lumen thrombosis	19 (100)
Change in maximum false lumen diameter, %	−71.9 ± 36.7

Data are presented as n (%) except where otherwise stated.
Reprinted from Jain A, Flohr TF, Johnston WF, et al. Staged hybrid repair of extensive thoracoabdominal aortic aneurysms secondary to chronic aortic dissection. *J Vasc Surg*. 2016;63:62-69, with permission from the Society for Vascular Surgery.

in all by using left heart bypass (n = 4) or partial cardiopulmonary bypass (n = 15). Table 3 summarizes the early outcomes of the stage approach. Short-term delayed paraplegia secondary to spinal cord ischemia was 5% (1 of 19). The median follow-up was 3.0 years (range, 6 months–6.2 years) and the outcomes are summarized in Table 4. Results of this study suggest that staged hybrid repair can be safely performed with acceptable results. Longer term data remain to be assessed and compared with the results of open repair.[1]

S. Shalhub, MD, MPH, FACS

Reference

1. Johnston WF, Upchurch GR Jr, Tracci MC, Cherry KJ, Ailawadi G, Kern JA. Staged hybrid approach using proximal thoracic endovascular aneurysm repair and distal open repair for the treatment of extensive thoracoabdominal aortic aneurysms. *J Vasc Surg*.. 2012;56:1495-1502.

Results of aberrant right subclavian artery aneurysm repair

Verzini F, for the Italian AARSA Collaborative Group (Univ of Perugia, Italy; et al)
J Vasc Surg 62:343-350, 2015

Objective.—The objective of this multicenter registry was to review current treatments and late results of repair of aneurysm of aberrant right subclavian artery (AARSA).

Methods.—All consecutive AARSA repairs from 2006 to 2013 in seven centers were reviewed. End points were 30-day and late mortality, reintervention rate, and AARSA-related death.

Results.—Twenty-one AARSA repairs were included (57% men; mean age, 67 years); 3 ruptures (14%) required emergent treatment; 12 (57%) were symptomatic for dysphagia (33%), dysphonia (24%), or pain (19%). Eight cases (38%) presented with thoracic aortic aneurysm, two with intramural hematoma, and one with acute type B aortic dissection. Mean AARSA diameter was 4.2 cm; a single bicarotid common trunk was present in 38% of cases. The majority of patients underwent hybrid intervention (n = 15; 71%) consisting of single (n = 2) or bilateral (n = 12) subclavian to carotid transposition or bypass or ascending aorta to subclavian bypass (n = 1) plus thoracic endovascular aortic repair (TEVAR); 19% of cases underwent open repair and 9% simple TEVAR with AARSA overstenting. Perioperative death occurred in two patients (9%): in one case after TEVAR in ruptured AARSA, requiring secondary sternotomy and aortic banding; and in an elective case due to multiorgan failure after a hybrid procedure. Median follow-up was 30 (interquartile range, 15-46) months. The Kaplan-Meier estimate of survival at 36 months was 90% (standard error, 0.64). Late AARSA-related death in one case was due to AARSA-esophageal fistula presenting with continuing backflow from distal AARSA and previous TEVAR. At computed tomography controls, one type I endoleak and one type II endoleak were detected; the latter required reintervention by aneurysm wrapping and ligature of collaterals. AARSA-related death was more frequent after TEVAR, a procedure reserved for ruptures, compared with elective open or hybrid repair.

Conclusions.—Hybrid repair is the preferred therapeutic option for patients presenting with AARSA. Midterm results show high rates of clinical success with low risk of reintervention. Simple endografting presents high risk of related death; these findings underline the importance of achieving complete sealing to avoid treatment failures (Figs 3 and 4).

▶ An aberrant right subclavian artery (AARSA) is a commonly seen congenital variant of the aortic arch and frequently develops aneurysmal degeneration at its

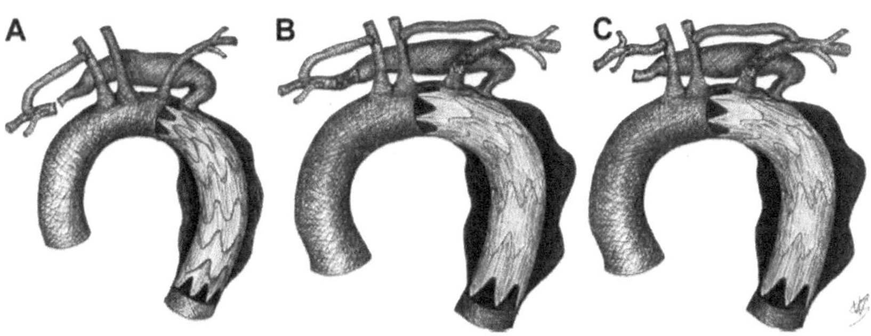

FIGURE 3.—Hybrid solutions for aneurysm of aberrant right subclavian artery (AARSA) repair. Details are listed in Table I. *Editor's Note*: Please refer to original journal article for full references. (Reprinted from Verzini F, for the Italian AARSA Collaborative Group. Results of aberrant right subclavian artery aneurysm repair. *J Vasc Surg*. 2015;62:343-350, with permission from the Society for Vascular Surgery.)

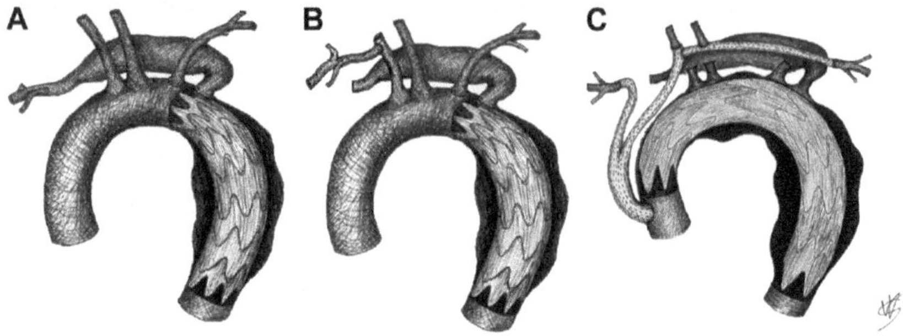

FIGURE 4.—Other hybrid solutions for aneurysm of aberrant right subclavian artery (AARSA) repair. Details are listed in Table I. *Editor's Note*: Please refer to original journal article for full references. (Reprinted from Verzini F, for the Italian AARSA Collaborative Group. Results of aberrant right subclavian artery aneurysm repair. *J Vasc Surg*. 2015;62:343-350, with permission from the Society for Vascular Surgery.)

origin off the descending thoracic aorta, known as a Kommerell diverticulum. It is an interesting anomaly because it can cause dysphagia lusoria, dysphonia, or substernal chest pain as it crosses left to right within the chest. Despite a well-described variant, there remains no standardized surgical treatment for these patients, especially for those patients with concomitant aortic aneurysm. Our Italian colleagues developed a multicenter registry for aneurysmal AARSA to review current treatments and late results of repair. Before the option of endovascular treatment, AARSA were treated with open repair, ordinarily replacement of aortic aneurysm, major branch vessel bypass or reimplantation, and ligation at the origin of the aberrant artery. However, over the 10 years reviewed here, a hybrid approach was the most routinely used contemporary technique. Multiple options exist for hybrid repair as described by Figs 3 and 4. More proximal coverage may be required to obtain adequate seal for the thoracic aortic aneurysm but can be accommodated by multivessel debranching. In this study, 2 patients died (1 hybrid and 1 simple thoracic endovascular aortic repair), comprising only 9% of the entire group. There were 3 endoleaks. The hybrid method was not employed in emergent cases to avoid prolonged operative times. In these instances, the authors admit that a simple TEVAR for rupture may provide reprieve but maintain that this should then be followed by a definitive repair to prevent continued perfusion of the AARSA. What is clear after this multicenter review is that repair of AARSA, whether open or hybrid, can be achieved with low mortality and long-term durability.

K. C. Orion, MD

7 Leg Ischemia

Impact of Hospital Volume on Outcomes of Lower Extremity Endovascular Interventions (Insights from the Nationwide Inpatient Sample [2006 to 2011])

Arora S, Panaich SS, Patel N, et al (Mt. Sinai St. Luke's Roosevelt Hosp Ctr, NY; Detroit Med Ctr, MI; Saint Peter's Univ Hosp, New Brunswick, NJ; et al)

Am J Cardiol 116:791-800, 2015

Our primary objective was to study postprocedural outcomes and hospitalization costs after peripheral endovascular interventions and the multivariate predictors affecting the outcomes with emphasis on hospital volume. The study cohort was derived from Healthcare Cost and Utilization Project Nationwide Inpatient Sample database (2006 to 2011). Peripheral endovascular interventions were identified using appropriate International Classification of Diseases, Ninth Revision diagnostic and procedural codes. Annual institutional volumes were calculated using unique identification numbers and then divided into quartiles. Two-level hierarchical multivariate mixed models were created. The primary outcome was inhospital mortality; secondary outcome was a composite of inhospital mortality and postprocedural complications. Amputation rates and hospitalization costs were also assessed. Multivariate analysis (odds ratio, 95% confidence interval, p value) revealed age (1.46, 1.37 to 1.55, $p < 0.001$), female gender (1.28, 1.12 to 1.46, $p < 0.001$), baseline co-morbidity status as depicted by a greater Charlson co-morbidity index score (≥2: 4.32, 3.45 to 5.40, $p < 0.001$), emergent or urgent admissions(2.48, 2.14 to 2.88, $p < 0.001$), and weekend admissions (1.53, 1.26 to 1.86, $p < 0.001$) to be significant predictors of primary outcome. An increasing hospital volume quartile was independently predictive of improved primary (0.65, 0.52 to 0.82, $p < 0.001$ for the fourth quartile) and secondary (0.85, 0.73 to 0.97, 0.02 for the fourth quartile) outcomes and lower amputation rates (0.52, 0.45 to 0.61, $p < 0.001$). A significant reduction hospitalization costs ($−3,889, −5,318 to −2,459, $p < 0.001$) was also seen in high volume centers. In conclusion, a greater hospital procedural volume is associated with superior outcomes after peripheral

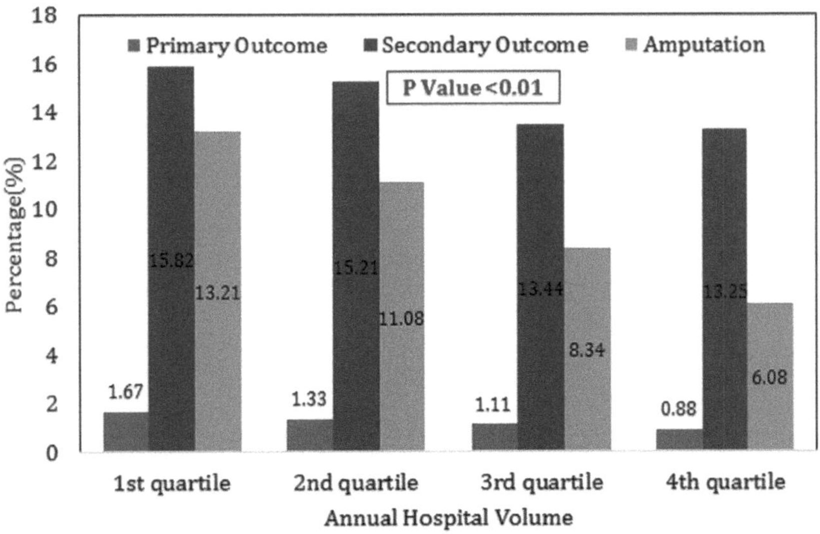

FIGURE 2.—Effect of annual hospital volume on different outcomes. (Reprinted from Arora S, Panaich SS, Patel N, et al. Impact of hospital volume on outcomes of lower extremity endovascular interventions (insights from the nationwide inpatient sample [2006 to 2011]). *Am J Cardiol.* 2015;116:791-800, with permission from Elsevier.)

endovascular interventions in terms of inhospital mortality, complications, and hospitalization costs (Fig 2).

▶ In-hospital mortality, the primary outcome of the study, was surprisingly common in this analysis of endovascular lower extremity procedures from the Nationwide Inpatient Sample (NIS). Most conversations between patients and providers are centered on symptomatic improvement and limb salvage as outcomes, and these results serve as a reminder that mortality is common among inpatients undergoing lower extremity revascularization. When interpreting the results, it is important to acknowledge that all patients in this study were admitted to the hospital and therefore might be expected to differ in a number of ways from patients undergoing outpatient endovascular procedures. Inpatients treated with endovascular procedures might be anticipated to have a increased rate of admission from the emergency department, decreased access to outpatient specialty care, greater prevalence of comorbid conditions, and a more severe disease (including ulcers or gangrene with infection) deemed unsafe or unsuitable for outpatient management. Interfacility transfer status was not evaluated as part of this analysis; because of selection bias, patients undergoing a posttransfer revascularization likely would be more complex, higher acuity, and more likely to have their procedure performed at a high-volume center.

High-volume hospitals may be distinguished by several attributes other than the practitioners performing the revascularization procedures. The lower mortality observed at high-volume centers may be partly attributable to a variety of factors outside the scope of this analysis (and the NIS data set), including multispecialty teams, intensive care and nursing units experienced with caring for patients with peripheral artery disease, and more organized resources dedicated to post-revascularization physical therapy and discharge planning. The authors suggest that the results of this study justify consideration of hospital volume as a competency metric, but several caveats warrant careful consideration before taking that step based on this analysis alone. It is important to remember that this analysis does not include any anatomic data or account for disease severity. It is therefore possible that higher volume centers may have used less selective criteria for performing inpatient endovascular interventions, particularly if the providers lack access to dedicated outpatient interventional suites (a common distinguishing factor between community practice and academic centers). Provider density might also be greater in areas where high-volume centers are located, resulting in less selective criteria for intervention in general. When analyzed based on procedure volume, the lowest complication rate was nearly 14% (Fig 2), suggesting that significant room for outcome improvement remains even at high-volume centers.

M. Corriere, MD, MS

Multidisciplinary care improves amputation-free survival in patients with chronic critical limb ischemia

Chung J, Modrall JG, Ahn C, et al (The Univ of Texas Southwestern Med Ctr, Dallas)

J Vasc Surg 61:162-169, 2015

Background.—This study was conducted to quantify the effect of multidisciplinary care (MDC) on amputation-free survival (AFS) and wound healing within a chronic critical limb ischemia (CLI) population.

Methods.—We performed a retrospective, single-center cohort study of consecutive CLI patients presenting to the Vascular Surgery Service. Patients who received initial and follow-up wound care from the MDC were compared with patients who received standard wound care (SWC). The MDC team consisted of vascular, plastic, and podiatric surgeons who jointly managed wound care and directed any other consults or services as deemed necessary. SWC consisted of an inconsistent mix of providers without a defined manager, including nurses, wound care midlevel providers, general surgeons, internists, or the patients themselves. The referring physician determined the allocation of patients. The primary outcome variable was AFS, with a secondary evaluation of wound healing. The effects of baseline demographics, comorbid medical conditions, laboratory values, ischemic lesion severity and location, Rutherford classification, and participation in MDC were assessed. Significant univariate predictors ($P < .10$) of AFS were entered into a multivariate Cox regression model and assessed at an $\alpha = .05$.

Results.—Between August 2010 and June 2012, 146 CLI patients (91 male [63%]) were evaluated by the Vascular Surgery Service and were followed up for a median of 539 days (interquartile range 314-679 days). Ischemic tissue loss was present in 85 patients (38 at Rutherford category 5, and 47 at Rutherford category 6). Within this cohort, 51 (60%) had MDC, and 34 (40%) had SWC. Fifty-eight patients (68%) underwent revascularization (open in 17, endovascular in 35, and hybrid in 6), 14 (8%) were managed with primary major amputation, and 13 (15%) declined revascularization. AFS was superior for patients in the MDC arm vs the SWC arm (593.3 ± 53.5 days vs 281.0 ± 38.2 days; log-rank, $P = .02$). Wound-healing times favored the MDC arm over the SWC arm (444.5 ± 33.2 days vs 625.2 ± 126.5 days), although this was not statistically significant (log-rank, $P = .74$). Multivariate modelling revealed that independent predictors of major amputation or death, or both, were nonrevascularized patients (hazard ratio [HR], 3.76; 95% confidence interval [CI], 1.78-8.02; χ^2, $P < .01$), treatment by SWC (HR, 2.664; 95% CI, 1.23-5.77; χ^2, $P = .012$), and baseline nonambulatory status (HR, 1.89; 95% CI, 1.17-2.85; χ^2, $P < .01$).

Conclusions.—MDC pathways for the management of a population of CLI patients improved AFS by greater than twofold and should be the standard of care for the CLI population. Baseline nonambulatory status and unrevascularized patients also predict worse AFS. Wound healing remains prolonged regardless of preoperative or postoperative wound care. Future study is required to evaluate the costs and functional outcomes for MDC in the management of CLI (Fig 1).

▶ Critical limb ischemia (CLI) is a huge challenge for quality improvement initiatives targeting readmission and unplanned reoperation as outcomes. As pointed out by Chung and colleagues, patients with CLI are resource-intensive, requiring input and receiving care from a variety of providers (including physicians, wound nurses, and therapists) and specialty backgrounds. When the approach to treatment decisions becomes fragmented and communication is poor (or absent), less efficient care often negatively affects clinical outcomes, cost, and patient satisfaction. The standard approach to CLI care used as the control group in this analysis is actually worse than the situation described by the idiom "too many cooks in the kitchen spoil the broth"; indeed, it might be more accurately described as too many cooks working in separate kitchens.

The multidisciplinary care approach is a promising concept with potential to streamline CLI care but requires dedication from all participating specialists and, ideally, a shared physical space where patients can be seen by the appropriate mix of specialists with direct access to the necessary diagnostic testing and treatment resources. The team in this analysis consisted of plastic, podiatric, and vascular surgeons and was defined from a vascular surgery perspective (patients receiving multidisciplinary care either presented to the vascular clinic or were seen as inpatient consults by vascular surgeons). The concept could be expanded, however, to include a much larger framework of physician and non-physician providers from both surgical and medical backgrounds (including primary care, vascular medicine, endocrinology, orthopedics, infectious diseases,

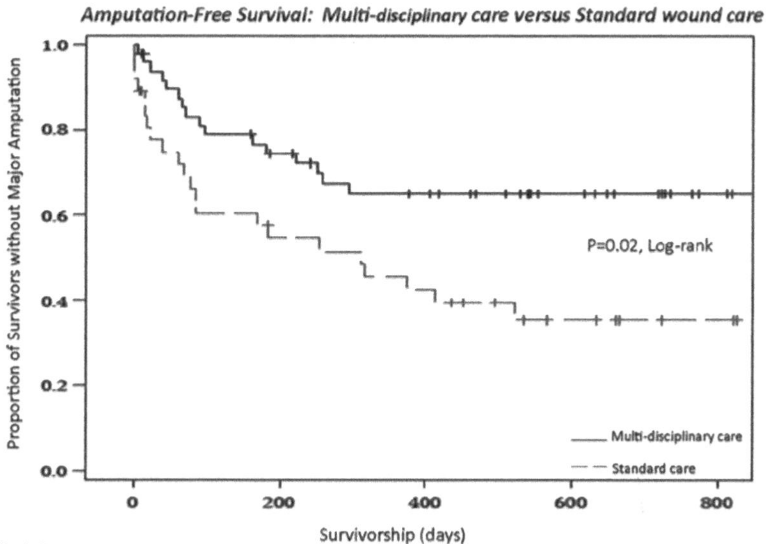

	0	200	400	600	800
Multi-disciplinary					
N	51	34	26	14	4
N Major amp/death	0	17	8	12	10
% SE	0	6	7	7	7
Standard					
N	34	18	14	7	3
N Major amp/death	0	16	4	7	4
% SE	0	8	8	8	8

FIGURE 1.—Kaplan-Meier analysis compares patients presenting with ischemic tissue loss and treated with multidisciplinary care (MDC) vs standard wound care (SWC). The standard error (SE) exceeds 10% at 848 days. (Reprinted from Chung J, Modrall JG, Ahn C, et al. Multidisciplinary care improves amputation-free survival in patients with chronic critical limb ischemia. *J Vasc Surg*. 2015;61:162-169, with permission from the Society for Vascular Surgery.)

cardiology, rehabilitation, neurology, etc). Although colocating all of these specialists into a shared clinical space would be difficult (if not impossible) from a logistical perspective, it is nonetheless helpful for the core provider group seeing most patients to establish working relationships with individuals from these disciplines who may not be physically present during the visit but contribute to a larger organized framework designed to improve CLI treatment efficiency and outcomes.

Regardless of which specialists comprise the ideal multidisciplinary team, the superior amputation-free survival among patients receiving multidisciplinary care in this analysis (Figure) provides strong support for the team-based approach. Chung et al observed a 2-fold higher rate of conversion to major amputation in the standard care group and in their discussion describe the considerable contributions that podiatric surgeons bring to CLI care, including experience with tendon lengthening and offloading procedures that are often unavailable within less comprehensive models. For providers seeking to establish a multidisciplinary care team at their center, these results will hopefully provide evidence to justify resources (the most important of which are space and personnel) necessary for these programs to succeed. Future guidance from model programs and/or medical societies regarding implementation, management, and organization of multispecialty models would likely be welcomed by both providers and health systems interested in advancing the quality of CLI care.

M. Corriere, MD, MS

Anatomic runoff score predicts cardiovascular outcomes in patients with lower extremity peripheral artery disease undergoing revascularization

Jones WS, Patel MR, Tsai TT, et al (Duke Univ Medi Ctr, Durham, NC; Kaiser Permanente Colorado, Denver; et al)

Am Heart J 170:400-408.e1, 2015

Background.—Although the presence, extent, and severity of obstruction in patients with lower extremity peripheral artery disease (LE PAD) affect their functional status, quality of life, and treatment, it is not known if these factors are associated with future cardiovascular events. We empirically created an anatomic runoff score (ARS) to approximate the burden of LE PAD and determined its association with clinical outcomes.

Methods.—We evaluated all patients with LE PAD and bilateral angiography undergoing revascularization in a community-based clinical study. Primary clinical outcomes of interest were (1) a composite of all-cause death, myocardial infarction (MI), and stroke and (2) amputation-free survival. Cox proportional hazards models were created to identify predictors of clinical outcomes.

Results.—We evaluated 908 patients undergoing angiography, and a total of 260 (28.0%) patients reached the composite end point (45 MI, 63 stroke, and 152 death) during the study period. Anatomic runoff score ranged from 0 to 15 (mean 4.7; SD 2.5) with higher scores indicating a higher burden of disease, and an optimal cutpoint analysis classified patients into low ARS (<5) and high ARS (≥5). The unadjusted rates of the primary composite end point and amputation-free survival were nearly 2-fold higher in patients with a high ARS when compared with patients with a low ARS. The most significant predictors of the composite end point (death/MI/stroke) were age (δ 10 years; hazard ratio [HR] 1.53; CI 1.32-1.78; $P < .001$), diabetes mellitus (HR 1.65; CI 1.26-2.18; $P < .001$), glomerular filtration rate <30 (HR 2.23; CI 1.44-3.44; $P < .001$), statin use (HR 0.66; CI 0.48-0.88; $P < .001$), and ARS (δ 2 points; HR 1.21; CI 1.08-1.35; $P < .001$).

Conclusions.—After adjustment for clinical factors, the LE PAD ARS was an independent predictor of future cardiovascular morbidity and mortality in a broadly representative patient population undergoing revascularization for symptomatic PAD. A clinically useful anatomic scoring system, if validated, may assist clinicians in risk stratification during the course of clinical decision making.

▶ All vascular specialists recognize that lower extremity peripheral artery disease (PAD) is often a marker for systemic disease. These patients are at increased risk for major cardiovascular events, major adverse limb events, and mortality. Although medical and interventional therapies continue to advance, patient selection for revascularization remains a priority for clinical investigation. There are multiple vascular scoring systems previously published that associate lower extremity peripheral vascular disease burden and anatomy with procedural success, patient symptom improvement, and limb salvage outcomes. These authors have created an anatomic lower extremity vascular runoff score based on preintervention imaging that serves as a prognostic tool for patient selection and risk stratification; it is similar to the Duke CAD index that associates coronary disease burden and treatment with cardiovascular mortality.[1]

This comprehensive observational analysis retrospectively evaluated the medical records and documentation of diagnostic angiography, CT-angiography or magnetic resonance angiography of 908 patients with complete bilateral imaging undergoing lower extremity revascularization in a community-based clinical setting. A 6-member multidisciplinary team reviewed data, but not direct imaging, to calculate a runoff score of 0 to 18 based on the degree of iliofemoral and popliteal arterial stenosis and tibial runoff. Sophisticated statistical modeling that considered comorbidities, intervention type (ie, open vs endovascular) and indication for procedure (ie, claudication vs critical limb ischemia) determined a score ≥5 to be an independent predictor of future cardiovascular morbidity and mortality (including all-cause mortality, myocardial infarction [MI], and stroke). Not surprisingly, those patients with an anatomic runoff score (ARS) ≥5 were more likely to have a history of prior MI, diabetes mellitus (DM), hypertension, and renal disease. In addition to ARS, after adjustment, the most significant predictors of the composite end point of all-cause mortality, MI, and stroke were age, DM, glomerular filtration rate < 30, and statin use.

On the surface, this scoring system represents a prognostic tool to aid with patient selection and risk stratification when considering revascularization. Despite certain limitations to the study design, additional value lies within the ability of a PAD "score" to risk adjust patients for future observational studies or stratify patients in the design of future randomized clinical trials. Going forward, a score that considers standardized anatomic imaging, more granular risk factor definition (such as hemoglobin A1C), specific medical therapies, and cohort validation across community- and academic-based practices will prove invaluable in the progress of PAD research and treatment.

D. Coleman, MD

Reference

1. Mark DB, Nelson CL, Califf RM, et al. Continuing evolution of therapy for coronary artery disease. Initial results from the era of coronary angioplasty. *Circulation.* 1994;89:2015-2025.

Cilostazol and freedom from amputation after lower extremity revascularization

Neel JD, Kruse RL, Dombrovskiy VY, et al (Univ of Missouri School of Medicine, Columbia; Rutgers-Robert Wood Johnson Med School, New Brunswick, NJ)

J Vasc Surg 61:960-964, 2015

Objective.—Cilostazol, an antiplatelet agent with vasodilating properties, has not been well evaluated in conjunction lower extremity revascularization (LER). We evaluated the association between cilostazol and limb salvage after endovascular or open surgery for LER.

Methods.—Patients aged ≥65 years undergoing LER were identified from 2007 to 2008 Medicare Provider Analysis and Review and Carrier files using International Classification of Diseases-9 Edition-Clinical Modification and Current Procedural Terminology-4 codes. Covariates included demographics, comorbidities, and disease severity. Use of cilostazol was identified using National Drug Codes and Part D files. Outcomes were compared using χ^2 and Kaplan-Meier analyses and Cox regression.

Results.—We identified 22,954 patients undergoing LER: 8128 (35.4%) with claudication, 3056 (13.3%) with rest pain, and 11,770 (51.3%) with ulceration/gangrene. Among them, 1999 patients (8.7%) used cilostazol before LER. More patients received endovascular (14,353) than open (8601) procedures. Cilostazol users had fewer amputations than nonusers at 30 days (7.8% vs 13.4%), 90 days (10.7% vs 18.0%), and 1 year (14.8% vs 24.0%; $P < .0001$ for all). Cox proportional hazards regression with adjustment for age, gender, race, comorbidities, type of procedure, and atherosclerosis severity showed noncilostazol users were more likely to undergo amputation ≤1 year after surgery (hazard ratio [HR], 1.15; 95% confidence interval [CI], 1.02-1.29; $P = .02$). Subgroup analyses using Cox proportional hazards models adjusted for age, gender, and comorbidities demonstrated significantly improved 1-year amputation-free survival for patients with renal failure (HR, 1.61; 95% CI, 1.28-2.02; $P < .001$) and diabetes (HR, 1.61; 95% CI, 1.36-1.92; $P < .001$) who were taking cilostazol.

Conclusions.—In patients undergoing LER, cilostazol use was associated with improved 1-year freedom from amputation. Patients with renal failure and diabetes also demonstrated a significant benefit from

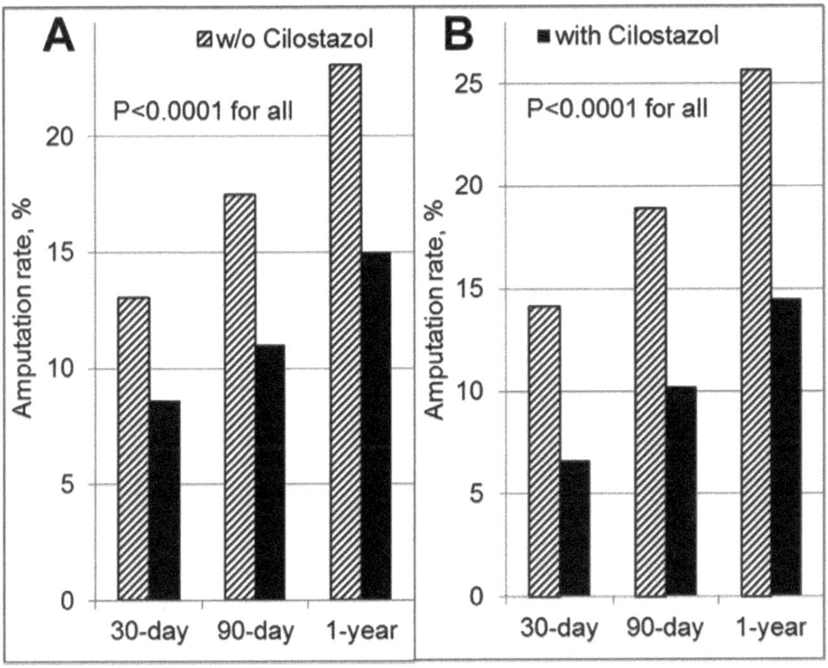

FIGURE 1.—Crude amputation rates after lower extremity revascularization (LER), with and without cilostazol, in patients undergoing (**A**) endovascular repair and (**B**) open surgery. (Reprinted from Neel JD, Kruse RL, Dombrovskiy VY, et al. Cilostazol and freedom from amputation after lower extremity revascularization. *J Vasc Surg*. 2015;61:960-964, with permission from the Society for Vascular Surgery.)

taking cilostazol. Further studies are needed to evaluate the benefits of cilostazol after LER (Fig 1).

▶ This analysis of Medicare beneficiaries includes patients with critical limb ischemia (CLI) as well as patients with claudication. Hospitalization for claudication is uncommon for anything other than open surgical revascularization. In this analysis of Medicare beneficiaries based on administrative data, it is therefore probable that at least some of the inpatient admissions identified involved atypical circumstances, unconventional management, or were not primarily related to the claudication diagnosis. The outcomes described for procedures performed for claudication in this analysis therefore may not be generalizable to outpatient procedures (which make up the majority of revascularizations for claudication and an expanding proportion of CLI procedures as well).

Cilostazol is US Food and Drug Administration—approved for symptomatic management of claudication and is considered a first-line therapy for this diagnosis. Patients with claudication therefore would be expected to have the highest rate of cilostazol utilization overall, as well as prerevascularization (assuming guideline-based therapy was used for the majority of patients). Given these considerations plus the major differences between claudication and CLI in terms of both amputation risk and survival, it is appropriate that amputation-free survival outcomes from this study were presented stratified by diagnosis. Although the authors observed a difference in crude amputation rates following both endovascular and surgical procedures based on cilostazol use (Fig 1), cilostazol was not associated with amputation risk in subgroup analyses based on indication, suggesting that the observed overall effect (which was statistically significant) may be at least partially attributable to differences in utilization based on disease severity. Given the size of the study cohort (more than 7000 patients with claudication , more than 2600 patients with rest pain, and more than 11 000 with tissue loss or gangrene as their indication), absence of a difference between groups based on indication is unlikely attributable to a type II error due to inadequate power. Subgroup analyses did suggest, however, that cilostazol may have specific benefits for patients with renal failure or diabetes (both of which are associated with unfavorable amputation-free survival) as well as those undergoing endovascular procedures. It seems reasonable to consider cilostazol therapy for patients in these subgroups regardless of the indication, given the high prevalence of infrapopliteal disease and inferior outcomes associated with these diagnoses.

When evaluating research based on administrative data, it is always important to consider not only the variables that were included but also potentially important ones that were absent. In this analysis, smoking comes to mind as a variable that has significant impact on PAD severity as well as revascularization outcomes, yet it was not accounted for. Likewise, it is important to point out that a cilostazol prescription is not always succeeded by long-term adherence. Intolerance is common with this medication, and the analysis did not account for which patients actually took the drug for an extended period of time; it is therefore possible that the effect on amputation-free survival was diminished because of nonadherence in some patients.

M. Corriere, MD, MS

Effect of Repetitive Intra-Arterial Infusion of Bone Marrow Mononuclear Cells in Patients With No-Option Limb Ischemia: The Randomized, Double-Blind, Placebo-Controlled Rejuvenating Endothelial Progenitor Cells via Transcutaneous Intra-arterial Supplementation (JUVENTAS) Trial

Teraa M, Sprengers RW, Schutgens REG, et al (Univ Med Ctr Utrecht, The Netherlands)

Circulation 131:851-860, 2015

Background.—Patients with severe limb ischemia may not be eligible for conventional therapeutic interventions. Pioneering clinical trials suggest that bone marrow–derived cell therapy enhances neovascularization, improves tissue perfusion, and prevents amputation. The objective of this trial was to determine whether repetitive intra-arterial infusion of bone marrow mononuclear cells (BMMNCs) in patients with severe, nonrevascularizable limb ischemia can prevent major amputation.

Methods and Results.—The Rejuvenating Endothelial Progenitor Cells via Transcutaneous Intra-arterial Supplementation (JUVENTAS) trial is a randomized, double-blind, placebo-controlled clinical trial in 160 patients with severe, nonrevascularizable limb ischemia. Patients were randomly assigned to repetitive (3 times; 3-week interval) intraarterial infusion of BMMNC or placebo. No significant differences were observed for the primary outcome, ie, major amputation at 6 months, with major amputation rates of 19% in the BMMNC versus 13% in the placebo group (relative risk, 1.46; 95% confidence interval, 0.62–3.42). The safety outcome (all-cause mortality, occurrence of malignancy, or hospitalization due to infection) was not significantly different between the groups (relative risk, 1.46; 95% confidence interval, 0.63–3.38), neither was all-cause mortality at 6 months with 5% versus 6% (relative risk, 0.78; 95% confidence interval, 0.22–2.80). Secondary outcomes quality of life, rest pain, ankle-brachial index, and transcutaneous oxygen pressure improved during follow-up, but there were no significant differences between the groups.

Conclusions.—Repetitive intra-arterial infusion of autologous BMMNCs into the common femoral artery did not reduce major amputation rates in patients with severe, nonrevascularizable limb ischemia in comparison with placebo. The general improvement in secondary outcomes during follow-up in both the BMMNC and the placebo group, as well, underlines the essential role for placebo-controlled design of future trials.

Clinical Trial Registration.—URL: http://www.clinicaltrials.gov. Unique identifier: NCT00371371 (Table 1).

▶ Some patients with critical limb ischemia (CLI) fall into the "no options" category at the time of initial presentation due to advanced tissue loss or lack of suitable runoff vessels to target, whereas others arrive there at the end of multiple revascularization procedures that ultimately failed. Approximately half of the randomized, double-blind, placebo-controlled, rejuvenating endothelial progenitor cells via transcutaneous intra-arterial supplementation (JUVENTAS) trial participants had previously undergone lower extremity bypass and more than 60% had been treated with lower extremity angioplasty, suggesting that many of them fell into the latter category (Table 1). Fifteen participants did not complete the scheduled bone marrow cell infusions before death or amputation, demonstrating that some participants had especially severe disease that might have progressed beyond salvage at the time of randomization.

This article also included a meta-analysis of preceding randomized controlled trials of bone marrow–derived cellular therapy for patients with CLI, which identified key limitations of previous studies (including statistical power, appropriate controls, and inclusion of clinically relevant endpoints) that informed design of the JUVENTAS trial. The meta-analysis demonstrated a "subtle, but significant" difference in major amputation associated with cellular therapy, but no difference was observed in a subgroup analysis limited to studies that used placebo controls. Bias favoring new treatments for no-options CLI is

TABLE 1.—Demographic and Clinical Characteristics

Characteristic	BMMNC (n = 81)	Placebo (n = 79)
Age, y	69 (57–76)	65 (55–74)
Male sex, n (%)	57 (70)	51 (65)
History of cardiovascular disease, n (%)		
Myocardial infarction or chest pain	33 (41)	33 (42)
TIA or stroke	10 (12)	13 (17)
Dialysis dependent renal disease	2 (3)	3 (4)
Angioplasty contralateral leg	18 (22)	19 (24)
Bypass contralateral leg	11 (14)	16 (20)
Major amputation contralateral leg	5 (6)	6 (8)
Body mass index, kg/m^2	26.2 ± 4.1	26.6 ± 5.1
Smoking, n (%)		
Currently	18 (23)	24 (31)
Past	47 (59)	46 (59)
Diabetes mellitus, n (%)	29 (36)	31 (39)
Nonfasting glucose, mmol/L	5.9 (5.2–7.1)	5.8 (5.1–6.9)
Hypertension, n (%)*	70 (86)	72 (91)
Systolic blood pressure, mm Hg	130 ± 19	132 ± 21
Diastolic blood pressure, mm Hg	73 ± 10	72 ± 10
Hyperlipidemia, n (%)†	74 (91)	71 (90)
Total cholesterol, mmol/L	4.3 ± 1.1	4.2 ± 1.1
LDL-cholesterol, mmol/L	2.4 ± 0.9	2.3 ± 1.0
HDL-cholesterol, mmol/L	1.17 (0.88–1.47)	1.11 (0.84–1.50)
Triglycerides, mmol/L	1.4 (1.0–2.0)	1.5 (0.9–1.9)
Renal insufficiency, n (%)‡	20 (25)	16 (20)
Creatinine, μmol/L	92 (74–122)	86 (74–110)
Cardioprotective drug use, n (%)		
Antiplatelet therapy	55 (68)	57 (72)
Coumadines	32 (39)	29 (37)
Statins	67 (83)	66 (84)
ACE inhibitors	31 (38)	31 (39)
Disease characteristics treated leg		
Right/ left limb treated, n (%)	47/34 (58/42)	45/34 (57/43)
Previous bypass ipsilateral, n (%)	37 (46)	43 (54)
Previous angioplasty ipsilateral, n (%)	48 (59)	47 (60)
Aorta to popliteal artery patent, n (%)	34 (42)	32 (41)
<2 patent crural vessels	67 (83)	70 (89)
Rutherford stage, n (%)		
3	4 (5)	4 (5)
4	26 (32)	25 (32)
5	46 (57)	46 (58)
6	5 (6)	4 (5)
Ulcer area, cm^2	2.0 (1.0–4.5)	1.7 (1.0–4.3)
Pain-free walking distance, m	50 (20–105)	50 (20–130)
Unreliable ankle-brachial index, n (%)§	28 (35)	28 (35)
Baseline ankle-brachial index‖	0.50 (0.36–0.66)	0.50 (0.39–0.77)
Baseline tco_2, mm Hg	35 ± 22	36 ± 22

Use of cardioprotective drugs was defined at time of inclusion. ACE indicates angiotensin-converting enzyme; BMMNC, bone marrow mononuclear cell; HDL, high-density lipoprotein; LDL, low-density lipoprotein; and TIA, transient ischemic attack.

*Hypertension was defined as having systolic blood pressure ≥140 mm Hg, or diastolic blood pressure ≥90 mm Hg, or antihypertensive drug use.

†Hyperlipidemia was defined as having blood levels of total cholesterol ≥6.50 mmol/L, triglycerides ≥2.3 mmol/L, or HDLcholesterol ≤1.0 mmol/L, or lipid-lowering drug use.

‡Renal insufficiency was defined as having creatinine blood levels >120 μmol/L.

§Unreliable ankle-brachial index was defined as incompressible arteries or an ankle-brachial index >0.6 not in proportion to the Fontaine classification.

‖Only patients with a reliable ankle-brachial index were included in the analysis (n = 53 in the BMMNC and n = 51 in the placebo group).

understandable given the unpleasant nature of alternatives to revascularization (which both patients and providers find unpalatable), and these findings demonstrate the importance of appropriate controls when interpreting results. The randomized trial results showed improvement of several outcomes in both the treatment and placebo groups, further supporting this notion. The treatment alternatives available to the "no-options" CLI patient are difficult to accept, and these patients and their providers therefore remain in desperate need of better options and outcomes when revascularization is not possible. Many have been hopeful that cell-based therapy is a potential answer to their dilemma.

M. Corriere, MD, MS

Gender differences following supervised exercise therapy in patients with intermittent claudication

Gommans LNM, Scheltinga MRM, van Sambeek MRHM, et al (Catharina Hosp, Eindhoven, The Netherlands; Maastricht Univ, The Netherlands; et al)
J Vasc Surg 62:681-688, 2015

Objective.—Prevalence of peripheral arterial disease is equal in men and women. However, women seem to suffer more from the burden of disease. Current studies on gender-related outcomes following supervised exercise therapy (SET) for intermittent claudication (IC) yield conflicting results.

Methods.—A follow-up analysis was performed on data from the 2010 Exercise Therapy in Peripheral Arterial Disease (EXITPAD) study, a multicenter randomized controlled trial including IC patients receiving SET or a walking advice. The SET program was supervised by physiotherapists and included interval-based treadmill walking approximating maximal pain combined with activities such as cycling and rowing. Patients usually started with three 30-minute sessions a week. Training frequency was adapted during the following year on the basis of individual needs. The primary outcome was gender differences regarding the change in absolute claudication distance (ACD) after SET. ACD was defined as the number of meters that a patient had covered just before he or she was forced to stop walking because of intolerable pain. Secondary outcomes were gender differences in change of functional walking distance, quality of life, and walking (dis) ability after SET. Walking distances were obtained by standardized treadmill testing according to the Gardner-Skinner protocol. Quality of life was measured by the 36-Item Short Form Health Survey, and walking (dis)ability was determined by the Walking Impairment Questionnaire (WIQ). Measurements were performed at baseline and after 3, 6, 9, and 12 months. Only patients who met the 12-month follow-up measure were included in the analysis.

Results.—A total of 113 men and 56 women were available for analysis. At baseline, groups were similar in terms of clinical characteristics and ACD walking distances (men, 250 meters; women, 270 meters; $P = .45$). ACD improved for both sexes. However, ACD increase was significantly lower for women than for men during the first 3 months of SET (Δ 280 meters for men vs Δ 220 meters for women; $P = .04$). Moreover, absolute walking distance was significantly shorter for women compared with men after 1 year (565 meters vs 660 meters; $P = .032$). Women also reported less on several WIQ subdomains, although total WIQ score was similar (0.69 for men vs 0.61 for women; $P = .592$). No differences in quality of life after SET were observed.

Conclusions.—Women with IC benefit less during the first 3 months of SET and have lower absolute walking distances after 12 months of follow-up compared with men. More research is needed to determine whether gender-based IC treatment strategies are required (Table 1).

▶ Numerous studies have demonstrated gender-based disparities related to peripheral arterial disease presentation and revascularization outcomes, with women having more advanced disease, older age at presentation, higher risk of perioperative adverse events, and inferior patency and amputation-free survival. These disparities are poorly understood and have prompted a call for focused investigation dedicated to understanding their etiology and developing strategies to overcome them.[1] It therefore seems reasonable to explore gender differences in supervised exercise therapy (SET) outcomes among patients with claudication, given that this treatment is one alternative to revascularization for this diagnosis (the other being cilostazol pharmacotherapy, which is often implemented simultaneously with SET but was not included as a treatment intervention in this trial). These investigators observed less benefit from SET in women during the first 3 months (the period of most dramatic walking improvement); women also had a lower absolute claudication distance at 12 months.

The superiority of SET over walking advice (WA) given during clinic, with the latter appropriately referred to as the "go home and walk" plan within this article. The SET protocol in this trial was both robust and comprehensive, including both rowing and cycling in addition to treadmill exercise as well as homework and regular evaluations (Table 1). The advantages of SET over WA may be related in part to the effect that coaching and scheduled expectations impart on adherence to the prescribed regimen. In the era of activity monitoring devices capable of tracking steps, stairs, distance, and speed, it will be interesting to see if incorporating these newer technologies into exercise therapy programs yields results that are more similar to SET or WA. Activity trackers are likely not equivalent to human therapists or exercise partners, and programs based on this technology may be best categorized as monitored but unsupervised. Patients with claudication certainly can use all the support they can get for exercise therapy, particularly in environments like the United States where SET is seldom covered by health care insurance, if it is available at all.

A third treatment group, those managed with WA, was not included in this analysis, although a gender-based evaluation of their outcomes would be of potential interest to providers attempting to choose between treatment options and also might provide additional insight into gender-specific patterns of adherence and patient activation. It would also be interesting to learn the fate of the 26 patients lost to follow-up postrandomization and whether their

TABLE 1.—Example of the Supervised Exercise Therapy (SET) Training Protocol for Intermittent Claudication (IC)

Frequency	Started at three times a week. Frequency is then adapted to the individual need, meaning that patients who perform well and comply with the exercise recommendations can phase down the therapy frequency sooner than other patients.
Duration	20-40 minutes per training session 40%-70% of Vo_2max or Borg RPE score 11-15
Intensity	Interval training: regimen included 2 to 5 minutes of walking (near to ACSM
Content	Claudication Pain Rating Scale score 2-3) and a subsequent 2 to 5 minutes of passive rest. Three to five cycles per training session Aerobic endurance training
Activities	Primarily walking (on a treadmill, with slope of 2 to 8 degrees) Combined with cycling, rowing, stepping, and sports activities in general
Progression	Duration (ie, amount of interval cycles) and intensity (ie, duration of interval cycles) of training are increased as based on individual progression. In general, first intensification takes place when a patient is able to exercise for 20 minutes (eg, five cycles of 4 minutes).
Home work	Moderate exercising for 30 minutes (in bouts of at least 10 minutes): 5 days per week
Evaluation	Continuous evaluation. Treadmill testing at least after 6 and 12 weeks
Termination	Program ends when patient is satisfied and the physiotherapist expects no further progression.

ACSM, American College of Sports Medicine (claudication pain scores range from 1 to 4: respectively, minimal discomfort to unbearable pain); *Borg RPE*, Borg Rating of Perceived Exertion (score ranges from 6 to 20: respectively, no exertion at all to maximal exertion); *Vo_2max*, maximal oxygen consumption (reflects the aerobic physical fitness).

Reprinted from Gommans LNM, Scheltinga MRM, van Sambeek MRHM, et al. Gender differences following supervised exercise therapy in patients with intermittent claudication. *J Vasc Surg*. 2015;62:681-688, with permission from the Society for Vascular Surgery.

dropout reflects rejection of the recommended SET plan. Although the dropout rate was fairly low in this clinical trial in which patients were screened and carefully selected, it might be higher in a clinical practice environment. Patients with claudication will often fail to verbally object to exercise therapy due to social response bias (or desire to avoid disagreeing with the provider's recommendation), even if they are unlikely to accept this treatment. When this happens, patients either return to the next visit having failed the program they did not commit to or instead seek another provider who might offer a different treatment that they will accept. Patient buy-in and acceptance of the treatment plan is particularly critical for SET to succeed because this treatment requires an active and sustained form of adherence (in contrast to pharmacotherapy and revascularization, in which the patient's role is more of a recipient of the treatment vs its delivery agent). Sustained SET is required for a sustained effect, and identifying patients likely to achieve long-term benefits requires understanding their level of engagement and managing contingencies related to their support and expectations.

M. Corriere, MD, MS

Angioplasty of Femoral-Popliteal Arteries With Drug-Coated Balloons: 5-Year Follow-Up of the THUNDER Trial

Tepe G, Schnorr B, Albrecht T, et al (RoMed Clinic Rosenheim, Rosenheim, Germany; Univ Hosp, Berlin, Germany; Vivantes Klinikum Neukölln, Berlin, Germany; et al)

JACC Cardiovasc Interv 8:102-108, 2015

Objectives.—The purpose of this study was to evaluate the 5-year follow-up (FU) data of the THUNDER (Local Taxan With Short Time Contact for Reduction of Restenosis in Distal Arteries).

Background.—The THUNDER trial was the first study to investigate the treatment of femoropopliteal arteries with a paclitaxel-coated balloon (PCB).

Methods.—In 154 patients, femoropopliteal arteries were treated with PCB, with angioplasty with paclitaxel in contrast medium, or no paclitaxel (control). The primary endpoint was 6-month late lumen loss (LLL). Secondary endpoints included freedom from target lesion revascularization (TLR), binary restenosis rate, and amputation. The 5-year FU compares outcomes in patients treated with PCB and control subjects. Additionally, LLL at 6 months and TLR up to 5-year FU were analyzed in terms of sex and lesion length.

Results.—Over the 5-year period, the cumulative number of patients with TLR remained significantly lower in the PCB group (21%) than in the control group (56%, $p = 0.0005$). In the small group of patients with angiographic and duplex sonographic follow-up, PCB was associated with a lower rate of binary restenosis (17% vs. 54%; $p = 0.04$). No signs of aneurysm formation or constrictive fibrosis were detected. Whereas LLL at 6-month FU did not differ between men and women in the PCB group, the TLR rate was lower in men than in women at 5-year FU. A benefit of PCB treatment in terms of LLL and TLR was seen independent of lesion length.

Conclusions.—The reduced TLR rate following PCB treatment was maintained over the 5-year FU period. No signs of drug-related local vessel abnormalities were detected. (Thunder Trial—Local Taxan With Short Time Contact for Reduction of Restenosis in Distal Arteries [THUNDER]; NCT00156624) (Fig 1).

▶ Clinical investigations into the efficacy and indications for drug-coated balloons in the treatment of peripheral artery disease are ongoing as efforts to advance peripheral artery disase (PAD) treatment and limit postinterventional restenosis continue with vigor. These authors provide limited 5-year follow-up on the previously published THUNDER trial (Local Taxan With Short Term Contact for Reduction of Restenosis in Distal Arteries), a pilot multicenter, randomized trial that demonstrated a benefit in late lumen loss and target lumen revascularization with a paclitaxel-coated balloon at 6 to 24 months.[1] The current study follows only 2 of the original 3 treatment arms of the THUNDER trial and concludes the benefit in freedom from target lesion

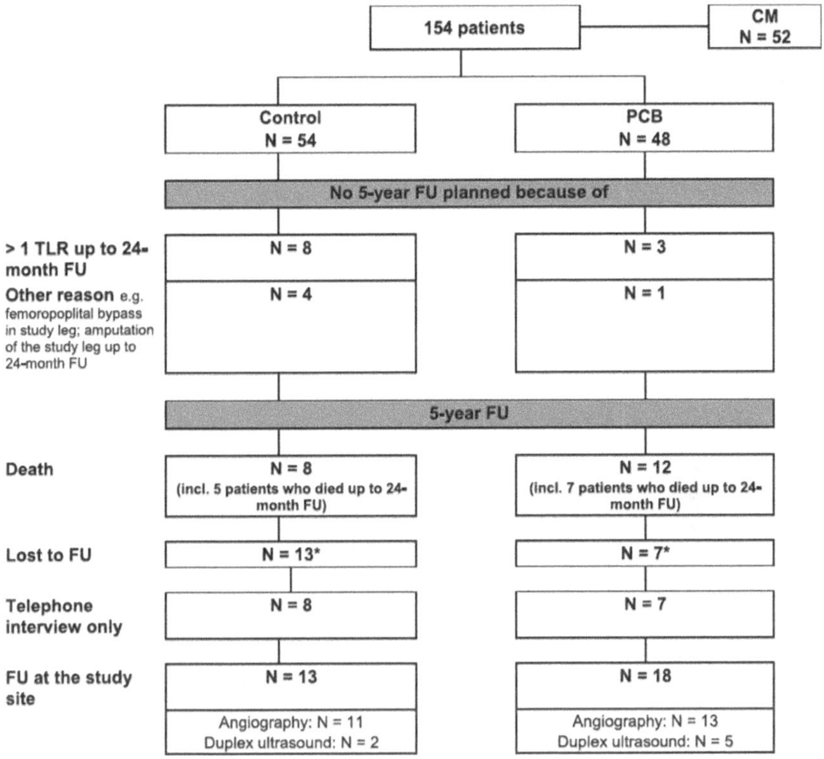

FIGURE 1.—Disposition of Patients at 5-Year FU. Chart presents the original THUNDER (Local Taxan With Short Time Contact for Reduction of Restenosis in Distal Arteries) population and the 5-year follow-up (FU) disposition. Only control patients and those treated with paclitaxel-coated balloon (PCB) were invited to a 5-year FU visit. Reasons for not performing the 5-year FU are listed. *1 study site dropped out (7 patients in the control group and 2 patients in the PCB group). CM = uncoated balloon plus paclitaxel in contrast medium; PCB = paclitaxel-coated balloon; TLR = target lesion revascularization. (Reprinted from Tepe G, Schnorr B, Albrecht T, et al. Angioplasty of femoral-popliteal arteries with drug-coated balloons: 5-year follow-up of the THUNDER trial. *JACC Cardiovasc Interv.* 2015;8:102-108, with permission from The American College of Cardiology Foundation.)

revascularization (TLR) and binary restenosis is maintained over the 5-year period in those patients treated with the paclitaxel-coated balloon (PCB) (Fig 1).

Caution is warranted when drawing conclusions from this study, however. Although the authors support long-term feasibility and safety, the original THUNDER trial was not powered to assess 5-year clinical outcomes. The current study is dramatically limited by sample size. Anatomic data derived by angiogram or duplex ultrasound was available for <40% of patients and was not interpreted by an independent core laboratory; additionally, a fair number of patients were followed with simply a telephone interview. The exclusion of those patients who required more than 1 target lesion revascularization or amputation of the study leg up to 24-month after their enrollment procedure introduced selection bias. Additionally, the THUNDER trial reported on the use of repeat balloon angioplasty and selective stenting for > 30% residual stenosis at the index procedure. Stenting was performed more frequently within the standard angioplasty group (compared with the PCB cohort), and, although relevant, this is not addressed in the current follow-up. Importantly, the majority of patients treated and studied in the THUNDER trial were claudicants (Rutherford class 1-3), and there is no analysis of primary and secondary outcomes that incorporates treatment indication.

These data do fuel support the ongoing investigation of drug-coated balloons to prevent restenosis in the treatment of PAD. This technology certainly has the potential to impact the care of PAD patients. Before drug-coated balloons can be endorsed by clinical guidelines, however, larger clinical trials that address the optimal drug and drug dosage for balloon coating, adjunctive patient medical therapy, and cost-effectiveness and that specifically compare the treatment of claudicants independently with best medical care and supervised exercise are absolutely necessary.

D. Coleman, MD

Reference

1. Tepe G, Zeller T, Albrecht T, et al. Local delivery of paclitaxel to inhibit restenosis during angioplasty of the leg. *N Engl J Med.* 2008;358:689-699.

Drug-Coated Balloon Versus Standard Percutaneous Transluminal Angioplasty for the Treatment of Superficial Femoral and Popliteal Peripheral Artery Disease 12-Month Results From the IN.PACT SFA Randomized Trial

Tepe G, for the IN.PACT SFA Trial Investigators (RodMed Klinikum, Rosenheim, Germany; et al)

Circulation 131:495-502, 2015

Background.—Drug-coated balloons (DCBs) have shown promise in improving the outcomes for patients with peripheral artery disease. We compared a paclitaxel-coated balloon with percutaneous transluminal angioplasty (PTA) for the treatment of symptomatic superficial femoral and popliteal artery disease.

Methods and Results.—The IN.PACT SFA Trial is a prospective, multicenter, single-blinded, randomized trial in which 331 patients with intermittent claudication or ischemic rest pain attributable to superficial femoral and popliteal peripheral artery disease were randomly assigned in a 2:1 ratio to treatment with DCB or PTA. The primary efficacy end point was primary patency, defined as freedom from restenosis or clinically driven target lesion revascularization at 12 months. Baseline characteristics were similar between the 2 groups. Mean lesion length and the percentage of total occlusions for the DCB and PTA arms were 8.94 ± 4.89 and 8.81 ± 5.12 cm ($P = 0.82$) and 25.8% and 19.5% ($P = 0.22$), respectively. DCB resulted in higher primary patency versus PTA (82.2% versus

52.4%; $P < 0.001$). The rate of clinically driven target lesion revascularization was 2.4% in the DCB arm in comparison with 20.6% in the PTA arm ($P < 0.001$). There was a low rate of vessel thrombosis in both arms (1.4% after DCB and 3.7% after PTA [$P = 0.10$]). There were no device- or procedure-related deaths and no major amputations.

Conclusions.—In this prospective, multicenter, randomized trial, DCB was superior to PTA and had a favorable safety profile for the treatment of patients with symptomatic femoropopliteal peripheral artery disease.

Clinical Trial Registration.—URL: http://www.clinicaltrials.gov. Unique Identifiers: NCT01175850 and NCT01566461.

▶ Local delivery of an antiproliferative drug during balloon angioplasty of peripheral arteries is meant to decrease the incidence of restenosis via intimal hyperplasia. Drug-coated balloons (DCBs), ideally, should improve vessel patency after intervention without the need for a permanent metallic stent implant, which may be subject to dynamic stresses in the femoropopliteal region. DCBs do not limit the options for future interventions and are simpler to use than atherectomy devices, which have not shown significant outcome improvement over PTA and stenting.

This study is a single-blinded, randomized, industry-sponsored, clinical trial that evaluated the impact of paclitaxel coating on femoropopliteal vessel patency after PTA of lesions >70% or short occlusions <10 cm. Improvements in primary patency and clinically driven revascularization (target lesions revascularization [TLR]) were noted to be significant at 12 months. As always, the inclusion of TLR in the primary patency end-point definition confuses the readers and may shift the focus from the follow-up duplex findings that were measured in the study but not reported in the article.

Although the DCB results of this trial are promising compared with plain old balloon angioplasty, they do not demonstrate an advantage over other therapeutic strategies in femoropopliteal lesions. A direct comparison between DCB and selective stenting, primary stenting, or atherectomy will be needed to make such a determination. Cost comparisons will also be essential in future studies. This study is an important addition to the literature but still does not answer the question about the efficacy of this strategy.

Y. Duwayri, MD

Drug-eluting balloons for femoropopliteal lesions show better performance in de novo stenosis or occlusion than in restenosis

Herten M, Torsello GB, Schönefeld E, et al (Univ of Münster, Germany)

J Vasc Surg 61:394-399, 2015

Objective.—Although drug-eluting balloons (DEBs) have shown promising results treating de novo (DN) atherosclerotic lesions and appear to have been widely adopted in Europe, their long-term efficacy in the broad spectrum of femoropopliteal restenosis (RE) remains to be proven.

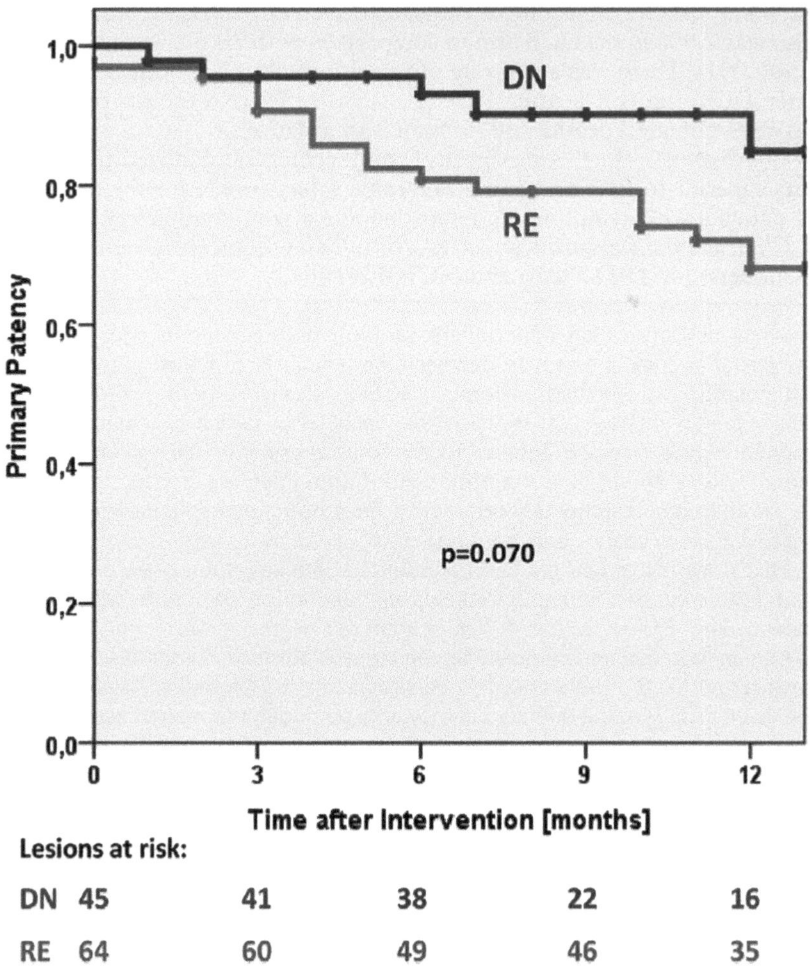

FIGURE 2.—Primary patency (PP) rate by Kaplan-Meier method after drug-eluting balloon (DEB) intervention of restenotic (*RE*) or de novo (*DN*) stenotic femoropopliteal arteries. Standard errors were ≤3.7% for RE and ≤6.4% for DN. (Reprinted from Herten M, Torsello GB, Schönefeld E, et al. Drug-eluting balloons for femoropopliteal lesions show better performance in de novo stenosis or occlusion than in restenosis. *J Vasc Surg*. 2015;61:394-399, with permission from Society for Vascular Surgery.)

The purpose of the study was to assess the efficacy of paclitaxel-DEBs in restenotic (stented and nonstented) vs DN stenotic femoropopliteal arteries.

Methods.—The study prospectively enrolled 100 patients undergoing femoropopliteal endovascular intervention by DEB for RE or DN stenosis. Patients who received additive atherectomy were excluded. The primary end point was the primary patency (PP) rate at 12 months. Secondary end points were sustained clinical improvement and clinically driven target lesion revascularization.

Results.—DEBs were used to treat 105 limbs for intermittent claudication (82 [78%]) or critical limb ischemia (23 [22%]) in 100 patients. Of these, 111 lesions were DN stenosis (46 [41%]) or RE (65 [59%]). The overall PP was 86% at 6 months and 74% at 12 months. PP of DN stenosis was higher at 6 months (93% vs 81%) and was significantly (P =.021) better than RE at 12 months (85% vs 68%). Sustained clinical improvement based on Rutherford classification was significant in both groups (P < .001). Target lesion revascularization was significantly lower in DN stenosis compared with RE at 12 months (15% vs 32%; P =.021).

Conclusions.—DEB angioplasty is an effective therapy for DN femoropopliteal lesions. The results of DEB angioplasty for RE are inferior compared with DN stenosis after 12 months. Nevertheless, results of DEB angioplasty for RE seem comparable with technically more demanding literature-derived strategies (Fig 2, Table 2).

▶ Randomized clinical trials of drug-eluting balloons (DEB) often restrict enrollment to de novo stenosis, which seems appropriate from the perspective of attempting to eliminate restenotic lesions as potentially confounding factor that would be anticipated to have inferior patency outcomes. One would expect restenotic lesions that were previously stented to be more complex than those which were successfully treated without the need for stenting, and this analysis indeed observed that restenosis lesions (of which the majority were previously stented) were indeed longer and more complex (Table 2). Subgroup comparisons between de novo lesions and restenotic lesions that were not previously stented would have permitted more direct comparisons of the restenosis effect independent of stenting or lesion length, but less than one-third of restenotic lesions fell into this category, and it is likely that statistical power would therefore be limited for this additional analysis.

TABLE 2.—Lesion Characteristics and Procedural Detail

Variable[a]	RE	DN	*P* value
Lesions (n = 111)	65 (59)	46 (41)	
In-stent RE	46 (71)		
Superficial femoral artery	49 (75)	29 (64)	.161
Popliteal artery involved	16 (24)	17 (37)	.161
Lesion length, mm	99 ± 76	77 ± 68	.050
Degree of stenosis, %	82 ± 16	81 ± 18	.900
Total occlusion	16 (25)	12 (27)	.935
DEB lesions, No.	1.2 ± 0.6	1.3 ± 0.7	.191
Length of PTX-DEB, mm	129 ± 71	122 ± 78	.289
PTX-DEB diameter, mm	4.9 ± 0.5	4.9 ± 0.6	.553
Inflation pressure, bar	13 ± 7	12 ± 6	.507
Inflation time, seconds	148 ± 80	159 ± 52	.223

DEB, Drug-eluting balloon; *DN*, de novo (the DN stenosis group included only native stenotic vessels); *PXT*, paclitaxel; *RE*, restenosis (the RE group included stented and nonstented restenotic arteries.

[a]Continuous variables are presented as mean ± standard deviation and categoric variables as number (%).

Reprinted from Herten M, Torsello GB, Schönefeld E, et al. Drug-eluting balloons for femoropopliteal lesions show better performance in de novo stenosis or occlusion than in restenosis. *J Vasc Surg*. 2015;61:394-399, with permission from Society for Vascular Surgery.

All other things being equal, the inferior patency associated with after DEB angioplasty of restenotic lesions (referred to by the authors using the regrettably confusing terminology of "primary" patency) observed (Fig 2) would therefore also be an anticipated finding. The same relative difference in patency would also be expected from a comparison between de novo and restenotic lesions treated with standard balloon angioplasty, save for the fact that the restenosis rates for both groups might be anticipated to be higher than observed with DEB angioplasty in this study. It is worth mentioning the higher smoking prevalence in the de novo versus restenosis group in this analysis (28% vs 7%, respectively), which may have resulted in a relatively conservative estimate of the patency difference between groups.

M. Corriere, MD, MS

Durability and Efficacy of Tibial Arterial Stent Placement for Critical Limb Ischemia

Silingardi R, Lauricella A, Coppi G, et al (Univ of Modena and Reggio Emilia, Baggiovara, Italy)

J Vasc Interv Radiol 26:475-483, 2015

Purpose.—To analyze the efficacy and durability of long-term tibioperoneal arterial stent placement for selected cases of symptomatic chronic limb ischemia (CLI).

Materials and Methods.—From January 2005 to June 2012, 168 limbs (155 patients) were treated with percutaneous transluminal angioplasty (PTA)/stent placement for de novo tibial stenosis or occlusion in at least one tibial artery. Most patients (92.9%) were classified with severe disease (Rutherford category 5/6). Concomitant interventions were performed in 58%. Bare metal (84%) and drug-eluting (16%) stents were used. Indications for stent placement were residual stenosis after PTA (>30%), elastic recoiling, and dissection. Primary endpoints were freedom from symptomatic intrastent restenosis, target lesion revascularization (TLR), major amputation, and overall survival (OS).

Results.—Technical success rate was 99%. Within 30 days, five deaths (3.2%) occurred, and a 1.8% (95% confidence interval [CI], 0.1%–27.2%) major adverse cardiac event rate, 3.6% (95% CI, 0.1%–22.1%) major adverse limb event rate, and 1.8% (95% CI, 0%–27.5%) amputation rate were recorded. Mean follow-up was 33 months (range, 1–96 mo). Symptomatic intrastent restenosis occurred in 20 limbs (12%) at a mean of 10.3 months ± 11.27; this was identified as a prognostic factor for limb loss ($P = .045$). TLR was necessary in 10.8% of limbs, for a limb salvage rate of 89.2%. OS was influenced by age (>75 y; $P < .001$), diabetes ($P = .048$), and renal insufficiency and/or dialysis ($P < .001$). Estimated survival rate was 63% at 36 months (hazard ratio, 1.63; 95% CI, 54%–70%).

Conclusions.—Stent placement offers promising short- to long-term restenosis and patency rates, even in cases of multilevel symptomatic disease. Rigorous follow-up is vital (Fig 2).

▶ Although the target lesion revascularization (TLR) in this study was low at 10.8%, the rate of "other" ipsilateral revascularizations (defined as treatment proximal or distal to the target vessel stent-implanted area or in arteries other than the target vessel) was much more common (28.3%). These rates considered in combination suggest that tibial stent placement was performed frequently in the setting of proximal or distal disease, which would be anticipated in a patient cohort defined based on critical limb ischemia (CLI) as the indication for intervention. It would be interesting to learn what proportion of the "other" repeat interventions were performed during follow-up also had a concomitant intervention (defined as an intervention on the ipsilateral leg at a separate anatomic location at the time of tibial stenting). If the 58% of patients who received a concomitant intervention at the time of the primary procedure also accounted for the majority of patients undergoing repeat intervention during follow-up, these findings would potentially support the notion that at least some of these patients might have been better served with a bypass due to extensive multilevel disease. The tibial lesions in this study were relatively short (mean length was 2.4 cm), but the tibial disease may have only

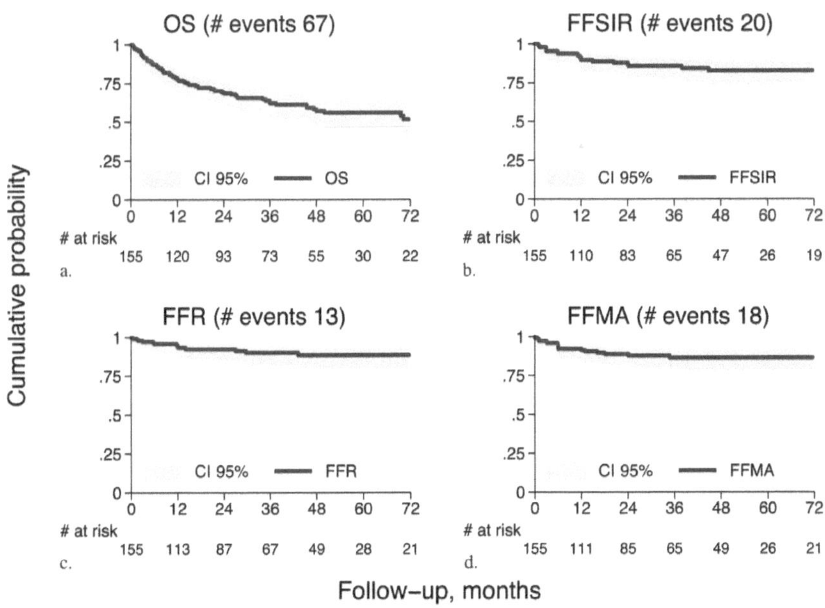

FIGURE 2.—Cumulative probability of the primary end points: (**a**) OS, (**b**) freedom from symptomatic intrastent restenosis (FFSIR), (**c**) freedom from repeat intervention (FFR), and (**d**) freedom from major amputation (FFMA), according to Kaplan–Meier analysis. (Available in color online at www.jvir.org.) (Reprinted from Silingardi R, Lauricella A, Coppi G, et al. Durability and efficacy of tibial arterial stent placement for critical limb ischemia. *J Vasc Interv Radiol.* 2015;26:475-483, with permission from SIR.)

represented part of the picture for many patients. Critical limb ischemia seldom occurs in the absence of multilevel disease, making it challenging to ascertain the impact of a procedural intervention defined based on a specific anatomic level when disease at other levels is treated simultaneously. Regardless of these challenges, freedom from symptomatic restenosis, repeat intervention, and major amputation were respectable in this group of patients with CLI (whose overall survival reflects this diagnosis) (Fig 2), although wound healing was achieved in only 40%. As the authors mention in the discussion, acceptable limb salvage can be achieved with tibial stenting at the expense of repeat interventions,[1] and this may be the best option when angioplasty yields suboptimal results and alternative revascularization strategies are limited.

M. Corriere, MD, MS

Reference

1. Lo RC, Darling J, Bensley RP, et al. Outcomes following infrapopliteal angioplasty for critical limb ischemia. *J Vasc Surg*. 2013;57:1455-1463.

Endovascular Revascularization and Supervised Exercise for Peripheral Artery Disease and Intermittent Claudication: A Randomized Clinical Trial

Fakhry F, Spronk S, van der Laan L, et al (Erasmus Univ Med Ctr, Rotterdam, the Netherlands; Dutch Health Care Inspectorate, Utrecht, the Netherlands; Amphia Hosp, Breda, the Netherlands; et al)

JAMA 314:1936-1944, 2015

Importance.—Supervised exercise is recommended as a first-line treatment for intermittent claudication. Combination therapy of endovascular revascularization plus supervised exercise may be more promising but few data comparing the 2 therapies are available.

Objective.—To assess the effectiveness of endovascular revascularization plus supervised exercise for intermittent claudication compared with supervised exercise only.

Design, Setting, and Participants.—Randomized clinical trial of 212 patients allocated to either endovascular revascularization plus supervised exercise or supervised exercise only. Data were collected between May 17, 2010, and February 16, 2013, in the Netherlands at 10 sites. Patients were followed up for 12 months and the data were analyzed according to the intention-to-treat principle.

Interventions.—A combination of endovascular revascularization (selective stenting) plus supervised exercise ($n = 106$) or supervised exercise only ($n = 106$).

Main Outcomes and Measures.—The primary end point was the difference in maximum treadmill walking distance at 12 months between the groups. Secondary end points included treadmill pain-free walking distance, vascular quality of life (VascuQol) score (1 [worst outcome] to 7 [best outcome]), and 36-item Short-Form Health Survey (SF-36) domain scores for physical functioning, physical role functioning, bodily pain, and general health perceptions (0 [severe limitation] to 100 [no limitation]).

Results.—Endovascular revascularization plus supervised exercise (combination therapy) was associated with significantly greater improvement in maximum walking distance (from 264 m to 1501 m for an improvement of 1237 m) compared with the supervised exercise only group (from 285 m to 1240 m for improvement of 955 m) (mean difference between groups, 282 m; 99% CI, 60-505 m) and in pain-free walking distance (from 117 m to 1237 m for an improvement of 1120 mvs from 135 m to 847 m for improvement of 712 m, respectively) (mean difference, 408 m; 99%CI, 195-622 m). Similarly, the combination therapy group demonstrated significantly greater improvement in the disease-specific VascuQol score (1.34 [99% CI, 1.04-1.64] in the combination therapy group vs 0.73 [99% CI, 0.43-1.03] in the exercise group; mean difference, 0.62 [99% CI, 0.20-1.03]) and in the score for the SF-36 physical functioning (22.4 [99% CI, 16.3-28.5] vs 12.6 [99% CI, 6.3-18.9], respectively; mean difference, 9.8 [99% CI, 1.4-18.2]). No significant differences were found for the SF-36 domains of physical role functioning, bodily pain, and general health perceptions.

Conclusions and Relevance.—Among patients with intermittent claudication after 1 year of follow-up, a combination therapy of endovascular revascularization followed by supervised exercise resulted in significantly greater improvement in walking distances and health-related quality-of-life scores compared with supervised exercise only.

Trial Registration.—Netherlands Trial Registry Identifier: NTR2249 (Fig 2, Tables 1 and 2).

▶ This randomized clinical trial compares 2 approaches: supervised exercise therapy (SET) alone versus SET in combination with endovascular revascularization. A greater clinical response was observed in the combined therapy group than with SET alone; this is not necessarily surprising, as one might anticipate that 2 treatments used together would potentially yield a greater symptomatic response than 1 alone. Although we often consider claudication treatment options from an "either—or" perspective (particularly in the research arena), in clinical practice, it is not unusual to implement more than 1 simultaneously. Exercise therapy plus cilostazol pharmacotherapy is probably the most common combination of treatments that are implemented at the same time, whereas revascularization is often reserved for patients who have an insufficient symptomatic response from 1 or both of these options. As acknowledged in the introduction, SET often performs well compared with revascularization in clinical trials but may not have similar effectiveness in clinical practice because of limited access, nonreimbursement, and poor patient adherence. If these barriers exist, then greater reliance on other treatments may not be underuse of SET (as the authors put it) but instead appropriate (or at least realistic) use. The SET protocol used in this trial had several unique aspects that may distinguish it from many real-world practice environments. Physiotherapists were available at either the practice site or in the patients' neighborhoods, were specifically

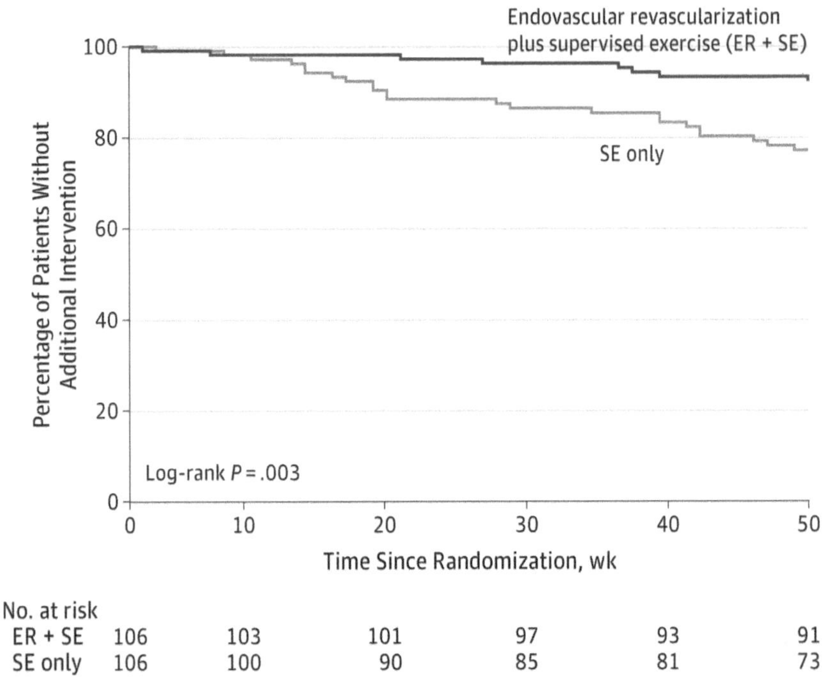

FIGURE 2.—Kaplan-Meier Estimates of the Proportion of Patients Without Additional Intervention During Follow-up. (Reprinted from Fakhry F, Spronk S, van der Laan L, et al. Endovascular revascularization and supervised exercise for peripheral artery disease and intermittent claudication: a randomized clinical trial. *JAMA*. 2015;314:1936-1944, with permission from American Medical Association.)

certified for claudication exercise therapy, and most participated in the ClaudicatioNet integrated national care network.[1]

The combination therapy group had superior outcomes for most clinical end points evaluated in this trial (including the primary outcome, maximum treadmill walking distance), but the gap between treatment groups appeared to diminish as the duration of follow-up increased (Table 2). Restenosis was identified in approximately one-third of patients in the revascularization group. Given that the majority of patients in both treatment groups were current smokers (Table 1), one might predict that the negative impact of smoking on post-revascularization patency rates would further diminish the long-term advantages of revascularization during more extended follow-up. Twenty-two percent of participants randomized to SET alone had some other treatment intervention during follow-up, whereas 8% of participants in the combination group had a secondary revascularization procedure (Fig 2). Revascularization procedures had a 7% minor complication rate and a 4% technical failure rate. These findings suggest that combination therapy was more definitive (at least in terms of short-term symptomatic response), but conversely, it is also worth considering that the less invasive, lower risk strategy of SET alone would potentially be adequate for nearly 80% of patients.

TABLE 1.—Baseline Characteristics

	Supervised Exercise (n = 106)	Endovascular Revascularization Plus Supervised Exercise (n = 106)
Age, mean (SD), y	66 (10)	64 (9)
Male sex, No. (%)	72 (68)	60 (57)
Race, No. (%)		
White	98 (92)	102 (96)
Black	2 (2)	2 (2)
Other[a]	6 (6)	2 (2)
Smoker, No. (%)		
Current	55 (52)	65 (61)
Former	42 (40)	33 (31)
Cholesterol, mean (SD), mg/dL		
Total	189 (46)	193 (58)
Low-density lipoprotein	108 (43)	112 (50)
High-density lipoprotein	50 (23)	54 (31)
Triglycerides, mean (SD), mg/dL	195 (133)	168 (133)
Hyperlipidemia, No. (%)[b]	44 (42)	47 (44)
Body mass index, mean (SD)[c]	26.2 (4.4)	27.0 (4.1)
Waist size, mean (SD), cm	102 (18)	102 (14)
Hypertension, No. (%)	66 (62)	62 (58)
History of disease, No. (%)		
Diabetes	27 (26)	17 (16)
Ischemic cardiac	42 (40)	35 (33)
Cerebrovascular	14 (13)	11 (10)
Pulmonary	17 (16)	15 (14)
Renal insufficiency, No. (%)	7 (7)	7 (7)
Lower limb osteoarthritis, No. (%)	12 (11)	11 (10)
Physical activity, median (IQR), h/w	4.0 (1.0-8.0)	4.0 (1.0-9.0)
Duration of intermittent claudication, median (IQR), mo	12.0 (6.0-24.0)	12.0 (5.0-24.0)
Fontaine stage, No. (%)[d]		
IIa	24 (23)	18 (17)
IIb	82 (77)	88 (83)
Dominant lesion, No. (%)		
Aortoiliac	54 (51)	58 (55)
Femoropopliteal	52 (49)	48 (45)
Walking distance, mean (SD), m		
Maximum	285 (165)	264 (145)
Pain free	135 (88)	117 (83)
Ankle brachial index, mean (SD)[e]		
At rest	0.68 (0.16)	0.71 (0.18)
After exercise	0.40 (0.24)	0.43 (0.21)
VascuQol score, mean (SD)[f]	4.51 (1.02)	4.48 (0.92)
Rating score, mean (SD)[g]	64.9 (17.8)	67.9 (17.8)
SF-36 score, mean (SD)[h]		
Physical functioning	52.7 (21.0)	51.4 (16.4)
Role physical	53.4 (40.9)	59.2 (40.2)
Bodily pain	53.1 (20.7)	52.7 (17.6)
General health	53.9 (20.3)	59.3 (15.4)

Abbreviations: IQR, interquartile range; SF-36, 36-item Short-Form Health Survey; VascuQol, Vascular Quality of Life Questionnaire. SI conversion factors: To convert low-density lipoprotein, high-density lipoprotein, and total cholesterol to mmol/L, multiply by 0.0259; triglycerides to mmol/L, multiply by 0.0113.

[a]Included Asian Indian, Chinese, and other Asian.

[b]Defined as a total cholesterol level of 193mg/dL or higher.

[c]Calculated as weight in kilograms divided by height in meters squared.

[d]IIa is defined as a pain-free walking distance of further than 200m; IIb, a pain-free walking distance of 200m or shorter.

[e]Minimum value for right and left legs.

[f]Composed of 25 questions in 5 domains, including activities, symptoms, pain, emotional, and social, which are scored on a scale from 1 (worst outcome) to 7 (best outcome).

[g]Composed of a single question in which patients score their health state on a scale from 0 (worst imaginable) to 100 (best imaginable).

[h]In this study, the SF-36 questionnaire is composed of 4 separate domain scores, which are the weighted sums of the questions in each domain. Each domain score is expressed on a scale from 0 (severe limitation) to 100 (no limitation).

TABLE 2.—Functional Performance Measures

Functional Performance Measures	Mean (99% CI) Supervised Exercise (n = 106)	Endovascular Revascularization Plus Supervised Exercise (n = 106)	Between-Group Difference	P Value[a]
Maximum walking distance, m				
At baseline	285 (244 to 326)	264 (228 to 300)		
1 mo	438 (282 to 595)[b]	1004 (835 to 1174)[b]	566 (358 to 774)	<.001
6 mo	851 (683 to 1018)[b]	1260 (1076 to 1444)[b]	409 (183 to 636)	<.001
12 mo	955 (786 to 1124)[b]	1237 (1058 to 1418)[b]	282 (60 to 505)	.001
Pain-free walking distance, m				
At baseline	135 (113 to 157)	117 (96 to 138)		
1 mo	181 (23 to 339)[b]	724 (561 to 886)[b]	543 (340 to 744)	<.001
6 mo	542 (378 to 707)[b]	1071 (900 to 1243)[b]	529 (315 to 743)	<.001
12 mo	712 (549 to 876)[b]	1120 (948 to 1293)[b]	408 (195 to 622)	<.001
Ankle brachial index at rest[c]				
At baseline	0.68 (0.64 to 0.72)	0.71 (0.67 to 0.76)		
1 mo	−0.02 (−0.07 to 0.02)[b]	0.19 (0.15 to 0.23)[b]	0.21 (0.15 to 0.27)	<.001
6 mo	0.04 (−0.01 to 0.09)[b]	0.16 (0.11 to 0.20)[b]	0.12 (0.05 to 0.17)	<.001
12 mo	0.03 (−0.02 to 0.08)[b]	0.16 (0.11 to 0.21)[b]	0.13 (0.06 to 0.19)	<.001
Ankle brachial index after exercise[c]				
At baseline	0.40 (0.34 to 0.46)	0.43 (0.38 to 0.48)		
1 mo	0.03 (−0.02 to 0.09)[b]	0.36 (0.30 to 0.42)[b]	0.33 (0.25 to 0.40)	<.001
6 mo	0.12 (0.06 to 0.18)[b]	0.33 (0.27 to 0.39)[b]	0.21 (0.13 to 0.29)	<.001
12 mo	0.11 (0.05 to 0.18)[b]	0.33 (0.27 to 0.40)[b]	0.22 (0.13 to 0.31)	<.001

[a]Calculated using the likelihood ratio test.
[b]Data are expressed as mean improvement compared with baseline.
[c]Minimum value for right and left legs.

Reprinted from Fakhry F, Spronk S, van der Laan L, et al. Endovascular revascularization and supervised exercise for peripheral artery disease and intermittent claudication: a randomized clinical trial. *JAMA*. 2015;314:1936-1944, with permission from American Medical Association.

Emerging evidence suggests that SET pays ongoing dividends, even if the symptomatic response to this treatment alone is unsatisfactory and revascularization is subsequently deemed necessary. Providers should keep this in mind and consider revascularization as an addition to (rather than substitution for) SET when it is necessary. In this trial, participants in the combined treatment group were less engaged in the SET component; the combined group completed a mean of 30 SET sessions versus 43 for participants randomized to SET alone. These findings suggest that simultaneous implementation may have had a negative impact on SET adherence, perhaps due to the need to recover from the procedure and/or a more immediate symptomatic response that possibly diminished the perceived additional benefit to be gained.

Perspective is important when defining how symptomatic response, cost, and risk of over- versus undertreatment of claudication should be prioritized. The investigators suggest that these results should reopen the debate related to revascularization for patients with claudication, and their findings are likely to increase enthusiasm for earlier consideration of revascularization among some providers. Ultimately, buy-in (pun intended) will be required from organizations that pay for health care. Hopefully, these investigators will share longer term follow-up data to provide insight into whether the outcomes are durable. When considering potential negative impacts of overtreatment, the long-term implications of more aggressive utilization of revascularization may extend well beyond recurrent claudication symptoms.

M. Corriere, MD, MS

Reference

1. www.claudicationet.nl/home/.

Percutaneous radial access for peripheral transluminal angioplasty

Coscas R, de Blic R, Capdevila C, et al (Hôpital Universitaire Ambroise Paré, Boulogne-Billancourt, France; Université Versailles Saint-Quentin en Yvelines, Montigny-le-Bretonneux, France)

J Vasc Surg 61:463-468, 2015

Objective.—The radial approach is currently gaining popularity in the setting of coronary percutaneous transluminal angioplasty (PTA) because it decreases the incidence of vascular complications. This study reports our initial results with radial access for peripheral PTA.

Methods.—Between November 2011 and January 2014, we performed peripheral PTA in 526 patients. PTA was performed through left radial access in 24 ambulatory patients (4.6%) presenting with TransAtlantic Inter-Society Consensus A or B lesions on preoperative computed tomography angiography. Materials included a 110-cm-long introducer, a 0.018-inch 400-cm-long wire, 150-cm-long angiography catheters, 180-cm-long shaft balloons and stents. Data were prospectively collected.

Results.—There were 22 men (92%), median age was 65 years (range, 45-88 years), and 38 target lesions were treated. Indication for revascularization was disabling claudication in 22 patients (92%) and critical ischemia in two (8%). Indication for choosing the radial approach was bilateral hostile groins in 12 patients (50%), bilateral infrainguinal lesions in 4 (17%), need for a contralateral femoral approach in the setting of kissing iliac stents or bifurcated surgical aortic grafts in 3 (13%), and elective in 5 (21%). Radial puncture failed in one patient (4%), and PTA was performed through brachial access. Technical success was 91% (20 of 22 patients). Thirty-seven stents were implanted. Total procedure duration was 45 minutes (range, 30-120 minutes). Fluoroscopy time was 9 minutes (range, 5-35 minutes), and 40 mL (range, 20-90 mL) of contrast was necessary. Radial artery rupture secondary to spasm was noted at the end of the procedure in two patients (8%). All patients could ambulate 2 hours after the procedure. No patient died. Median follow-up was 8 months (range, 1-23 months). Three radial arteries (13%) were occluded at the last follow-up. At 6 months, freedom from target lesion revascularization and target vessel revascularization were 91% and 91%, respectively, for iliac lesions and 93% and 86%, respectively, for infrainguinal lesions.

Conclusions.—This study demonstrates the feasibility of radial access for peripheral PTA. Radial access could represent an alternative to brachial access for peripheral and visceral interventions. Although complication rates of the present series are concerning, larger studies are needed to determine the role of transradial PTA once the learning curve is overcome. A wider diffusion of the technique mandates (1) smaller-diameter sheaths, (2) longer shaft devices, and (3) the development of specifically designed rescue devices such as covered stents and thromboaspiration catheters.

▶ Percutaneous transfemoral arterial access is currently the most popular method of arterial and coronary imaging. Advantages of this technique include its ease, interventionalist familiarity, and relatively low complication rate. However, use of this technique can be limited in patients with morbid obesity, severe iliofemoral occlusive disease, and aortic bifurcation implants. Major and minor bleeding complications are common (3% to 5%), although this incidence can be lowered with the use of ultrasound guidance and arterial closure devices. The alternative brachial access is fraught with a higher morbidity risk due to bleeding, thrombosis, or nerve injury.

In this retrospective study, the authors present their transradial access experience in selected patients undergoing peripheral arterial interventions. Transradial access was used in only 4.6% of patients undergoing lower extremity interventions in the study period. All patients had TASC A and B lesions by preoperative computed tomography. Although the presence of bilateral hostile groins was the most common indication for this technique, transradial access was used for other indications including simultaneous bilateral lower extremity interventions and unfavorable anatomy of the aortic bifurcation. Patients with extensive atherosclerosis of the aortic arch or a negative Allen test were not offered this procedure. Five- and six-French sheath sizes were used. The technique resulted in 13% (3 patients) incidence of radial artery occlusions on follow-up and 1 perioperative minor stroke (4%).

Despite the small number of patients and the low complexity of the lesions treated, this small European series proves feasibility of this technique for supra-inguinal and infrainguinal lower extremity angioplasty and stenting procedures. The limited availability of the long delivery sheathes, balloon shafts, and stent delivery systems, particularly in the United States, may restrict the rapid adoption of transradial access. Also, the complications encountered in this series prove that a learning curve must be overcome. Regardless, based on the experience from the world of coronary interventions, it is likely that this technique will have a role as an alternative to brachial and femoral access in selected patients.

Y. Duwayri, MD

Randomized Controlled Study of Excimer Laser Atherectomy for Treatment of Femoropopliteal In-Stent Restenosis: Initial Results From the EXCITE ISR Trial (EXCImer Laser Randomized Controlled Study for Treatment of FemoropopliTEal In-Stent Restenosis)

Dippel EJ, on behalf of the EXCITE ISR Investigators (Genesis Med Ctr, Davenport, IA; et al)

JACC Cadiovasc Interv 8:92-101, 2015

Objectives.—The purpose of this study was to evaluate the safety and efficacy of excimer laser atherectomy (ELA) with adjunctive percutaneous transluminal angioplasty (PTA) versus PTA alone for treating patients with chronic peripheral artery disease with femoropopliteal bare nitinol in-stent restenosis (ISR).

Background.—Femoropopliteal stenting has shown superiority to PTA for lifestyle-limiting claudication and critical limb ischemia, although treating post-stenting artery reobstruction, or ISR, remains challenging.

Methods.—The multicenter, prospective, randomized, controlled EXCITE ISR (EXCImer Laser Randomized Controlled Study for Treatment of FemoropopliTEal In-Stent Restenosis) trial was conducted across 40 U.S. centers. Patients with Rutherford Class 1 to 4 and lesions of target lesion length ≥4 cm, vessel diameter 5 to 7 mm were enrolled and randomly divided into ELA + PTA and PTA groups by a 2:1 ratio. The primary efficacy endpoint was target lesion revascularization (TLR) at 6-month follow up. The primary safety endpoint was major adverse event (death, amputation, or TLR) at 30 days post-procedure.

Results.—Study enrollment was stopped at 250 patients due to early efficacy demonstrated at a prospectively-specified interim analysis. A total of 169 ELA + PTA subjects (62.7% male; mean age 68.5 ± 9.8 years) and 81 PTA patients (61.7% male; mean age 67.8 ± 10.3 years) were enrolled. Mean lesion length was 19.6 ± 12.0 cm versus 19.3 ± 11.9 cm, and 30.5% versus 36.8% of patients exhibited total occlusion. ELA + PTA subjects demonstrated superior procedural success (93.5% vs. 82.7%; $p = 0.01$) with significantly fewer procedural complications. ELA + PTA and PTA subject 6-month freedom from TLR was 73.5% versus 51.8% ($p < 0.005$), and 30-day major adverse event rates were 5.8% versus 20.5% ($p < 0.001$), respectively. ELA + PTA was associated with a 52% reduction in TLR (hazard ratio: 0.48; 95% confidence interval: 0.31 to 0.74).

Conclusions.—The EXCITE ISR trial is the first large, prospective, randomized study to demonstrate superiority of ELA + PTA versus PTA alone for treating femoropopliteal ISR. (Randomized Study of Laser and Balloon Angioplasty Versus Balloon Angioplasty to Treat Peripheral In-stent Restenosis [EXCITE ISR]; NCT01330628) (Fig 2, Table 3).

▶ In-stent restenosis (ISR) is a common problem after endovascular femoropopliteal intervention that frequently leads to loss of patency, loss of symptomatic response, and repeat intervention. This analysis compared conventional percutaneous transluminal balloon angioplasty (PTA) alone versus in combination with excimer laser atherectomy (ELA) for ISR. The trial, which was supported by the excimer laser atherectomy catheter manufacturers, demonstrated advantages with its use for most study end points including the

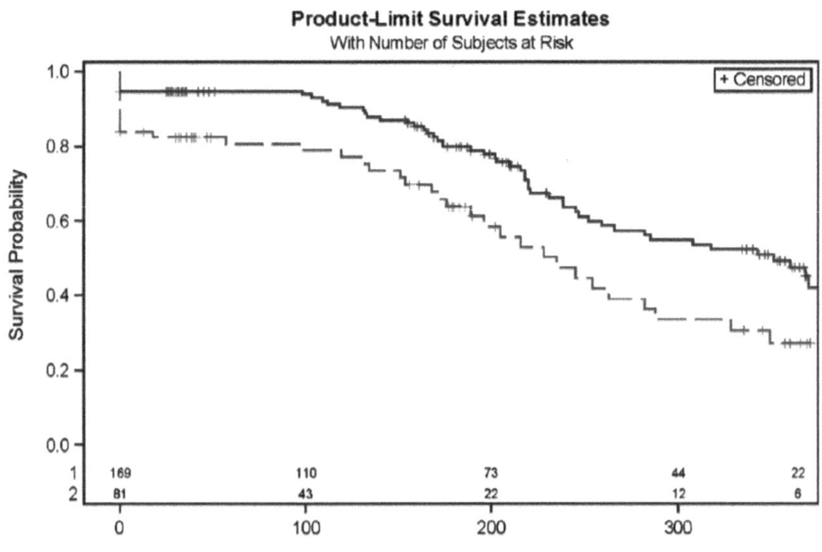

FIGURE 2.—Freedom from TLR through 1 year. Kaplan-Meier survival curve up to 1 year is shown for TLR. Number of subjects at risk is shown at the bottom of the graph ($p < 0.003$). Abbreviations as in Figure 1. *Editor's Note*: Please refer to original journal article for full references. (Reprinted from Dippel EJ, on behalf of the EXCITE ISR Investigators. Randomized controlled study of excimer laser atherectomy for treatment of femoropopliteal in-stent restenosis: initial results from the EXCITE ISR Trial (EXCImer Laser Randomized Controlled Study for Treatment of FemoropopliTEal In-Stent Restenosis). *JACC Cardiovasc Interv.* 2015;8:92-101, with permission from American College of Cardiology Foundation.)

TABLE 3.—Procedural Outcomes

	ELA + PTA (n = 169)	PTA (n = 81)	*p* Value
Turbo Elite used	79.9	—	—
Distal protection	40.2	30.9	0.16
% diameter stenosis*	23.9 ± 9.3	25.5 ± 10.9	0.24
Residual stenosis >30%	4.7	13.6	0.02
Dissection grade			
Any	7.7	17.2	0.03
≥Grade C	2.4	7.4	0.08
Embolism	8.3	4.9	0.44
Bailout stenting	4.1	11.1	0.05
Procedural TLR	5.3	16.0	0.008

Values are % or mean ± SD.
TLR = target lesion revascularization; other abbreviations as in Table 1 in the original article.
*Post-assigned treatment.
Reprinted from Dippel EJ, on behalf of the EXCITE ISR Investigators. Randomized controlled study of excimer laser atherectomy for treatment of femoropopliteal in-stent restenosis: initial results from the EXCITE ISR Trial (EXCImer Laser Randomized Controlled Study for Treatment of FemoropopliTEal In-Stent Restenosis). *JACC Cardiovasc Interv.* 2015;8:92-101, with permission from American College of Cardiology Foundation.

primary outcome, target lesion revascularization (TLR) at 6 months. TLR is an outcome that is not consistently associated with clinical sequelae in PAD and may be subject to bias in trials such as this one, where the study investigators were unblinded and no standardized criteria for repeat intervention were specified. More objective end points (such as change in maximum walking distance or ankle brachial index) were not included. Procedural TLR (presumably meaning adjunctive revascularization interventions during the index procedure) accounted for a considerable gap between PTA versus PTA-ELA at time zero (Fig 2), which remained fairly stable during follow-up. Procedural TLR was nearly 3-fold higher in the PTA alone group, but it is unclear what factors prompted procedural TLR and whether operators used consistent definitions for residual stenosis and similar criteria for bailout stenting or other adjunctive procedures.

Approximately 80% of ELA procedures utilized 2 separate catheters, the first of which was used selectively to create a pilot channel when necessary (Table 3). This might increase device-related costs (and necessary inventory) considerably, as it seems that the "selective" utilization applied to the vast majority of cases. For providers considering whether ELA should be used as a matter of routine for ISR, it would have been useful to see comparisons with other techniques that are more aggressive than standard PTA (including mechanical atherectomy, cutting/scoring balloons, drug-coated balloons, and restenting) and are therefore often used for treating ISR lesions. Perhaps investigator-initiated studies will provide some of these more relevant comparisons in the future.

M. Corriere, MD, MS

Safety, Clinical Outcome, and Fracture Rate of Femoropopliteal Stenting Using a 4F Compatible Delivery System

Sarkadi H, Bérczi V, Kollár A, et al (Semmelweis Univ, Budapest, Hungary)

Eur J Vasc Endovasc Surg 49:199-204, 2015

Objective.—To determine the safety, clinical outcome, and fracture rate of femoropopliteal interventions using 4F stents.

Methods.—Between January 2010 and December 2011, 112 symptomatic patients were treated by stent implantation. Ten patients were lost to follow up; therefore, 102 patients (62 men; mean age 66.4 ± 10.1 years) were retrospectively analyzed. The indication for femoropopliteal revascularization was severe claudication (Rutherford–Becker score = 3) in 63 (62%) patients and chronic critical limb ischemia (Rutherford–Becker score = 4–6) in 39 (38%). Follow up included palpation of peripheral pulses and measurement of ankle brachial index. In patients with suspected in-stent restenosis duplex ultrasonography was performed. In 2013, patients were asked to return for a fluoroscopic examination of the stents.

Results.—114 lesions (Trans-Atlantic InterSociety Consensus-C and D, $n = 45$) were treated with 119 stents (Astron Pulsar, $n = 42$; Pulsar-18, $n = 77$). Lesions were long (≥100 mm) in 49 cases and heavily calcified in 35. Stents were long (≥120 mm) in 46 cases. Ten stents were partially overlapped. The technical and clinical success rates were 100%. Two puncture related complications were noted, neither of which required surgical repair. Eleven patients died (myocardial infarction, $n = 4$; stroke, $n = 2$; cancer, $n = 5$) and nine patients underwent major amputation (above knee, $n = 4$). The primary patency rate was 83% at 6 months and 80% at 12 months. The primary assisted patency rate was 97% at 6 months and 94% at 12 months. The secondary patency rate was 86% at 6 months and 85% at 12 months. The prevalence of fractures was 26% (type III and IV, 10%) after an average follow up of 25 months.

Conclusion.—Femoropopliteal stenting using a 4F compatible delivery system can be accomplished with a low complication rate, acceptable fracture rate, and with similar 12 month patency and revascularization rates as their 6F counterparts.

▶ Percutaneous lower extremity intervention has become the dominant first-line treatment for peripheral artery disease (PAD) patients who require revascularization. Sheath diameter is a known predictor of access site complications (including hematoma, pseudoaneurysm, and need for surgical repair),[1] prompting device manufacturers to develop smaller profile systems to minimize risk. A key consideration with smaller profile systems, however, is whether the diameter reduction comes at the cost of technical success (including ability to cross the target lesion and deliver the therapeutic intervention (self-expanding stent placement in this case) to the intended location when required). These investigators seem to be adept at using the 4-Fr self-expanding stent system described in this study (which may not yet be available to many providers), and the advantages associated with reduced diameter access will expand if other technologies (including balloon-expandable stents, drug-eluting balloons, and atherectomy) can also be used without the need to depend on a more restricted array of treatment options.

The 100% technical success rate reported in this analysis is impressive, particularly considering that antegrade ipsilateral access was used in the majority of procedures (79 vs 31 with a contralateral up-and-over approach) in a group of patients with a 43% prevalence of obesity (although body mass index was not included among descriptive statistics). The authors also reported symptom resolution or improvement in all patients (38% of whom were treated for critical limb ischemia). Providers who perform PAD interventions for severe disease may these technical and symptomatic outcomes seem too good to be true. These results may indicate that the patients were selected or screened with alternative imaging before intervention; this seems likely given that no patients in the series had significant common femoral or iliac disease. Additionally, symptomatic results were not evaluated using a standardized measure, and duplex imaging was used selectively, allowing for the possibility that investigator bias might also have affected the reported outcomes.

The discussion asserts that "no comprehensive data have been published in patients with femoropopliteal disease," but without a direct comparison to a larger profile system, it is difficult to determine the potential benefit that would be derived from switching to 4-Fr-compatible technology. Although the discussion refers to potential advantages over 6-Fr systems, perhaps 5-Fr self-expanding stents (now widely available in a variety of diameters and lengths) would be a more appropriate comparison group. The value of 4-Fr systems (and presumably even smaller systems in the not-so-distant future) will be greater if the diameter reduction does not come with trade-offs related to treatment options and technical success.

M. Corriere, MD, MS

Reference

1. Corriere MA, Guzman RJ. True and false aneurysms of the femoral artery. *Semin Vasc Surg*. 2005;18:216-223.

Sustained Benefit at 2 Years for Covered Stents Versus Bare-Metal Stents in Long SFA Lesions: The VIASTAR Trial

Lammer J, Zeller T, Hausegger KA, et al (Med Univ Vienna, Austria; Universitaets-Herzzentrum Freiburg-Bad Krozingen, Germany; Klinikum Klagenfurt, Austria; et al)

Cardiovasc Intervent Radiol 38:25-32, 2015

Purpose.—The hypothesis that covered stents are superior to bare-metal stents (BMS) in long femoropopliteal artery disease was tested. The one-year results of the VIASTAR trial revealed a patency benefit of covered stents in the treatment-per-protocol (TPP) analysis only.

Methods.—A prospective, randomized, single-blind, multicenter study evaluated 141 patients with symptomatic peripheral arterial disease (PAD) after treatment with heparin-bonded covered stents (VIABAHN® Endoprosthesis) or BMS. Clinical outcomes and patency rates were assessed at 1, 6, 12, and 24 months. Mean lesion length was 19.0 ± 6.3 cm in the VIABAHN® versus 17.3 ± 6.6 cm in the BMS group.

Results.—The 24-month primary patency rates in the VIABAHN® and BMS group were: intention-to-treat 63.1 (95 % CI 0.52–0.76) versus 41.2 % (95 % CI 0.29–0.57; log rank $p = 0.04$) and TPP 69.4 (95 % CI 0.58–0.83) versus 40.0 % (95 % CI 0.28–0.56; log rank $p = 0.004$). Freedom from target-lesion-revascularization (TLR) was 79.4 (95 % CI 0.70–0.90) versus 73.0 % (95 % CI 0.63–0.85) for VIABAHN® versus BMS (log rank $p = 0.37$). For the TPP group in lesions ≥20 cm, the 24-month patency rates were 65.2 (95 % CI 0.50–0.85) versus 26.7 % (95 % CI 0.12–0.59; log rank $p = 0.004$) for VIABAHN® versus BMS, and freedom from TLR was 80.0 (95 % CI 0.68–0.94) versus 61.9 % (95 % CI 0.44–0.87; log rank $p = 0.13$). The ankle brachial index was 0.89 ± 0.18 versus 0.91 ± 0.17 ($p = 0.76$) at 24-month in the VIABAHN® versus the BMS group, respectively.

Conclusion.—At 24-month, this trial in PAD patients with long femoropopliteal lesions demonstrated a significantly improved primary patency rate for heparin-bonded covered stents compared to BMS, however, without a significant impact on clinical outcomes and TLR rate (Reg. Nr. ISRCTN48164244).

▶ Antiplatelet therapy in the trial was not standardized beyond the first 6 post-procedural months; all participants received aspirin indefinitely plus clopidogrel for at least 6 months. The rate of clopidogrel use was lower among participants in the bare-metal stents (BMS) group during late follow-up; these participants also had a lower rate of dual antiplatelet therapy as well as aspirin use (although statistical tests were not provided for these comparisons). These differences in medical therapy may reflect biases of unblinded providers toward more aggressive therapy for covered stents and may have affected the patency outcomes. An additional element of the study design that may have influenced results is the use of 3 BMS were used in this study versus a single covered stent, introducing device and procedure variability among the former group.

In the current atmosphere of value-based care, providers face resource constraints and increasing scrutiny for low-value procedures. Providers treating peripheral artery disease have a wide array of endovascular options, including balloon angioplasty, drug-coated balloon angioplasty, BMS, drug-eluting stents, covered stents, and atherectomy. They may also choose endoluminal versus subintimal approaches to recanalization, with the latter of these approaches often requiring special techniques and devices for distal reentry. These treatments can be used individually or in combination, allowing a variety of alternatives to consider if the first-line approach fails before abandoning endovascular treatment. Costs can add up rapidly because additional techniques (and related equipment) are attempted after others have failed, however, and deciding when to call it quits instead of trying that third, fourth, or fifth option becomes important for avoiding waste. An endovascular procedure that exhausts available inventory but provides little or no benefit to the patient fits the definition of low-value care,[1] a concept that providers should take heed of as quality initiatives increasingly evaluate outcomes based on both clinical and cost end points. Selecting the appropriate outcomes and defining what constitutes a meaningful improvement are key considerations when evaluating the value of new (and more expensive) technologies. Although covered stents had superior patency compared with BMS in this analysis (and this difference was even more pronounced in the subgroup of participants with lesions greater than 20 cm in length), there were no significant differences in clinical end points, including ankle brachial index, walking distance based on the Walking Impairment Questionnaire, or freedom from target lesion revascularization. The "sustained benefit" mentioned in the article title therefore may not have been evident to the patients who received covered stents, and the patency advantage (although statistically significant) may not be sufficient to justify routine use of covered stents. Value is in the eye of the beholder.

M. Corriere, MD, MS

Reference

1. Schwartz AL, Landon BE, Elshaug AG, Chernew ME, McWilliams JM. Measuring low-value care in Medicare. *JAMA Intern Med.* 2014;174:1067-1076.

Technical and Early Outcomes Using Ultrasound-Guided Reentry for Chronic Total Occlusions

Baker AC, Humphries MD, Noll RE Jr, et al (Univ of California Davis Med Ctr, Sacramento)
Ann Vasc Surg 29:55-62, 2015

Background.—Subintimal angioplasty is a common treatment for chronic total occlusions (CTOs) in the iliac and infrainguinal arteries. Although technical success has been described using intravascular ultrasound-guided reentry devices (IVUS-RED), outcomes are still not well defined. This report describes the technical aspects and longitudinal follow-up after intravascular ultrasound-guided reentry of iliac and infrainguinal CTOs.

Methods.—A retrospective review was performed of 20 patients with lower extremity CTO treated with IVUS-RED from 2011 to 2013. A matched cohort of patients who underwent lower extremity interventions without the use of IVUS-RED was also identified. Procedural success, patency estimates, ankle-brachial indices (ABIs), complications, and limb salvage were analyzed.

Results.—Twenty patients (mean age, 69 ± 13 years), including 11 men and 9 women, underwent attempted IVUS-RED–guided recanalization. Median follow-up was 4.3 months (range, 0.4–24). Eleven patients presented with critical limb ischemia (CLI), and 9 presented with claudication. Technical success was achieved in 18 (90%) patients. Ten common iliac arteries, 3 external iliac arteries, and 5 superficial femoral arteries (SFA) were treated. No intraoperative complications resulted from device use. After procedure, ABIs significantly increased (0.5–0.9; $P < 0.01$) in the 13 patients with follow-up. Primary patency for the entire cohort was 62% at 12 months. No patient treated for claudication required reintervention, whereas 3 (27%) of those treated for CLI required repeat interventions. During follow-up, 2 patients died unrelated to the procedure, 1 patient required an amputation, and 1 patient eventually required open revascularization. When the IVUS-RED group was compared with a cohort matched on Trans-Atlantic Inter-Society Consensus and age, no difference was found in runoff scores and patency between the 2 groups during follow-up ($P > 0.05$).

Conclusions.—Recanalization of CTO using IVUS-RED is safe and effective. Use of IVUS-RED does not adversely impact outcomes in conjunction with other endovascular techniques. Early follow-up demonstrates acceptable patency, especially in patients with claudication, and freedom from reintervention (Fig 1).

▶ This analysis describes outcomes associated with use of ultrasound-guided reentry device (IVUS-RED), the Pioneer catheter, during subintimal angioplasty for chronic total occlusions (CTO). Outcomes were generally similar between patients treated with IVUS-RED and a retrospectively identified control cohort treated with other endovascular techniques. The methods used to treat CTO in the control group were not described in detail, making it unclear whether any of these patients had conventional endoluminal treatment versus subintimal angioplasty (either using fluoroscopy-guided reentry or no reentry device at all). Although the control patients were matched based on anatomic location of the target lesions, disease severity, and comorbidity, the technical success comparison is a bit artificial because the procedures were not consecutive and included 2 patients with acute limb ischemia. Of the 20 procedures, 17 were first-time attempts, and 3 were repeat attempts after initial failure of a previous procedure using other techniques (which were not specified). The IVUS-RED cohort was a mix of claudicant patients and patients with critical limb ischemia, as well as (in decreasing order of frequency) a mix of common iliac, superficial femoral artery, and superficial femoral artery CTO lesions.

Ability to gain access to the true lumen distal to a CTO is essential for successful subintimal angioplasty. The technical success rate using IVUS-RED was 90%, and the 2 technical failures were attributed to inability to deliver the reentry device to the intended distal location. This is a common technical limitation that can often be anticipated if a 4-Fr catheter will not track through the subintimal plane to the site of planned reentry. It would be of interest to learn whether any IVUS characteristics (Fig 1) could be identified that might

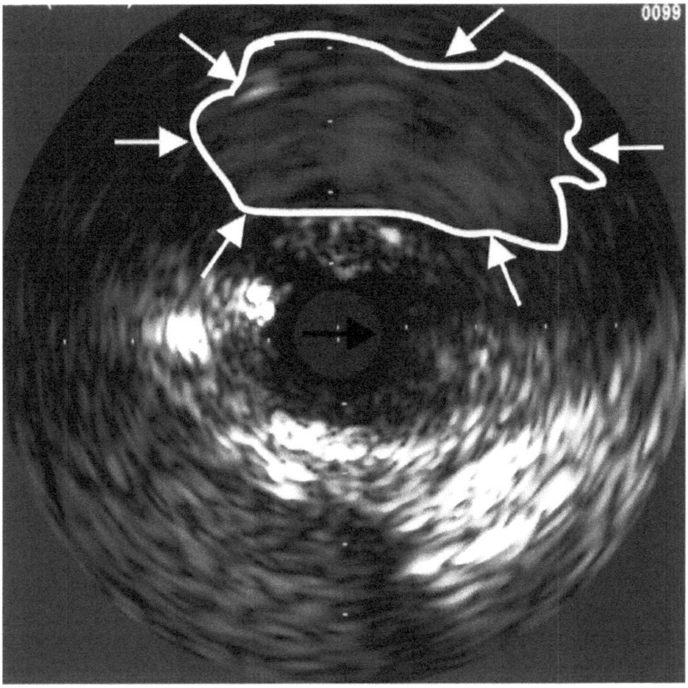

FIGURE 1.—The true lumen is visualized by using chromoflow imaging (*white arrows/outlined*) and IVUS. The reentry needle (*black arrow*) is then positioned at the 12-o'clock position and deployed into the true lumen. (Reprinted from Baker AC, Humphries MD, Noll RE Jr, et al. Technical and early outcomes using ultrasound-guided reentry for chronic total occlusions. *Ann Vasc Surg*. 2015;29:55-62, with permission from Elsevier.)

be useful in distinguishing lesions as favorable versus unfavorable for subintimal angioplasty. Angiogram or CTA characteristics predictive of technical failure might be even more useful because reentry catheters (either fluoroscopy or IVUS-guided) are expensive and potentially require sheath upsizing. The agony of defeat is therefore worsened when endovascular treatment is abandoned after opening this additional equipment before conceding technical failure. Although not specifically indicated in the Methods section, the article gives the impression that subintimal angioplasty was performed as a fallback technique rather than the preferred primary mode of CTO treatment. There is no question that subintimal angioplasty is a valuable technique, even after other approaches have been attempted but proven unsuccessful. The value of reentry devices will be maximized when providers are able to identify circumstances where the odds of technical success are high, and a potential advantage of IVUS-RED over fluoroscopy-guided approaches may prove to be the additional imaging data that informs the technique.

M. Corriere, MD, MS

Trial of a Paclitaxel-Coated Balloon for Femoropopliteal Artery Disease

Rosenfield K, for the LEVANT 2 Investigators (Massachusetts General Hosp, Boston; et al)

N Engl J Med 373:145-153, 2015

Background.—The treatment of peripheral artery disease with percutaneous transluminal angioplasty is limited by the occurrence of vessel recoil and restenosis. Drug-coated angioplasty balloons deliver antiproliferative agents directly to the artery, potentially improving vessel patency by reducing restenosis.

Methods.—In this single-blind, randomized trial conducted at 54 sites, we assigned, in a 2:1 ratio, 476 patients with symptomatic intermittent claudication or ischemic pain while at rest and angiographically significant atherosclerotic lesions to angioplasty with a paclitaxel-coated balloon or to standard angioplasty. The primary efficacy end point was primary patency of the target lesion at 12 months (defined as freedom from binary restenosis or from the need for target-lesion revascularization). The primary safety end point was a composite of freedom from perioperative death from any cause and freedom at 12 months from limb-related death (i.e., death from a medical complication related to a limb), amputation, and reintervention.

Results.—The two groups were well matched at baseline; 42.9% of the patients had diabetes, and 34.7% were current smokers. At 12 months, the rate of primary patency among patients who had undergone angioplasty with the drug-coated balloon was superior to that among patients who had undergone conventional angioplasty (65.2% vs. 52.6%, $P = 0.02$). The proportion of patients free from primary safety events was 83.9% with the drug-coated balloon and 79.0% with standard angioplasty ($P = 0.005$ for noninferiority). There were no significant between-group differences in functional outcomes or in the rates of death, amputation, thrombosis, or reintervention.

Conclusions.—Among patients with symptomatic femoropopliteal peripheral artery disease, percutaneous transluminal angioplasty with a paclitaxel-coated balloon resulted in a rate of primary patency at 12 months that was higher than the rate with angioplasty with a standard balloon. The drug-coated balloon was noninferior to the standard balloon with respect to safety. (Funded by Lutonix–Bard; LEVANT 2 ClinicalTrials.gov number, NCT01412541.) (Fig 1).

▶ Restenosis remains a major undefeated challenge for peripheral artery disease (PAD), a chronic disease that is managed over the patient's lifetime without ever being cured. Restenosis has major implications for treatment decision making in the modern era of value-based care, particularly among claudicants, in whom postintervention symptomatic improvement may be short-lived and repeat intervention is likely for patients with expected survival of 5 years or more. The femoral-popliteal arterial segment also undergoes changes in both length and diameter during walking; these forces inflict repetitive trauma on

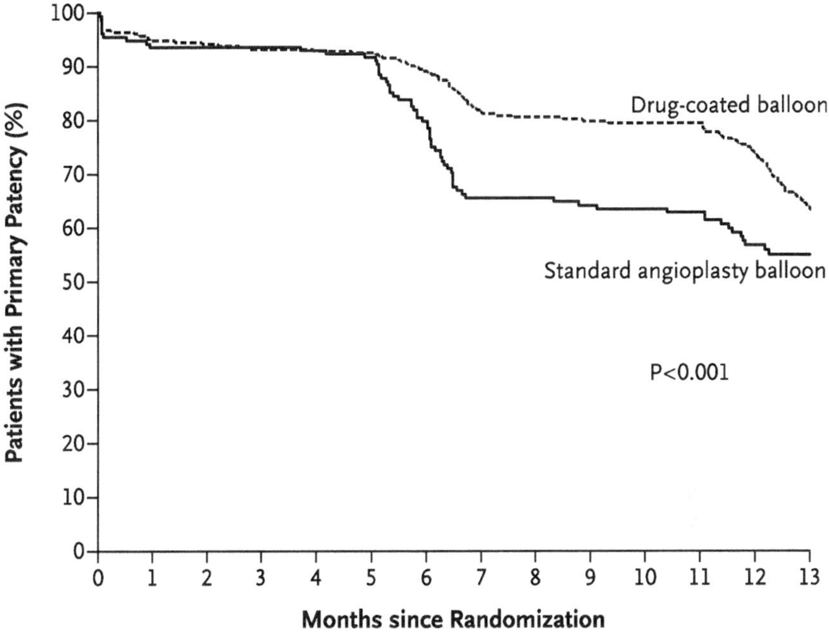

FIGURE 1.—Kaplan–Meier Curves for Primary Patency at 12 Months. Primary patency was defined as the absence of target-lesion restenosis (defined by core-laboratory adjudication) and target-lesion revascularization (adjudicated by the clinical-events committee). (Reprinted from Rosenfield K, for the LEVANT 2 Investigators. Trial of a paclitaxel-coated balloon for femoropopliteal artery disease. *N Engl J Med.* 2015;373:145-153, with permission from Massachusetts Medical Society.)

stents used to treat occlusive disease, leading to stent fracture and reduced patency over time. Given these considerations, a drug-eluting balloon with better patency would have potential for major impact on PAD treatment.

This randomized comparison between standard vs paclitaxel-coated balloon angioplasty noted improved primary patency at 12 months among patients randomized to the paclitaxel-coated balloon group. The patency difference, however, was modest at best (65% vs 52%; Fig 1) and was not accompanied by a difference in functional outcomes, reintervention, or thrombosis. Given the relatively strict anatomic inclusion criteria (including total lesion length of 15 cm or less), the impact of the drug-eluting balloon would be more appropriately described as a small incremental improvement rather than a game-changer. Providers attempting to justify use of this new technology (which is more expensive than standard angioplasty, although this study did not include cost data) therefore may encounter barriers based on value that may, in fact, be completely justified. The authors concede that their trial "does not provide definitive guidance concerning the potential role of this paclitaxel-coated balloon in clinical practice." Nonetheless, the fight against restenosis is clearly shaping up to be a war rather than a single battle, and small incremental changes in revascularization techniques accompanied by similar advances in medical management and risk-factor reduction may be the ultimate path to meaningful improvement in outcomes.

M. Corriere, MD, MS

Fusion Guidance in Endovascular Peripheral Artery Interventions: A Feasibility Study

Sailer AM, de Haan MW, de Graaf R, et al (Maastricht Univ Med Ctr, The Netherlands)

Cardiovasc Intervent Radiol 38:314-321, 2015

Purpose.—This study was designed to evaluate the feasibility of endovascular guidance by means of live fluoroscopy fusion with magnetic resonance angiography (MRA) and computed tomography angiography (CTA).

Methods.—Fusion guidance was evaluated in 20 endovascular peripheral artery interventions in 17 patients. Fifteen patients had received pre-interventional diagnostic MRA and two patients had undergone CTA. Time for fluoroscopy with MRA/CTA coregistration was recorded. Feasibility of fusion guidance was evaluated according to the following criteria: for every procedure the executing interventional radiologists recorded whether 3D road-mapping provided added value (yes vs. no) and whether PTA and/or stenting could be performed relying on the fusion road-map without need for diagnostic contrast-enhanced angiogram series (CEAS) (yes vs. no). Precision of the fusion road-map was evaluated by recording maximum differences between the position of the vasculature on the virtual CTA/MRA images and conventional angiography.

Results.—Average time needed for image coregistration was 5 ± 2 min. Three-dimensional road-map added value was experienced in 15 procedures in 12 patients. In half of the patients (8/17), intervention was performed relying on the fusion road-map only, without diagnostic CEAS. In two patients, MRA roadmap showed a false-positive lesion. Excluding three patients with inordinate movements, mean difference in position of vasculature on angiography and MRA/CTA road-map was 1.86 ± 0.95 mm, implying that approximately 95 % of differences were between 0 and 3.72 mm (2 ± 1.96 standard deviation).

Conclusions.—Fluoroscopy with MRA/CTA fusion guidance for peripheral artery interventions is feasible. By reducing the number of CEAS, this technology may contribute to enhance procedural safety.

▶ As endovascular interventions for peripheral artery disease (PAD) continue to advance and increase in frequency, cumulative radiation exposure and risk of contrast-induced nephropathy warrant consideration. These authors have demonstrated the feasibility of "fusion-guided" endovascular peripheral artery interventions. The use of fusion image road mapping has been reported previously in the context of endovascular aneurysm repair, resulting in both decreased fluoroscopy time and decreased iodinated contrast volume with fusion guidance.[1,2] Simply put, preintervention magnetic resonance angiogram (MRA) or computed tomography angiogram is coregistered with live, dynamic fluoroscopic imaging based on vessel wall calcification, bony landmarks, and organ borders that are visible in both datasets. As a result, real-time catheter and guidewire movements overlay the preacquired background dataset.

These authors evaluated 20 endovascular iliofemoral and popliteal procedures in 17 patients with claudication; in 8 of 17 patients (nearly half) intervention was performed relying on the fusion road map alone ("diagnostic contrast-enhanced angiogram was not required"). Notably 11 of 13 interventions involved stenting of the aorta, iliofemoral, and popliteal arteries. It is unclear from the study details whether these stents were deployed empirically based on the fusion road map alone or selectively based on postangioplasty angiography. There is no obvious direct comparison of the preacquired road map image to a preprocedure arteriogram. Additionally, there is reference to postprocedure angiography, but limited information provided regarding balloon or stent sizing and technical success.

There are important limitations to this technology. Specifically, there is a potential difference in vascular position between preacquired (ie, MRA) and dynamic (ie, fluoroscopic) imaging that can be profound with major leg and pelvic movement during the procedure (up to 17 mm in this study). Additionally, although MRA offers > 90% sensitivity and specificity, artifact or "pseudo" lesions should be considered. Two patients in this cohort with "severe" iliac stenosis by MRA were determined to have pseudo lesions and in fact required no intervention after diagnostic arteriogram. Fusion image road mapping may offer benefits for PAD patients; however, much more study is necessary for proof of concept, including prospective randomized controlled trials that focus on technical precision and procedural details, procedural radiation dose, procedure length, and iodinated contrast volume while also considering the learning curve required to master this emerging technology.

D. Coleman, MD

References

1. Sailer AM, de Haan MW, Peppelenbosch AG, Jacobs MJ, Wildberger JE, Schurink GW. CTA with fluoroscopy image fusion guidance in endovascular complex aortic aneurysm repair. *Eur J Vasc Endovasc Surg*. 2014;47:349-356.
2. McNally MM, Scali ST, Feezor RJ, Neal D, Huber TS, Beck AW. Three-dimensional fusion computed tomography decreases radiation exposure, procedure time, and contrast use during fenestrated endovascular aortic repair. *J Vasc Surg*. 2015;61:309-316.

Routine use of ultrasound-guided access reduces access site-related complications after lower extremity percutaneous revascularization

Lo RC, Fokkema MTM, Curran T, et al (Beth Israel Deaconess Med Ctr, Boston, MA)

J Vasc Surg 61:405-412, 2015

Objective.—We sought to elucidate the risks for access site-related complications (ASCs) after percutaneous lower extremity revascularization and to evaluate the benefit of routine ultrasound-guided access (RUS) in decreasing ASCs.

Methods.—We reviewed all consecutive percutaneous revascularizations (percutaneous transluminal angioplasty or stent) performed for lower extremity atherosclerosis at our institution from 2002 to 2012. RUS began in September 2007. Primary outcome was any ASC (bleeding, groin or retroperitoneal hematoma, vessel rupture, or thrombosis). Multivariable logistic regression was used to determine predictors of ASC.

Results.—A total of 1371 punctures were performed on 877 patients (43% women; median age, 69 [interquartile range, 60- 78] years) for claudication (29%), critical limb ischemia (59%), or bypass graft stenosis (12%) with 4F to 8F sheaths. There were 72 ASCs (5%): 52 instances of bleeding or groin hematoma, nine pseudoaneurysms, eight retroperitoneal hematomas, two artery lacerations, and one thrombosis. ASCs were less frequent when RUS was used (4% vs 7%; $P = .02$). Multivariable predictors of ASC were age >75 years (odds ratio [OR], 2.0; 95% confidence interval [CI], 1.1-3.7; $P = .03$), congestive heart failure (OR, 1.9; 95% CI, 1.1-1.3; $P = .02$), preoperative warfarin use (OR, 2.0; 95% CI, 1.1-3.5; $P = .02$), and RUS (OR, 0.4; 95% CI, 0.2-0.7; $P < .01$). Vascular closure devices (VCDs) were not associated with lower rates of ASCs (OR, 1.1; 95% CI, 0.6-1.9; $P = .79$). RUS lowered ASCs in those >75 years (5% vs 12%; $P < .01$) but not in those taking warfarin preoperatively (10% vs 13%; $P = .47$). RUS did not decrease VCD failure (6% vs 4%; $P = .79$).

Conclusions.—We were able to decrease the rate of ASCs during lower extremity revascularization with the implementation of RUS. VCDs did not affect ASCs. Particular care should be taken with patients >75 years old, those with congestive heart failure, and those taking warfarin (Fig 1).

► Access site–related complications (ASCs) are common after percutaneous endovascular interventions and may result in prolonged hospital length of stay, patient discomfort, increased health care costs, and even increased mortality. Two previous multicenter randomized controlled trials have demonstrated fewer attempts, reduced time to access, higher first pass rates, and decreased risk of vascular access complications with ultrasound-guided access compared with fluoroscopic- and palpation-guided access. These trials were conducted within interventional cardiology and interventional radiology practices however, with interventions toward peripheral artery disease representing a minority of the procedures assessed.[1,2]

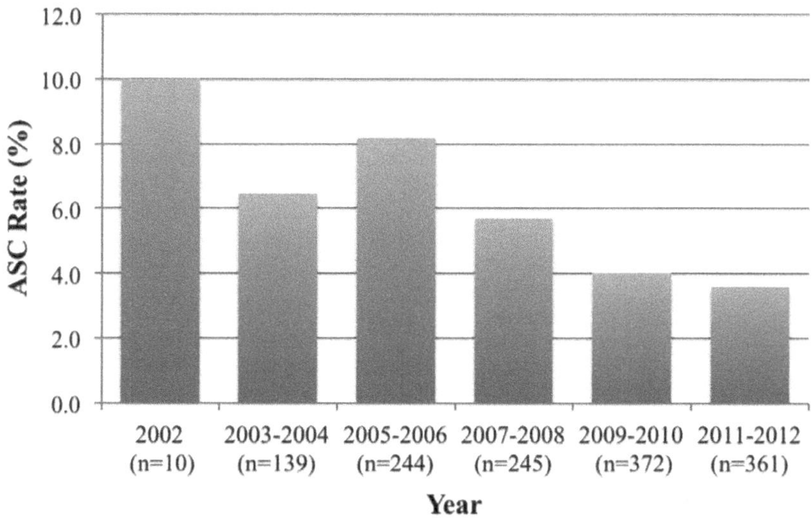

FIGURE 1.—Access site-related complication (*ASC*) rates by year of study. The total number of procedures per period is indicated in parentheses. Routine ultrasound-guided access (RUS) was initiated in September of 2007. (Reprinted from Lo RC, Fokkema MTM, Curran T, et al. Routine use of ultrasound-guided access reduces access site-related complications after lower extremity percutaneous revascularization. *J Vasc Surg*. 2015;61:405-412, with permission from the Society for Vascular Surgery.)

Lo et al have published on a topic that most vascular specialists may find intuitive: that ultrasound-guided access for common femoral arterial puncture with fluoroscopic confirmation to exclude a high puncture decreases the rate of ASCs following elective lower extremity percutaneous revascularization for claudication, critical limb ischemia, and stenosis or impending graft failure of an existing bypass graft (4% vs 7%, $P = 0.02$). Moreover, trending percutaneous vascular interventions over time, the number and proportion of punctures obtained under ultrasound guidance increased and ACSs continued to decrease each year (2007-2012) after the institution of routine ultrasound-guided access (Fig 1). Advanced age (> 75 years), congestive heart failure and preoperative warfarin use were independent risk factors for ASC by multivariate analysis, whereas gender, body mass index, tobacco use, and preoperative antiplatelet therapy did not have a significant association with ASC. Importantly, among the high-risk groups, ultrasound-guided access decreased ASC rates, specifically for elderly patients. The authors also went as far as to report that operator experience had no effect on the rate of ASC by comparing procedures between the first and second halves of the academic year. Finally, vascular closures devices (VCDs) were used in approximately half of patients in lieu of manual pressure. Not only was VCD use not associated with a decrease in ASC rates, but VCD failure was associated with an increase in ASC rates (15%). These failures were not influenced by the use of ultrasound-guided access.

Ultrasound-guided access should be considered standard of care for percutaneous endovascular procedures across disciplines. Although this study excluded revascularization procedures for acute limb ischemia, trauma, aneurysms, and the use of platforms > 8 Fr, it seems reasonable to extrapolate results to these more advanced cases and those cases of nontraditional access (ie, superficial femoral artery and brachial artery access). Education to this end and perhaps institutional standards will be increasingly important as the number of endovascular diagnostic procedures and interventions continues to increase.

D. Coleman, MD

References

1. Seto AH, Abu-Fadel MS, Sparling JM, et al. Real-time ultrasound guidance facilitates femoral artery access and reduces vascular complications: FAUST (Femoral Artery Access With Ultrasound Trial). *JACC Cardiovasc Interv.* 2010;3:751-758.
2. Gedikoglu M, Oguzkurt L, Gur S, Andic C, Sariturk C, Ozkan U. Comparison of ultrasound guidance with the traditional palpation and fluoroscopy method for the common femoral artery puncture. *Catheter Cardiovasc Interv.* 2013;82: 1187-1192.

Arm Veins versus Contralateral Greater Saphenous Veins for Lower Extremity Bypass Reconstruction: Preliminary Data of a Randomized Study

Linni K, Aspalter M, Butturini E, et al (PMU, Salzburg, Austria)
Ann Vasc Surg 29:551-559, 2015

Background.—The aim of this randomized study was to determine whether arm vein (AV) or contralateral greater saphenous vein (CGSV) is the better alternative vein source for lower extremity bypass reconstruction.

Methods.—Consecutive patients with absent ipsilateral greater saphenous vein undergoing lower extremity revascularization were allocated to group A (AV bypass) or B (CGSV bypass).

Results.—From 6, 2010, to 11, 2013, 64 patients (32 each group) were randomized. In all, 29 of 93 patients had to be excluded for various reasons.Median age was 76 years vs. 71 years ($P = 0.01$) for group A and B patients. There were no statistically significant differences regarding gender, cardiovascular risk factors, redo bypass procedures ($P = 0.77$), below-knee bypass procedures ($P = 0.61$), median bypass length ($P = 0.6$), and median length of incision on ipsilateral leg to perform anastomoses ($P = 0.2$) between group A and B patients, respectively. Incisions for vein harvest were longer in group A ($P = 0.003$). Overall surgical site infections (SSIs, $P = 1.0$) and SSI from vein harvest ($P = 1.0$) were equally distributed. No patient was lost to follow-up (17 vs. 18 months, $P = 0.74$). There was no statistically significant difference regarding primary ($P = 0.77$) and secondary ($P = 0.25$) patency rates at 1 year (group A: 52% vs. group B: 54% and group A: 72% vs. group B: 61%) and at 2 years (52%vs. 48%and 64%vs. 61%), respectively. There were 4 vs. 6

major amputations ($P = 0.23$) and 5 vs. 2 deaths ($P = 0.1$) in groups A and B during follow-up.

Conclusions.—Preliminary results suggest that both AV and CGSV may serve as a secondary vein bypass graft equally well.

▶ The dilemma of choosing between contralateral great saphenous vein (CGSV) versus arm vein (AV) for use as lower extremity bypass conduit is not uncommon. The situation may arise in redo situations in which the ipsilateral vein was used in a previous procedure on the same leg or when the vein was harvested for use in a remote anatomic location (usually for coronary bypass). Peripheral artery disease (PAD) is almost never a unilateral process, and CGSV harvest places a wound on an extremity that may be at risk for impaired wound healing while simultaneously eliminating the possibility of using that conduit if contralateral leg revascularization is required in the future. Conversely, arm vein harvest can be challenging from a technical perspective, potentially requiring a spliced vein graft if adequate length cannot be obtained from a single segment. Although the authors used a diameter cutpoint of 2.5 mm to define adequate vein conduit, providers considering a choice between these 2 conduit options might lean toward the largest diameter conduit available (likely CGSV more often than AV).

Above-knee popliteal bypass grafts were included in this analysis. Although autogenous conduit is preferred (and supported by evidence) in this location, many surgeons would potentially consider a prosthetic graft as a reasonable alternative to vein harvest (and related risk of wound complications) on an extremity other than the one being bypassed. An additional factor influencing the choice between prosthetic versus CGSV or AV conduit is the time commitment: exposure of the vein graft located in another extremity and closure at the end of the case can easily double the duration of the procedure, potentially increasing risk of infection and other complications. The fact that these investigators performed CGSV and AV bypass for above-knee popliteal artery bypasses indicates their commitment to achieving excellent outcomes. Their approach, which utilized 2 operative teams, has the advantage of avoiding prolonged procedure times but may not be feasible for many practitioners who lack the personnel or institutional commitment to support a 2-team approach.

The authors provide detailed descriptions of the vein harvest approaches, including the types of incisions and methods of dissection. It is interesting to note that continuous incisions were used to harvest AV, whereas skip incisions with intervening skin bridges were used to harvest CGSV. Graft orientation (ie, reversed vs in situ) was left to the discretion of the operating surgeon and may have had an impact on outcomes related to diameter mismatch between proximal and distal ends of the bypass graft with the inflow and target vessels. Participants in this study were randomized using sealed envelopes. Although the time of randomization was not specifically mentioned in the article, it must have occurred well in advance of the bypass procedure to allow appropriate IV access (allowing avoidance of arm intravenous access ipsilateral to planned AV harvest among participants randomized to this conduit).

Power calculations for this trial determined that more than 300 participants per group would be needed to achieve 80% power to detect an 11% or greater difference in patency between AV and CGSV. After more than 3 years since the study was initiated, approximately 10% of the targeted enrollment has been achieved. Given the pace, it is likely that the study will fail to achieve adequate power without transitioning to a multicenter design (unless the investigators have adequate persistence to continue at the current pace for several decades). They mention that their initial plan was to use a multicenter design, but lack of familiarity with both techniques among surgeons in Austria prevented this approach from moving forward. Perhaps it would be worthwhile to expand the study to collaborators in other countries; the question they are attempting to answer is certainly important enough to justify an international multicenter study.

M. Corriere, MD, MS

Comparison of risk factors for length of stay and readmission following lower extremity bypass surgery

Damrauer SM, Gaffey AC, DeBord Smith A, et al (Hosp of the Univ of Pennsylvania, Philadelphia; Brigham and Women's Hosp, Boston, MA)
J Vasc Surg 62:1192-1200, 2015

Objective.—Recent initiatives to improve health care quality have focused attention on length of stay (LOS) and readmission rates for surgical patients, yet these two outcomes may be inversely related. This study was designed to elucidate the risk factors for both outcomes and to clarify the relationship between them in patients undergoing lower extremity bypass (LEB).

Methods.—Peripheral arterial disease (PAD) patients who underwent LEB were identified from the 2007-2010 California State Inpatient Database. LOS and risk factors were analyzed using Poisson regression. Risk factors for 30-day readmission were analyzed using logistic regression.

Results.—There were 6307 patients who underwent LEB, and 1291 (20%) were readmitted. The average index LOS was 8.3 days for those who were readmitted and 5.5 days for those who were not ($P < .0001$) and was an independent risk factor for 30-day readmission. The significant factors with the largest effect estimates for increased LOS reflected disease severity and postoperative complications: emergency department admission; advanced PAD; postoperative pneumonia, respiratory failure, urinary tract infection, wound/graft infection, graft complication, and discharge to a nursing facility. Independent predictors of readmission, other than LOS, reflected underlying patient factors: advanced PAD, chronic lung disease, diabetes, renal failure, postoperative congestive heart failure, and discharge status. Age, Medicaid or private insurance, and low income were protective. Of the 1291 readmissions, 453 (35%) were for definitive complications.

Conclusions.—In patients undergoing LEB, LOS is primarily associated with the occurrence of postoperative complications, whereas 30-day readmission is largely explained by underlying patient illness. Additionally, increased LOS is an independent risk factor for readmission. These findings suggest that efforts to reduce both LOS and readmission will be complementary. Furthermore, they support the notion that both LOS and 30-day readmission rates should be risk-adjusted (Fig 2).

▶ The California State Inpatient Database (SID) was the data source for this analysis. The authors cite advantages of this data set as inclusion of a large, diverse geographic area with a well-contained health care delivery system where patient migration to out-of-state sites is unusual. These advantages are all legitimate but should also be regarded as caveats by providers outside California practicing in areas with distinctly different patient populations, demographics, and state-administered health care plans (this last point is particularly relevant because Medicaid coverage, a distinctly state-specific

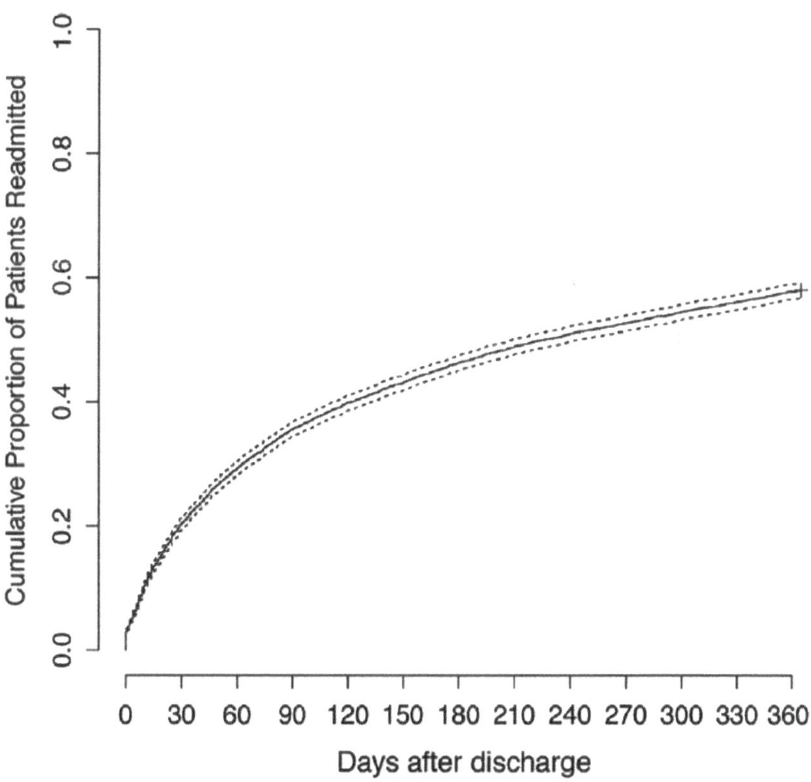

FIGURE 2.—Risk of readmission for the year following discharge after lower extremity bypass (LEB) surgery. The dashed lines represent 95% confidence intervals (CIs). (Reprinted from Damrauer SM, Gaffey AC, DeBord Smith A, et al. Comparison of risk factors for length of stay and readmission following lower extremity bypass surgery. *J Vasc Surg*. 2015;62:1192-1200, with permission from Elsevier.)

consideration, was found to be protective against readmission). The results therefore cannot be assumed representative of the United States or other geographic areas. Cost, convenience, availability, or other factors also may have contributed to selection of the California SID over larger, more extensive datasets. These limitations aside, this analysis provides useful information about risk factors associated with length of stay (LOS) and readmission as well as important insight into how these outcomes are related. The analytic approach included robust methodology, including Poisson regression and time-dependent covariates, and the results were both impressive and concerning. Twenty percent of patients were readmitted within 30 days, and nearly 60% were readmitted within 1 year. Interestingly, there appeared to be an inflection point where readmission risk leveled off between 60 and 90 days (Fig 2). Claudication was the most frequent primary diagnosis in this analysis, so these results therefore may not be consistent with series where critical limb ischemia is more predominant as the procedural indication (in other words, these readmission rates may be conservatively biased).

As alluded to in this article's discussion, LOS and 30-day readmission are not independent outcomes.[1-3] Providers making discharge decisions often struggle with the concern that these outcomes are reciprocal in nature (ie, pushing one lower may come at the expense of a corresponding increase in the other). Results of this study demonstrated, however, that increasing LOS is associated with increased risk of readmission. The results contradict the notion that a longer window of inpatient observation has potential benefit by allowing problems that might otherwise occur in the early post-discharge period to be identified sooner and preemptively addressed. The variables that were associated with LOS and readmission in this study reflect many scenarios where discharge might be delayed by severe disease at presentation, lack of insurance or other resources needed at the time of discharge, postoperative complications, or all of the above. Given these findings, the key to avoiding readmission might be more careful patient selection (particularly when claudication is the indication) and perhaps more aggressive follow-up during the first few months after the procedure. Heart failure was the only patient comorbidity independently associated with both LOS and readmission, suggesting that development of specific screening and management strategies directed toward this subgroup of patients might represent a risk reduction opportunity when they require lower extremity bypass.

M. Corriere, MD, MS

References

1. Bueno H, Ross JS, Wang Y, Chen J, et al. Trends in length of stay and short-term outcomes among Medicare patients hospitalized for heart failure, 1993–2006. *JAMA*. 2010;303:2141-2147.
2. Heidenreich PA, Sahay A, Kapoor JR, Pham MX, Massie B. Divergent trends in survival and readmission following a hospitalization for heart failure in the Veterans Affairs health care system 2002 to 2006. *J Am Coll Cardiol*. 2010;56:362-368.
3. O'Connor CM, Fiuzat M. Is rehospitalization after heart failure admission a marker of poor quality? Time for re-evaluation. *J Am Coll Cardiol*. 2010;56:369-371.

Differential Impact of Bypass Surgery and Angioplasty on Angiosome-Targeted Infrapopliteal Revascularization

Spillerova K, Biancari F, Leppäniemi A, et al (Helsinki Univ Central Hosp, Finland; Oulu Univ, Finland)

Eur J Vasc Endovasc Surg 49:412-419, 2015

Objective.—The aim of this study was to evaluate the impact of angiosome targeted revascularization according to the revascularization method.

Design.—Retrospective observational study.

Materials and Methods.—This study cohort comprised 744 consecutive patients who underwent infrapopliteal endovascular or surgical revascularization between January 2010 and July 2013. Differences in outcomes after bypass surgery and PTA were adjusted by estimating a propensity score, which was employed for one to one matching as well as adjusted analysis.

Results.—Cox proportional hazards analysis showed that angiosome-targeted revascularization (HR 1.29, 95% CI 1.02–1.65), bypass surgery (HR 1.79, 95% CI 1.41–2.27), C-reactive protein ≤10 mg/dL (HR 1.42, 95% CI 1.11–1.81), and the number of affected angiosomes (HR 0.85, 95% CI 0.74–0.98) were independent predictors of improved wound healing. When adjusted for the number of affected angiosomes and C-reactive protein ≤10 mg/dL, angiosome-targeted bypass surgery was associated with a significantly higher rate of wound healing than non-angiosome-targeted angioplasty (HR 2.27, 95% CI 1.61–3.20). This was confirmed in propensity score adjusted analysis (HR 1.72, 95% CI 1.35–2.16). Among patients who underwent angiosome-targeted revascularization, the propensity score adjusted analysis showed that bypass surgery was associated with a significantly better rate of wound healing (HR 154, 95% CI 1.09–2.16) but similar limb salvage rates when compared with angioplasty (HR 0.79, 95% CI 0.44–1.43).

Conclusion.—Rates of wound healing and limb salvage in patients with critical limb ischemia (CLI) were significantly better after angiosome-targeted revascularization, bypass surgery achieving significantly better wound healing than angioplasty (Fig 3).

▶ Providers choosing between revascularization alternatives (when alternatives exist) must often consider compromises among risk, invasiveness, and durability. Although establishing direct inline flow to the wound bed is always a key guiding principle in planning revascularization, patients with foot wounds commonly have multilevel disease that makes achievement of this goal unlikely with an "endovascular-first" approach. Providers may therefore face a difficult decision between performing an endovascular procedure that may be inadequate to achieve wound healing versus a more invasive surgical bypass that may be overkill. The former approach risks additional time and tissue loss and may lower the odds of a subsequent procedure's success, whereas the latter involves increased risk procedure-related adverse events in a patient population with

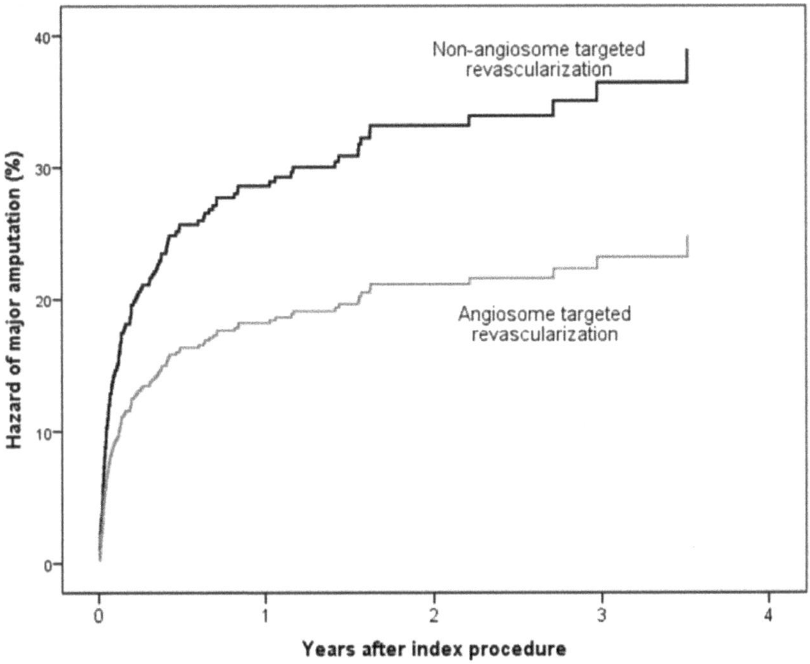

FIGURE 3.—Propensity score adjusted hazard of major amputation according to angiosome-targeted and non-targeted revascularization ($p = .010$, HR 0.637, 95% CI 0.452–0.897). (Reprinted from Spillerova K, Biancari F, Leppäniemi A, et al. Differential impact of bypass surgery and angioplasty on angiosome-targeted infrapopliteal revascularization. *Eur J Vasc Endovasc Surg*. 2015;49:412-419, with permission from European Society for Vascular Surgery.)

poor survival and a significant prevalence of comorbid conditions. Consistent with the approach of many providers who care for critical limb ischemia (CLI) and can offer either endovascular or surgical revascularization options, these authors favor an endovascular-first approach in the absence of unfavorable anatomic factors (such as long-segment occlusions or extensive atherosclerosis).

Among patients with CLI, angiosome-targeted revascularization comes into consideration for patients who have tissue loss and revascularization options that would primarily target different outflow vessels. Although the concept of angiosome-targeted revascularization makes sense, evidence supporting angiosome-specific approaches is scant. In propensity-adjusted analyses, this study identified associations between angiosome-targeted revascularization and improved amputation-free survival (Fig 3), although wound healing was not significantly different between approaches. Interestingly, when adjusted for propensity score and treatment method (bypass vs angioplasty) bypass surgery was also an independent predictor of a higher rate of wound healing. The authors attempted to control for selection bias using propensity score adjustment, it is important to remember that all patients who received a bypass were deemed appropriate candidates to have one. Although the methods indicate that patients who were demented, immobile, had extremely short life expectancy, or were not candidates for revascularization, it remains possible that some patients received nonangiosome targeted revascularization because of their operative risk, quality of the target angiosome vessel, available bypass conduit, or other factors.

These results support pursuit of angiosome-targeted therapy when possible, but this retrospective analysis leaves several important questions unanswered. Perioperative adverse events were not included among outcomes and are an important consideration, along with quality of available autogenous bypass conduit, degree of tissue loss, and qualitative characteristics of the lesion and target vessel. Although a randomized trial that included standardized medical management (medical therapy, by the way, was neither standardized nor mentioned in this analysis) would have potential to provide additional information to guide decision making, a randomized trial would likely be quite challenging to conduct due to lack of equipoise between randomization to angiosome-targeted versus nontargeted revascularization among patients who are candidates for either approach. In the meantime, outcomes from comparative effectiveness studies will remain important to providers and patients attempting to individualize CLI revascularization strategies.

M. Corriere, MD, MS

Outcomes of completion imaging for lower extremity bypass in the Vascular Quality Initiative

Woo K, Palmer OP, Weaver FA, et al (Univ of Southern California, Los Angeles)
J Vasc Surg 62:412-416, 2015

Objective.—The objective of this study was to determine the association of intraoperative completion imaging (CI) for lower extremity vein bypass to a below-knee target with primary patency in the Vascular Quality Initiative.

Methods.—The Vascular Quality Initiative database was queried from January 2003 to October 2013 for lower extremity bypass (LEB) procedures that were elective, had an indication of occlusive disease, used a single-segment greater saphenous vein conduit, and had a below-knee target. LEBs with inflow arteries above the knee and below the knee were included. LEBs with concomitant endovascular procedures were excluded. CI was defined as completion angiography, completion duplex ultrasound, or both. The end points were primary patency at discharge and at 1 year. Multivariable analysis was performed controlling for patient demographics, comorbidities, bypass characteristics, and center.

Results.—Of 14,284 LEBs that were performed during the study period, 3147 satisfied the inclusion and exclusion criteria. Of 1457 (46%) that underwent CI, 287 (20%) underwent duplex ultrasound, 1116 (77%) underwent angiography, and 54 (3.7%) underwent both duplex ultrasound and angiography. There were more patients in the CI group with a history of smoking and a bypass graft crossing the knee. There was no difference in primary patency at discharge between the two groups (CI, 93.2% vs no CI, 93.8%; $P = .52$). Of the patients who underwent CI, the discharge primary patency was 95.1% for completion duplex ultrasound vs 92.8% for completion angiography ($P = .17$). On multivariable analysis, there was no significant association of CI with discharge primary patency ($P = .69$). The 1-year primary patency was 63% in the CI group vs 68% in the no CI group ($P = .051$). The 1-year primary patency was 60% for the duplex ultrasound group vs 65% for the angiography group ($P = .61$). On multivariable analysis, there was no significant association of CI with 1-year primary patency ($P = .69$).

Conclusions.—In electively performed LEBs using single-segment saphenous vein to a below-knee target artery for occlusive disease, CI does not influence primary graft patency at discharge or at 1 year.

▶ The early identification and correction of technical defects in bypass grafts can influence short- and long-term graft performance. Previous reports have demonstrated that routine intraoperative completion imaging (CI) can detect correctible defects in up to 8% of patients.[1] On the other hand, results from other studies have not identified benefits of intraoperative imaging over simpler methods such as palpation or continuous wave Doppler evaluation in predicting subsequent graft-related outcomes.[2]

This study uses the database from the Vascular Quality Initiative (VQI) to try to answer the value question of intraoperative imaging in elective infrapopliteal bypass procedures using single-segment vein conduits. Short-term and mid-term (1-year) patency rates were evaluated. Almost half of the procedures ($n = 1457$) underwent CI. Multivariable analysis showed that CI did not influence discharge or 1-year patency rates.

One of the major limitations of the VQI database is that it does not differentiate between selective imagers and routine imagers; therefore, potentially resulting in bias in favor of disadvantaged conduits that underwent CI and achieved improved patency. In addition, the study does not provide detail about the proportion of patients in which CI resulted in bypass revision. With the limited information provided in the VQI registry about the intraoperative findings of completion imaging, the study failed to prove the value of this additional step. However, it is important to recognize that this study, as is, is a descriptive study of physician behavior toward CI rather than a comparative effectiveness study.

Y. Duwayri, MD

References

1. Mills JL, Fujitani RM, Taylor SM. Contribution of routine intraoperative completion arteriography to early infrainguinal bypass patency. *Am J Surg*. 1992;164:506-511.
2. Dalman RL, Harris EJ, Zarins CK. Is completion arteriography mandatory after reversed-vein bypass grafting? *J Vasc Surg*. 1996;23:637-644.

Outcomes of infrainguinal bypass determined by age in the Vascular Study Group of New England

Dermody M, for the Vascular Study Group of New England (Lancaster General Health Physicians Surgical Group, PA; et al)

J Vasc Surg 62:83-92, 2015

Background.—Many believe extremes of age correlate with poorer outcomes in treatment for lower extremity peripheral arterial disease (PAD). We hypothesized that the youngest patients would have significantly poorer outcomes compared with older cohorts due to the precocious nature of their PAD.

Methods.—We studied all patients in the Vascular Study Group of New England database undergoing infrainguinal bypass for PAD between 2003 and 2013. Age was grouped by <50 years, 50 to 79 years, and ≥80 years. Our primary outcomes were 1-year freedom from a major adverse limb event (MALE), defined as ipsilateral amputation or need for secondary intervention, and amputation-free survival. A second analysis was performed to analyze the subgroup of patients aged <50 years with critical limb ischemia (CLI), which included a Cox regression model to determine risk factors for MALE or death at 1 year.

Results.—Of 5265 patients who were treated with infrainguinal bypass for PAD, 324 (6.2%) were aged <50 years. The mean age was 44.6 years, and 66.4% were male. The proportion of African Americans was significantly higher in the youngest age group (<50 years: 6.8% vs 50-79 years: 3.5%, $P = .002$; vs ≥80 years: 3.5%, $P = .013$). More bypasses were done for claudication than acute limb ischemia in patients aged <50 years (33.3% vs 11.4%). More vein grafts were used vs prosthetic (<50 years: 72.1% vs 50-79 years: 65.9%, $P = .024$; vs ≥80 years: 62.6%, $P = .002$). Fewer concomitant proximal procedures were performed compared with the older groups (<50 years: 37.7% vs 50-79 years: 51.1%, $P < .001$; vs ≥80 years: 39.5%, $P = .045$). More young patients returned to the operating room within their initial hospitalization for early graft thrombosis (<50 years: 5.6% vs 50-79 years: 2.9%, $P = .001$; vs ≥80 years: 2.4%, $P = .009$) and revision (<50 years: 4.7% vs 50-79 years: 2.2%, $P = .012$; vs ≥80 years: 1.4%, $P = .002$) compared with the older patients. Overall, MALE-free survival was similar across age groups ($P = .323$), as were patency and amputation rates. When considering only patients with CLI, MALE-free survival in the youngest patients was again similar ($P = .171$) but with significantly more major amputations at 1 year ($P = .022$).

Conclusions.—For patients aged <50 undergoing infrainguinal bypass surgery, this large series demonstrates similar overall medium-term graft-related outcomes compared with older cohorts. Further, although the youngest patients with CLI have similar MALEs, their amputation rates are higher than in older cohorts (Tables 1 and 3).

▶ When interpreting the results presented from this analysis of infrainguinal lower extremity bypasses (LEB) from the Vascular Study Group of New

TABLE 1.—Patients Demographics by Age

Variables	<50 Years	50-79 Years	P Values[a]	≥80 Years	P Values[a]
Patients, No.[b]	324	4058		883	
Age, mean years	44.56	65.82		84.09	
Height, mean cm	172.94	171.44		168.38	
Weight, mean kg	85.57	81.07		70.71	
Male, No. (%)	215 (66.4)	2781 (68.5)	.227	498 (56.4)	.001
Race, No. (%)					
White	291 (89.8)	3835 (94.5)	.001	840 (95.1)	.001
Black	22 (6.8)	140 (3.5)	.002	31 (3.5)	.013
Asian	0	4 (0.1)		0	
Other	11 (3.4)	79 (2)		12 (1.4)	
BLE symptoms, No. (%)					
Claudication	108 (33.3)	1146 (28.2)	.008	93 (10.5)	<.001
CLI (rest pain, tissue loss)	171 (52.8)	2501 (61.6)	.001	703 (79.6)	<.001
Acute ischemia	37 (11.4)	305 (7.5)	.004	72 (8.2)	.018
Diabetes, No. (%)	135 (41.7)	2119 (52.2)	<.001	401 (45.4)	.137
Dialysis, No. (%)	20 (6.2)	291 (7.2)	.075	48 (5.4)	.097
COPD, No. (%)	57 (17.6)	1150 (28.3)	<.001	201 (22.8)	.03
CAD, No. (%)	62 (19.1)	1459 (36)	<.001	343 (38.9)	<.001
CHF, No. (%)	16 (4.9)	643 (15.9)	<.001	208 (23.6)	<.001
Prior PCI or CABG, No. (%)	45 (13.9)	1365 (33.6)	<.001	258 (29.2)	<.001
Hypertension, No. (%)	206 (63.6)	3544 (87.3)	<.001	790 (89.5)	<.001
Smoking history, No. (%)	290 (89.5)	3561 (87.8)	.201	585 (66.3)	<.001
Prior PVI, No. (%)					
Total interventions	95 (29.3)	1272 (31.3)	.245	196 (22.3)	.007
Ipsilateral inflow PVI	31 (9.6)	551 (13.6)	.041	78 (8.8)	.734
Ipsilateral infrainguinal PVI	58 (17.9)	584 (14.4)	.102	108 (12.2)	.014

BLE, Bilateral lower extremities; *CABG*, coronary artery bypass graft; *CAD*, coronary artery disease; *CHF*, congestive heart failure; *CLI*, critical limb ischemia; *COPD*, chronic obstructive pulmonary disease; *PCI*, percutaneous coronary intervention; *PVI*, percutaneous vascular intervention.

[a]Missing in variables were not included in analysis, percentage was referred to column percentage; *P* values are from the Fisher exact test (all values converted to categoric variables), and $P < .05$ is statistically significant.

[b]Patients receiving bypass for popliteal aneurysms were eliminated; the first procedure per patient was counted in the analysis.

TABLE 3.—Secondary Outcomes by Age at the 1-Year Follow-up

Secondary Outcomes[a]	<50 Years, No. (%)	50-79 Years, No. (%)	P Values[b]	≥80 Years, No. (%)	P Values[b]
Patency					
Primary	158/220 (71.8)	1953/2706 (72.2)	.938	333/470 (70.9)	.857
Primary-assisted	14/220 (6.4)	243/2706 (9)	.216	39/470 (8.3)	.444
Secondary	5/220 (2.3)	64/2706 (2.4)	1	7/470 (1.5)	.534
Occluded	43/220 (19.6)	446/2706 (16.5)	.259	91/470 (19.4)	1
Major amputation	28/306 (9.2)	250/3801 (6.6)	.097	55/772 (7.1)	.257
Mortality	13/219 (5.9)	268/2824 (9.5)	.089	147/573 (25.7)	<.001

[a]Patients receiving bypass for popliteal aneurysms were eliminated; the first procedure per patient was counted in the analysis.

[b]Missing in variables were not included in analysis, percentage was referred to column percentage. *P* values are from the Fisher exact test, and $P < .05$ is statistically significant.

England (VSGNE), several important caveats warrant consideration. This study was not a randomized trial; biases therefore likely affected patient and procedure selection and were probably most influential at the extremes of age. From a symptomatic presentation perspective, patients aged <50 years with claudication likely have a more severe form of disease (and perhaps the accompanying risk factors), whereas those >80 have obviously survived into old age and remain functional enough to seek care for their symptoms. In a one way of thinking, patients >80 years old versus those <50 years old in this study likely represent the best of the best and the worst of the worst, respectively, in terms of both disease severity and selection bias among patients undergoing LEB for claudication. Among patients <50 years old, a lower threshold for performing LEB might have existed due to unique considerations in this age group, such as employment and the potentially longer duration of symptoms over the patient's lifetime. Conversely, patients >80 may face more barriers to receiving LEB, some of which may be unjustified and/or unfair. Providers may be willing to accept greater functional impairment in octogenarians, perceive them as higher risk for procedure-related complications, and wonder whether a major procedure should be undertaken given their anticipated survival. These biases are apparent from the study results; patients <50 had a much higher prevalence of claudication as their indication for LEB (33% vs 10% among those >80; Table 1).

The introduction of this article includes the assertion that "the literature on PAD [peripheral artery disease] is outdated," with reference to the fact that much of the evidence used to guide PAD care was published more than a decade ago. This may be a bit of an overstatement because it implies that previous findings based on sound data must be reproven periodically after an arbitrary period of time to determine whether they remain valid. This rationale is questionable in the absence of novel factors that might affect the outcomes or comparators based on existing evidence (such as significant advances in medical therapy or procedural interventions). Readers should also note that other studies (in addition to those referenced in this article) suggest inferior LEB outcomes in younger patients, although some include aortofemoral bypass (which was excluded from this analysis).[1-3] Functional outcomes were conspicuously absent from the end points included in this study, a major limitation for an analysis in which claudication was the most common indication for LEB in the <50-year-old subgroup of interest. Anticipated amputation-free survival would be high among claudicant patients, even if their interventions failed, and this end point therefore represents only part of the picture. A subgroup analysis limited to patients with critical limb ischemia was also included, but exclusion of all patients with incomplete 1 year follow-up from analysis might have resulted in amputation-free survival estimates that were still conservatively biased.

Although results for younger versus older patients were similar at 1 year for many outcomes included in this analysis (Table 3), the results do not necessarily mean that an age-specific perspective should be abandoned during treatment selection. Considering that a patient <50 years would have similar outcomes to one >80 years perhaps should inspire hesitation when the LEB is elective and being performed for claudication. If anticipated survival is longer for patients < 50 years but the patency outcomes are no better, younger patients undergoing LEB might therefore expect a higher rate of graft failure and/or repeat intervention over their lifetime, particularly if failure is accompanied by progression to more severe symptoms. Conversely, these findings suggest that the higher rate of prosthetic grafts used in elderly patients might be reasonable considering their shorter anticipated survival.

M. Corriere, MD, MS

References

1. Green RM, Abbott WM, Matsumoto T, et al. Prosthetic above-knee femoropopliteal bypass grafting: five-year results of a randomized trial. *J Vasc Surg*. 2000;31: 417-425.
2. Olsen PS, Gustafsen J, Rasmussen L, Lorentzen JE. Long-term results after arterial surgery for arteriosclerosis of the lower limbs in young adults. *Eur J Vasc Surg*. 1988;2:15-18.
3. Reed AB, Conte MS, Donaldson MC, Mannick JA, Whittemore AD, Belkin M. The impact of patient age and aortic size on the results of aortobifemoral bypass grafting. *J Vasc Surg*. 2003;37:1219-1225.

Outcomes of lower extremity revascularization among the hemodialysis dependent

Fallon JM, for the Vascular Study Group of New England (Dartmouth-Hitchcock Med Ctr, Lebanon, NH; et al)

J Vasc Surg 62:1183-1191, 2015

Objective.—Optimal patient selection for lower extremity revascularization remains a clinical challenge among the hemodialysis-dependent (HD). The purpose of this study was to examine contemporary real world open and endovascular outcomes of HD patients to better facilitate patient selection for intervention.

Methods.—A regional multicenter registry was queried between 2003 and 2013 for HD patients (N = 689) undergoing open surgical bypass (n = 295) or endovascular intervention (n = 394) for lower extremity revascularization. Patient demographics and comorbidities were recorded. The primary outcome was overall survival. Secondary outcomes included graft patency, freedom from major adverse limb events, and amputation-free survival (AFS). Multivariate analysis was performed to identify independent risk factors for death and amputation.

Results.—Among the 689 HD patients undergoing lower extremity revascularization, 66% were male, and 83% were white. Ninety percent of revascularizations were performed for critical limb ischemia and 8% for claudication. Overall survival at 1, 2, and 5 years survival remained low at 60%, 43%, and 21%, respectively. Overall 1- and 2-year AFS was 40% and 17%. Mortality accounted for the primary mode of failure for both open bypass (78%) and endovascular interventions (80%) at two years. Survival, AFS, and freedom from major adverse limb event outcomes did not differ significantly between revascularization techniques.

At 2 years, endovascular patency was higher than open bypass (76% vs 26%; 95% confidence interval [CI], 0.28-0.71; $P = .02$). Multivariate analysis identified age ≥80 years (hazard ratio [HR], 1.9; 95% CI, 1.4-2.5; $P < .01$), indication of rest pain or tissue loss (HR, 1.8; 95% CI, 1.3-2.6; $P < .01$), preoperative wheelchair/bedridden status (HR, 1.5; 95% CI, 1.1-2.1; $P < .01$), coronary artery disease (HR, 1.5; 95% CI, 1.2-1.9; $P < .01$), and chronic obstructive pulmonary disease (HR, 1.4; 95% CI, 1.1-1.8; $P = .01$) as independent predictors of death. The presence of three or more risk factors resulted in predicted 1-year mortality of 64%.

Conclusions.—Overall survival and AFS among HD patients remains poor, irrespective of revascularization strategy. Mortality remains the primary driver for these findings and justifies a prudent approach to patient selection. Focus for improved results should emphasize predictors of survival to better identify those most likely to benefit from revascularization (Fig 5, Table 4).

▶ The results of this study are sobering in terms of both the outcomes reported and the seeming lack of meaningful interval improvement in this "contemporary" (as the authors put it) analysis relative to previous series. Data for this study came from the Vascular Study Group of New England (VSGNE), and this analysis is a great example of why quality registries like the VSGNE (and overarching Vascular Quality Initiative) are important. Quality registries allow health care providers to overcome the negative publication bias that might prevent an analysis such as this, in which the results do not inspire celebration, from being published from a single-center series. These results suggest that

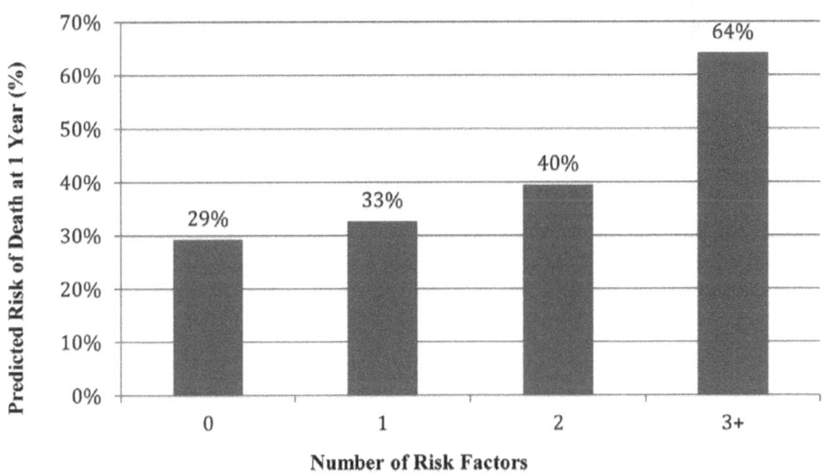

FIGURE 5.—Predicted risk of 1-year mortality by number of risk factors present. (Reprinted from Fallon JM, for the Vascular Study Group of New England. Outcomes of lower extremity revascularization among the hemodialysis dependent. *J Vasc Surg*. 2015;62:1183-1191, with permission from the Society for Vascular Surgery.)

TABLE 4.—Cox Proportional Hazard Regression Model for Death in Patients Without Amputation, Overall Cohort (N = 512)

Variable	HR	95% CI	*P* Value
Age ≥80	1.9	1.4-2.5	<.01
Any CAD	1.5	1.2-1.9	<.01
Any COPD	1.4	1.1-1.8	.01
Preoperative ambulatory status - wheelchair/bedridden	1.5	1.1-2.1	.01
Indication - rest pain/tissue loss	1.8	1.3-2.5	<.01

CAD, Coronary artery disease; *CI*, confidence interval; *COPD*, chronic obstructive pulmonary disease; *HR*, hazard ratio.
Reprinted from Fallon JM, for the Vascular Study Group of New England. Outcomes of lower extremity revascularization among the hemodialysis dependent. *J Vasc Surg*. 2015;62:1183-1191, with permission from the Society for Vascular Surgery.

overutilization of revascularization among hemodialysis-dependent patients warrants critical appraisal. This is an important observation that has been validated in other recent studies[1,2] and is likely to spark heated debate related to treatment selection for a patient population with significant comorbidity and poor survival.

Mortality was the primary mode of revascularization failure in this analysis, with a 2-year amputation-free survival of 17%. The authors concluded that these results "justify a prudent approach to patient selection" and suggest that their risk models for death and failed limb salvage may help to identify "when to avoid revascularization entirely and consider primary amputation or continued medical or palliative therapy." Although the VSGNE deserves commendation for publishing this analysis, which is likely to prompt controversial and difficult discussion, applying population-based analyses to treatment choices for individual patients is often challenging. This is particularly true for critical limb ischemia (CLI) in hemodialysis, where the stakes are high and none of the available options are particularly desirable. Medical or palliative therapy for patients with CLI, particularly those with tissue loss, is hardly an attractive alternative in most cases. Palliative care specialists are often in short supply, and many patients who initially opt for a palliative management strategy eventually present to the emergency department when symptoms worsen or another provider is uncomfortable accepting responsibility for failing to escalate care. Palliative care therefore often proves to be a resource-intensive experiment that is short-lived and fails due to pain, sleeplessness, or a wound that progresses or becomes infected. When palliative options are not acceptable, patients and providers face a choice between primary amputation and revascularization; this analysis suggests that the latter may be overkill in some patients.

Given that mortality was the most common cause for loss of amputation-free survival (rather than graft thrombosis or amputation in the setting of a patent revascularization), it is not clear that patients undergoing revascularization did not benefit from symptomatic and/or functional perspectives between the procedure and their death. Although a 40% 1-year amputation-free survival rate is too low to justify offering all patients on hemodialysis a leg revascularization, it is also too high to justify the conclusion that amputation and palliative medical management are the only options that should be considered for these patients. The multivariable model from this study may provide some guidance for patients with PAD on hemodialysis regarding treatment choices and expectations (Table 4); the key considerations will be where to draw the line in terms of expected survival and what alternative management should be pursued if revascularization is not. The best approach to this difficult conversation should not be based on selecting the acceptable 1-year mortality cutpoint between 29% and 64% (Fig 5), but instead on a conversation with the patient centered on his or her quality of life, functional status, and individual goals and values.

M. Corriere, MD, MS

References

1. Kumada Y, Nogaki H, Ishii H, et al. Clinical outcome after infrapopliteal bypass surgery in chronic hemodialysis patients with critical limb ischemia. *J Vasc Surg.* 2015;61:400-404.
2. Kodama A, Sugimoto M, Kuma S, Okazaki J, Mii S, Komori K. Clinical outcomes after infrainguinal bypass grafting for critical limb ischaemia in patients with dialysis-dependent end-stage renal failure. *Eur J Vasc Endovasc Surg.* 2014;48: 695-702.

Postoperative complications after common femoral endarterectomy

Nguyen B-N, Amdur RL, Abugideiri M, et al (George Washington Univ, DC)
J Vasc Surg 61:1489-1494, 2015

Background.—Common femoral endarterectomy (CFE) for limited arterial occlusive disease is considered a fairly low-risk operation of short duration. This study investigated the timing of 30-day outcomes as they related to hospital discharge and predicted the risk of operative mortality of this procedure.

Methods.—All patients in the National Surgical Quality Improvement Program database who underwent isolated CFE between 2005 and 2010 were selected for the test sample. We identified postoperative mortality and morbidities occurring before and after hospital discharge. A risk calculator for 30-day mortality, developed in the test sample using logistic regression, was validated in a new sample of cases from 2011 to 2012.

Results.—A total of 1843 CFEs reported from 2005 to 2010 met the inclusion and exclusion criteria. The average operative time was 146 ± 69.5 minutes (median, 133; interquartile range, 98-179 minutes), and 10% of patients needed to return to the operating room. The average length of stay was 4 ± 7.5 days (median, 3; interquartile range, 2-5 days); 91% of patients were discharged ≤1 week of surgery. Occurrences of cardiovascular events, renal dysfunction, and pulmonary complication were relatively low. There was 3.4% mortality and 8% wound-related complications, 30% and 86% of which occurred after hospital discharge, respectively. Overall, there was a 15% risk of combined mortality/morbidity, and >60% of these events occurred after discharge. The independent predictors of 30-day mortality were age, nonindependent functional status, preoperative dialysis, sepsis, emergency status, and American Society of Anesthesiologists Physical Status Classification 4 or 5, and the association between risk strata and death in the validation sample was strong ($\varphi = 0.29$) and significant ($P < .001$).

Conclusions.—CFE is not as "benign" a procedure as previously believed. The risks of death and wound complications are not insignificant, and a high percentage of these complications occurred after patients were discharged from the hospital. Patients should be carefully selected, especially in the elderly population, and close postoperative follow-up should be considered.

▶ Although common femoral endarterectomy (CFE) is often viewed as a less invasive and lower risk alternative to a distal bypass, these results reinforce the notion that this procedure is neither minor nor low risk. The 10% rate of reoperation was particularly impressive among outcomes considering the complex and resource-intensive nature of managing groin wound complications. These results may fuel the growing enthusiasm for endovascular common femoral artery intervention, including common femoral stenting. Many providers have traditionally regarded the common femoral artery as off limits for endovascular treatment (barring unusual circumstances), primarily because of concerns related to the dynamic changes that occur with hip flexion and during ambulation, resulting in stent deformation and related concerns for deep femoral artery occlusion in the setting of stent thrombosis. As difficult as groin complications can be to manage, this challenge would probably preferred over deep femoral artery thrombosis among providers who manage both problems.

Only 9% of wound complications occurred during the first week after CFE, meaning that the vast majority was identified after hospital discharge. Although the authors repeatedly advocate close follow-up based on the study findings, this strategy addresses earlier detection of complications but does not provide an actionable strategy for preventing them. Rotational muscle flaps are sometimes considered for preemptive avoidance of groin wound complications, but the subgroup analysis of the minority of patients who had this additional procedure performed at the time of CFE experienced a higher complication rate. It is unclear whether the rotational muscle flaps were performed in the setting of redo groin exposures or other circumstances that would prompt consideration of this more involved approach to coverage and closure. Drain use, which is another predictor of groin wound complications, was also omitted from this analysis. Lack of anatomic and technical details related to the procedure are a commonly cited limitation of the American College of Surgeons National Surgery Quality Improvement (NSQIP) data file. Anesthesia type has been identified as a predictor of mortality following for lower extremity revascularization procedures within NSQIP[1] but was not included as a covariate in this analysis.

M. Corriere, MD, MS

Reference

1. Ghanami RJ, Hurie J, Andrews JS, et al. Anesthesia-based evaluation of outcomes of lower extremity vascular bypass procedures. *Ann Vasc Surg*. 2013;27:199-207.

Results of combined vascular reconstruction and free flap transfer for limb salvage in patients with critical limb ischemia

Meyer A, Goller K, Horch RE, et al (Univ Hosp Erlangen, Germany)

J Vasc Surg 61:1239-1248, 2015

Objective.—Combined vascular reconstruction and free flap transfer has been established in centers as a feasible therapeutic option in cases with critical limb ischemia (CLI) and large tissue defects otherwise destined for major amputation. However, the number of patients treated with this combined approach is limited, and data regarding long-term follow-up and functional outcome are scarce. We therefore report our 10-year experience in free flap transplantation after vascular reconstruction as a last attempt for limb salvage, with special emphasis of complication rate, limb salvage, and postoperative mobility.

Methods.—CLI patients undergoing combined vascular reconstruction and consequent free flap transfer from 2003 to 2013 were retrospectively observed. Of 80 cases in total, patients with traumatic and oncologic indications were excluded; 33 (mean age, 66 years; range, 51-82 years) of these cases were performed for limb salvage and were included in this study. Long-term follow-up was possible in 32 of 33 patients (mean, 58 months; range, 2-126 months).

Results.—Thirty-three patients were analyzed. We performed arterial revascularization with 9 arteriovenous loops, 23 bypass grafts (10 popliteal-pedal, 9 femoral-crural, and 4 femoral-popliteal), and 1 venous interposition graft. For defect coverage, tissue transfer was comprised of six different flap entities (10 latissimus dorsi, 2 gracilis, 1 anterior lateral thigh, 7 rectus abdominis, 11 radialis, and 2 greater omentum flaps). Complications occurred in 16 of 33 patients (49%). Early complications included eight acute occlusions of arterial reconstructions; major bleedings were seen in eight patients as well. There were two flap losses and one major amputation in the early postoperative period. No in-hospital deaths were observed. Late results revealed a limb salvage rate of 87% after 1 year and 83% after 5 years. Amputation-free survival was 87% after 1 year and 75% after 5 years. Overall survival was 100% and 87% after 1 year and 5 years, respectively. Follow-up showed 42% of patients with no limitations in ambulation, 54% with maintained preoperative ambulatory status, and one bedridden patient.

Conclusions.—The combined approach for limb salvage in CLI patients is associated with excellent results in limb salvage and functional outcome in patients who would otherwise be candidates for major amputation, despite an initially elevated complication rate. The option of combined

revascularization with free tissue transfer should be evaluated in all mobile patients with CLI, large tissue defects, and exposed tendon or bone structures before major amputation. However, further studies are required to support these results.

▶ Although the clinical effectiveness of open revascularization is often judged by bypass graft patency, the most important outcomes in patients with for critical limb ischemia (CLI) are limb salvage and restoring mobility. Patients with large ischemic tissue defects in the foot are frequently denied revascularization because of the low likelihood of healing by secondary intention alone. Limb salvage carries improved long-term mortality and health-related quality of life compared with primary amputation.

The study is a retrospective review of a small number (33) of CLI patient with large tissue defects who underwent combined revascularization and free flap tissue coverage of the ischemic wounds. The procedures were done in 1 or 2 stages. Free flap arterial perfusion was based on an end-to-side anastomosis to the saphenous vein bypass graft conduit or an end-to-end anastomosis to the arterial end of a saphenous vein arteriovenous (AV) loop. Venous outflow was dependent on a tibial vein or the venous limb of the AV loop. The operative candidates were carefully selected, and patients who were nonambulatory or with severe comorbidities were not offered the combined procedures. Early reoperation was necessary in half the patients for early flap compromise. However, early flap loss occurred in only 2 patients and the 5-year limb salvage rate was exemplary at 83%.

Despite the relatively small number of patients in this series, the high early complication rate and lengthy initial operations, the study shows a highly effective approach in the management of challenging ischemic wounds in CLI patients. Compared with similar previous series, the limb salvage rates are slightly improved due to the highly selective approach this group has taken in offering these procedures. Revascularization procedures with prosthetic grafts and endovascular means were not offered, likely contributing to the improved long-term outcome as well.

In summary, CLI patients with extensive tissue loss should be considered for a combined multidisciplinary approach of free flap coverage (with revascularization) if vacuum-assisted closure is not thought to be possible. Careful selection is essential, and management of early complications should allow for an excellent long-term outcome.

Y. Duwayri, MD

Spliced Arm Vein Grafts Are a Durable Conduit for Lower Extremity Bypass

McGinigle KL, Pascarella L, Shortell CK, et al (Duke Univ, Durham, NC)

Ann Vasc Surg 29:716-721, 2015

Background.—Many patients with peripheral vascular disease (PAD) requiring revascularization do not have adequate ipsilateral great saphenous vein (GSV) for constructing a bypass because of intrinsic vein disease or prior harvesting for limb or coronary bypass. Prosthetic conduits have poor long-term patency, especially for distal bypass. With advancing endovascular sophistication, tibial angioplasty may be a good revascularization option, but we hypothesize that using spliced arm vein for distal lower extremity bypass is still a well-tolerated and more durable solution.

Methods.—A retrospective chart review was conducted of all PAD patients undergoing lower extremity bypass or tibial angioplasty for lifestyle-limiting claudication or critical limb ischemia at a single institution over a 7-year period. Statistical analysis was conducted by Kaplan–Meier survival analysis and Cox proportional hazards model. Statistical significance was set at $P = 0.05$.

Results.—From 2005 to 2012, there were 120 patients who underwent infrageniculate revascularization with conduit other than GSV. Over half of the patients (66 patients, 71.2% male, mean age 62 years) underwent bypass operations using arm vein conduit, and 88% of those bypasses were to tibial vessels. Patency was 100% at 1 year and 85% at 2 years. There was no impact on patency or amputation rate based on the source of vein or the number of splices. Forty-three patients underwent tibial angioplasty and patency was 70% at 1 year and 50% at 2 years.

Conclusions.—When GSV is not available, spliced arm vein grafts provide durable lower extremity revascularization with favorable patency and limb preservation rates. Spliced arm vein grafts should be considered over prosthetic grafts and angioplasty alone in patients with distal occlusive disease (Table 3).

▶ This study exemplifies many of the challenges inherent to conducting comparative effectiveness research on lower extremity revascularization outcomes. The cohort for this study was defined based on a combination of procedural and anatomic characteristics; analyses included both claudicants and patients with critical limb ischemia and both single and spliced vein conduit bypasses to popliteal, tibial, and pedal targets (Table 3). A technical description is given for the approach to bypass (including vein harvest and spliced graft creation), but none is provided for the endovascular procedures. Approximately 75% of patients in the tibial angioplasty group had a femoral-popliteal intervention at the same time, but the details (in terms of exactly which treatments were performed in addition to the tibial angioplasty) are not included. Medical management, a key determinant of patency and survival outcomes, was not described or analyzed. The resulting array of interventions, targets, and indications makes it challenging to draw definitive conclusions from treatment comparisons, but it is nonetheless informative to consider the outcomes associated

TABLE 3.—Comparison of the Inflow Vessels and Distal Target Vessels

	Single Arm Vein Bypass	Spliced Arm Vein Bypass	Angioplasty	*P* Value
Inflow vessel				
Common femoral artery (%)	78.3	86.0	27.5	0.000
Profunda femoris artery (%)	13.0	11.6	0	0.059
Above-knee popliteal artery (%)	8.7	2.3	72.5	0.000
Target vessel				
Below-knee popliteal artery (%)	4.4	16.3	4.6	0.097
Posterior tibial artery (%)	47.8	46.5	44.2	0.080
Peroneal artery (%)	8.7	18.8	20.9	0.443
Anterior tibial artery (%)	17.4	16.3	30.2	0.246
Dorsalis pedis artery (%)	21.7	2.3	0	0.461

Reprinted from McGinigle KL, Pascarella L, Shortell CK, et al. Spliced arm vein grafts are a durable conduit for lower extremity bypass. *Ann Vasc Surg*. 2015;29:716-721, with permission from Elsevier.

with use of arm vein grafts from a group of investigators experienced with this technique.

Spliced arm vein bypasses outnumbered single-segment arm vein bypasses by nearly 2 to 1 in this retrospective study, highlighting the importance of conduit length (which can be a disadvantage when using arm vein vs leg vein). Many providers would think twice about performing a bypass to a tibial target with single-segment ipsilateral great saphenous vein for claudication, let alone an arm vein conduit potentially requiring a spliced graft (as described in this study). The 3-mm diameter cutpoint used by the authors to define suitable vein conduit would certainly be acceptable to most surgeons who perform lower extremity bypass, but many providers would likely also accept 2.5-mm conduit, particularly if this flexibility meant the difference between using ipsilateral great saphenous vein (GSV) versus conduit from a separate location. When ipsilateral GSV is inadequate, another common dilemma is whether to use contralateral GSV versus arm vein when both are comparable. Small saphenous vein is an additional option for patients requiring infrapopliteal bypass that might be worthy of comparison to arm vein, although the positioning issues related to vein harvest probably make it the third choice (if providers are willing to consider it at all).

M. Corriere, MD, MS

Technique and results of femoral bifurcation endarterectomy by eversion

Dufranc J, Palcau L, Heyndrickx M, et al (Hospitalier Universitaire de Caen, France)

J Vasc Surg 61:728-733, 2015

Objective.—This study evaluated, in a contemporary prospective series, the safety and efficacy of femoral endarterectomy using the eversion technique and compared our results with results obtained in the literature for the standard endarterectomy with patch closure.

Methods.—Between 2010 and 2012, 121 patients (76% male; mean age, 68.7 years; diabetes, 28%; renal insufficiency, 20%) underwent 147 consecutive femoral bifurcation endarterectomies using the eversion technique, associating or not inflow or outflow concomitant revascularization. The indications were claudication in 89 procedures (60%) and critical limb ischemia in 58 (40%). Primary, primary assisted, and secondary patency of the femoral bifurcation, clinical improvement, limb salvage, and survival were assessed using Kaplan-Meier life-table analysis. Factors associated with those primary endpoints were evaluated with univariate analysis.

Results.—The technical success of eversion was of 93.2%. The 30-day mortality was 0%, and the complication rate was 8.2%; of which, half were local and benign. Median follow-up was 16 months (range, 1.6-31.2 months). Primary, primary assisted, and secondary patencies were, respectively, 93.2%, 97.2%, and 98.6% at 2 years. Primary, primary assisted, and secondary maintenance of clinical improvement were, respectively, 79.9%, 94.6%, and 98.6% at 2 years. The predictive factors for clinical degradation were clinical stage (Rutherford category 5 or 6, $P = .024$), platelet aggregation inhibitor treatment other than clopidogrel ($P = .005$), malnutrition ($P = .025$), and bad tibial runoff ($P = .0016$). A reintervention was necessary in 18.3% of limbs at 2 years: 2% involving femoral bifurcation, 6.1% inflow improvement, and 9.5% outflow improvement. The risk factors of reintervention were platelet aggregation inhibitor (other than clopidogrel, $P = .049$) and cancer ($P = .011$). Limb preservation at 2 years was 100% in the claudicant population. Limb salvage was 88.6% in the critical limb ischemia population, with a statistically higher rate for patients with malnutrition ($P = .029$), preoperative platelet count $>450 \times 10^9$/L ($P = .0071$), platelet aggregation inhibitor treatment other than clopidogrel ($P = .022$), preoperative deep femoral artery occlusion or stenosis >75% ($P = .0064$), and poor tibial runoff ($P = .00042$).

Conclusions.—Eversion femoral bifurcation endarterectomy is a safe, efficient, and reproducible technique for the treatment of atherosclerotic femoral lesions. Advantages are notable, especially the lack of need for prosthetic angioplasty, eliminating the risk of patch infection or pseudoaneurysms and permitting direct puncture if endovascular procedures are needed for assisted patency.

▶ Endarterectomy of the common femoral artery is commonly performed for claudication and critical limb ischemia. Not infrequently, the procedure is performed with concomitant inflow and outflow revascularization procedures. In isolation, the procedure is usually performed through standard longitudinal or transverse groin incisions, and arterial closure is performed with a prosthetic patch. Deep and superficial wound complications are the main morbidity of standard endarterectomy resulting in frequent rehospitalzation and reoperation due to fear of underlying patch involvement.

This study is a retrospective review of a single center's experience with a modified endarterectomy procedure using the eversion technique, adopted from treatment of the carotid bifurcation. The authors describe their technique and address the reader's questions about the proximal and distal ends of the endarterectomy flap. The series included 147 procedures, out of which 18% were performed in isolation. Technical failure was encountered in 7%, and managed with a short interposition graft. Due to the absence of foreign material, the local wound complications that occurred in 4% of patients were managed conservatively. Restenosis occurred in 4%. The results were favorable and reflect durability of this procedure.

This case series provides evidence that supports eversion endarterectomy of the femoral bifurcation as a safe alternative to patch angioplasty, therefore eliminating the risk of foreign graft infection and preserving the native common femoral artery for future percutaneous access. It is not likely that this technique will gain wide acceptance among vascular surgeons in standard risk patients because of the challenges in managing the distal plaque extension. However, it can potentially become a valuable option in patients who carry a higher risk of groin wound complications.

Y. Duwayri, MD

The Society for Vascular Surgery's objective performance goals for lower extremity revascularization are not generalizable to many open surgical bypass patients encountered in contemporary surgical practice

Saraidaridis JT, Ergul E, Patel VI, et al (Massachusetts General Hosp, Boston; et al)

J Vasc Surg 62:392-400, 2015

Objective.—In 2009, the Society for Vascular Surgery (SVS) established objective performance goals (OPG) for lower extremity bypass (LEB) in patients with critical limb ischemia (CLI) based on pooled data from previously performed prospective studies in an effort to provide a benchmark and historical control for future trials. However, patients with a prosthetic conduit and end-stage renal disease were excluded from this cohort. In contemporary practice, many patients do not meet the criteria for SVS OPG inclusion, making generalization of the SVS OPG difficult. The goal of this study was to establish safety and efficacy measures for patients who were excluded from the original SVS OPG analysis.

Methods.—All patients who underwent LEB for CLI in the Vascular Study Group of New England (VSGNE) from 2003 to 2013 were identified. Patients were stratified into OPG-eligible and non-OPG-eligible cohorts. Outcomes included 30-day major adverse limb events, 30-day major adverse cardiovascular events, 1-year survival, and 1-year freedom from amputation. The SVS OPG methodology was used to create new performance goals for the non-OPG-eligible patients.

Results.—We identified 3609 patients: 2360 OPG (65%) vs 1249 non-OPG (35%), and overall results were stratified as a function of OPG status. The 30-day major adverse limb event rate was 5.0% (5.5% non-OPG vs 4.4% OPG; $P = .34$), and the 30-day major adverse cardiovascular event rate was 7.3% (9.2% non-OPG vs 6.2% OPG; $P = .001$). At 1 year, survival was 84% (75.9% non-OPG vs 88.3% OPG; $P < .001$), and freedom from amputation was 86.9% (80.9% non-OPG vs 90.1% OPG; $P < .001$).

Conclusions.—The SVS OPG were attainable in New England for the population of patients who would have met SVS OPG study cohort inclusion criteria. However, 35% of the patients who underwent LEB for CLI in the last 10 years fell outside of these criteria by having end-stage renal disease or requiring a prosthetic conduit. We therefore suggest new benchmarks for these high-risk populations (Tables 2 and 3).

▶ Appropriate risk adjustment is a critical element of benchmarking, and performance goals are potentially inappropriate if they are applied to patient populations or circumstances where the evidence used to create them may not be valid. As the lengthy but informative title of this article points out quite clearly, the Society for Vascular Surgery Objective Performance Goals (SVS-OPG) for lower extremity revascularization may not be valid for a substantial proportion of patients with CLI. Participants in the clinical trials used to develop the SVS-OPG[1-4] were excluded from the pooled data set if they had end-stage renal disease (ESRD) or required prosthetic conduit. Although this approach allowed development of more specific and appropriate benchmarks against future therapies for CLI, this selection bias is important to consider when comparing treatment outcomes or using the SVS-OPG as a quality assessment metric. It is also important to remember that in addition to the preceding exclusion criteria, the pooled data set also excluded patients who were screened for the clinical trials but did not participate. Additional selection biases that might have affected the pooled data set therefore may also include volunteer bias and, for at least some trial participants, an element of equipoise between treatment alternatives that is often absent in contemporary clinical practice.

This analysis leveraged the Vascular Surgery Group of New England data set, making the results more generalizable than would have been the case if this analysis had been based on a cohort from a single center (although generalizability to other regions and countries might still raise potential validity concerns). Thirty-five percent of patients undergoing lower extremity bypass (LEB) during the study period fell into the non-OPG group, including 28% who had prosthetic conduit and the remainder of whom had ESRD. The investigators were not likely surprised to observe that the non-OPG group had more severe disease and a higher prevalence of other comorbid conditions (Table 2). Safety and efficacy outcomes between the OPG and non-OPG groups were also significantly different in most cases, although (to the credit of the VSGNE surgeons) major adverse cardiovascular events were the only safety or efficacy outcome where the non-OPG group crossed the threshold suggested by the SVS (Table 3).

TABLE 2.—Demographics for the Nonobjective Performance Goals (*Non-OPG*)-Eligible Group and the OPG-Eligible Group

Demographic	Non-OPG (n = 1249), No. (%)	OPG (n = 2360), No. (%)	*P* Value
Age, years	69.2	68.8	.34
Female sex	502 (40.2)	788 (33.4)	<.001
Nonwhite	99 (7.9)	159 (6.4)	.19
Any smoking	1030 (82.5)	1915 (81.0)	.33
Current smoking	423 (33.9)	887 (37.6)	.03
Hypertension	1142 (91.4)	2054 (87.0)	<.001
Diabetes	771 (61.7)	1328 (56.3)	.002
Diabetes requiring insulin	483 (38.7)	691 (29.3)	<.001
CAD	560 (44.8)	783 (33.2)	<.001
History of coronary artery bypass grafting	73 (5.8)	68 (2.9)	<.001
Congestive heart failure	323 (25.9)	414 (17.5)	<.001
Chronic obstructive pulmonary disease	372 (29.8)	593 (25.1)	.003
History of previous			
Ipsilateral bypass	220 (17.6)	240 (10.2)	<.001
Ipsilateral PVI	171 (13.7)	358 (15.2)	.23
Carotid endarterectomy/carotid artery stenting	147 (11.8)	209 (8.9)	.005
Major amputation	86 (6.9)	104 (4.4)	.002
Preoperative aspirin	930 (74.5)	1779 (75.4)	.54
Preoperative statin	865 (69.3)	1601 (67.8)	.38
Popliteal distal target			
Above the knee	441 (35.3)	233 (9.9)	<.001
Below the knee	323 (25.9)	768 (32.5)	<.001
Tibial distal target	328 (26.3)	991 (42.0)	<.001
Pedal distal target	117 (9.4)	349 (14.8)	<.001
Prosthetic conduit	1001 (80.1)	–	–
ESRD	343 (27.5)	–	–

CAD, Coronary artery disease; *ESRD*, end-stage renal disease; *PVI*, peripheral vascular intervention.
Reprinted from Saraidaridis JT, Ergul E, Patel VI, et al. The Society for Vascular Surgery's objective performance goals for lower extremity revascularization are not generalizable to many open surgical bypass patients encountered in contemporary surgical practice. *J Vasc Surg*. 2015;62:392-400, with permission from the Society for Vascular Surgery.

One-year survival was 75.9% in the non-OPG group versus 88.3% in the SVS-OPG group. One-year survival among patients with both prosthetic conduit and ESRD was especially poor at 58% (which also happened to be the rate of limb salvage in this patient subgroup). Survival as an efficacy measure within the SVS-OPG[4] is curious given that death among this population is most often due to coronary disease and stroke; LEB may alleviate symptoms and lower amputation risk but is unlikely to have a positive impact on survival in patients with CLI. Perhaps the survival efficacy outcome was intended to be used as a selection criterion based on the premise that LEB should be avoided when near-term anticipated survival is poor. Although this idea seems reasonable from a general population perspective, it is difficult to tell an individual patient who has rest pain or tissue loss that they will need to spend 6 months or more with severe (and potentially progressive) symptoms because they may not survive long enough to benefit from the procedure. The results of the study clearly demonstrate that patients with ESRD and prosthetic conduit are least likely to benefit from LEB, but the alternatives (primary amputation

TABLE 3.—Safety and Efficacy Outcomes for the Nonobjective Performance Goals (*Non-OPG*)-Eligible Group vs the OPG-Eligible Group

Outcome Measures	Non-OPG Group (n = 1249)	OPG Group (n = 2360)	*P* Value	SVS OPG, %
Safety outcomes at 30 days, No. (%)				
MALE	69 (5.5)	113 (4.8)	.34	<8
MACE	115 (9.2)	147 (6.2)	.001	<8
Myocardial infarction	67 (5.4)	110 (4.7)	.35	
Death	65 (5.2)	46 (2.0)	<.001	
Amputation	32 (2.6)	21 (0.9)	<.001	<3
Efficacy outcomes at 1 year, % (SE)				
Survival	75.9 (1.3)	88.3 (.7)	<.001	>80
Freedom from amputation	80.9 (1.6)	90.1 (.8)	<.001	>84

MACE, Major adverse cardiovascular event; *MALE*, major adverse limb event; *SE*, standard error; *SVS*, Society for Vascular Surgery.

Reprinted from Saraidaridis JT, Ergul E, Patel VI, et al. The Society for Vascular Surgery's objective performance goals for lower extremity revascularization are not generalizable to many open surgical bypass patients encountered in contemporary surgical practice. *J Vasc Surg*. 2015;62:392-400, with permission from the Society for Vascular Surgery.

or palliative pain management) are often hard to accept for ambulatory patients, leaving patients and providers with difficult conversations and tough choices.

M. Corriere, MD, MS

References

1. Adam DJ, Beard JD, Cleveland T, et al. Bypass versus angioplasty in severe ischaemia of the leg (BASIL): multicentre, randomised controlled trial. *Lancet*. 2005; 366:1925-1934.
2. Conte MS, Bandyk DF, Clowes AW, et al. Results of PREVENT III: a multicenter, randomized trial of edifoligide for the prevention of vein graft failure in lower extremity bypass surgery. *J Vasc Surg*. 2006;43:742-751.
3. Nehler MR, Brass EP, Anthony R, et al. Adjunctive parenteral therapy with lipoecraprost, a prostaglandin E1 analog, in patients with critical limb ischemia undergoing distal revascularization does not improve 6-month outcomes. *J Vasc Surg*. 2007;45:953-960.
4. Conte MS, Geraghty PJ, Bradbury AW, et al. Suggested objective performance goals and clinical trial design for evaluating catheter-based treatment of critical limb ischemia. *J Vasc Surg*. 2009;50:1462-1473.

Nasal methicillin-resistant *Staphylococcus aureus* colonization is associated with increased wound occurrence after major lower extremity amputation

Azarbal AF, Harris S, Mitchell EL, et al (Oregon Health and Science Univ, Portland)

J Vasc Surg 62:401-405, 2015

Objective.—Wound occurrence (WO) after major lower extremity amputation (MLEA) can be due to wound infection or sterile dehiscence. We sought to determine the association of nasal methicillin-resistant

Staphylococcus aureus (MRSA) colonization and other patient factors with overall WO, WO due to wound infection, and WO due to sterile dehiscence.

Methods.—The medical records of all patients undergoing MLEA from August 1, 2011, to November 1, 2013, were reviewed. Demographic data, hemoglobin A1c level, albumin concentration, dialysis dependence, peripheral vascular disease (PVD), nasal MRSA colonization, and diabetes mellitus (DM) were examined as variables. The overall WO rate was determined, and the cause of WO was categorized as either a sterile dehiscence or a wound infection.

Results.—Eighty-three patients underwent 96 MLEAs during a 27-month period. The rates of overall WO, WO due to infection, and WO due to sterile dehiscence were 39%, 19%, and 19%, respectively (1% developed a traumatic wound). On univariate analysis, PVD, MRSA colonization, DM, and dialysis dependence were all associated with higher rates of overall WO ($P < .05$). On multivariate analysis, MRSA colonization was associated with higher rates of overall WO ($P = .03$) and WO due to wound infection (11% vs 45%; $P < .01$). DM and PVD were associated with higher rates of overall WO and WO due to sterile dehiscence on both univariate and multivariate analysis ($P < .05$).

Conclusions.—Nasal MRSA colonization is associated with higher rates of overall WO and WO due to wound infection. DM and PVD are associated with higher rates of overall WO and WO due to sterile dehiscence but are not associated with WO due to wound infection. Further studies addressing the effect of nasal MRSA eradication on postoperative wound outcomes after MLEA are warranted.

▶ "Wound occurrence" was used in this article to refer to either infection or sterile dehiscence after leg amputation. This terminology is not used widely in either clinical practice or outcomes reporting and may have been adopted to establish 2 mutually exclusive outcomes for the purpose of analysis. Referring to any amputation wound dehiscence as sterile is a bit incorrect, however, and these 2 categories really distinguish wound complications attributed to infectious versus other etiologies. Accepting this misnomer for the sake of discussion, sterile dehiscence can result from a variety of attributable etiologies, including pressure ulceration, ischemia, wound tension, or tissue handling. Although amputations are usually less technically demanding than lower extremity bypasses, careful planning and attention to technique (including tissue handling, wound closure, and postoperative care) are nonetheless critical to avoid wound complications. Amputation in the setting of peripheral vascular disease (PVD) usually means that revascularization either failed or was never attempted, so the association between PVD and wound occurrence identified in this analysis is not unexpected. It is also interesting to note that higher wound complication rates were observed for below- versus above-knee amputations, although infection rates were similar between these procedure categories. The choice of amputation level is sometimes difficult, particularly among patients who may be borderline in terms of their likelihood to heal a below-knee amputation but were also recently ambulatory.

Methicillin-resistant *Staphylococcus aureus* (MRSA) colonization was associated with higher rates of overall wound occurrence and infection in this analysis. Critical limb ischemia can be a setup for MRSA colonization in many ways, particularly for patients with ulcers or gangrene who often receive inpatient care over a period of several hospital stays when revascularization and/or debridement are performed in a staged fashion before amputation. Having identified an association between MRSA colonization and wound complications, the next logical step would be to attempt to identify an intervention that reduces associated risk. The discussion points out that MRSA colonization was not associated with wound complications in a previous analysis performed at another center where patients received perioperative prophylactic antibiotics that cover MRSA[1] (not the case in this study), suggesting that this practice may be advisable for patients known to be colonized. Alternative interventions include skin and/or nasal decontamination, although these may pose greater challenges in terms of successful implementation, particularly when attempted in the outpatient setting.

M. Corriere, MD, MS

Reference

1. Richards T, Pittathankel AA, Pursell R, Magee TR, Galland RB. MRSA in lower limb amputation and the role of antibiotic prophylaxis. *J Cardiovasc Surg*. 2005; 46:37-41.

Outcomes of Neuroischemic Wounds Treated by a Multidisciplinary Amputation Prevention Service

Vartanian SM, Robinson KD, Ofili K, et al (Univ of California, San Francisco)
Ann Vasc Surg 29:534-542, 2015

Background.—Multidisciplinary amputation prevention teams decrease the frequency of major amputations by increasing the use of revascularization procedures and minor amputations. The outcomes of wound healing, wound recurrence, and ambulatory status are assumed to be improved but are not routinely reported. This study investigates the midterm outcomes of neuroischemic wounds treated by our multidisciplinary team.

Methods.—A retrospective review of patients with neuroischemic wounds treated at a single institution amputation prevention clinic from March 2012 to July 2013. Patient demographics, wound characteristics, procedural details, and clinical and functional outcomes were reviewed. Clinical end points under study included time to wound healing, reulceration rate, and ambulatory status.

Results.—Over 16 months, there were 202 new patients and 1,355 clinic visits. Ninety-one limbs from 89 patients were treated for complex neuroischemic wounds. In 67% (61 of 91) of limbs, wounds were present for >6 weeks before referral. A history of previous revascularization was present in 39% (31 of 91), and 28% (22 of 91) had a previous minor amputation. Forty-one percent of wounds (38 of 91) were limited to the toes or the forefoot whereas 24% (22 of 91) involved the hindfoot or ankle. A total of 151 podiatric and 86 vascular interventions were performed, with an equal distribution of endovascular and open revascularizations. Complete healing was observed for 59% of wounds (54 of 91) over the observation period (median follow up, 207 days; range 56–561 days), and the average time to full healing was 12 weeks. Hindfoot wounds were predictive of failure to heal (odds ratio, 0.21; $P < 0.01$; 95% confidence interval, 0.06–0.68). Nineteen percent of patients (17 of 91) developed a new wound in the ipsilateral leg during follow-up. Three major amputations were performed (2 below-knee amputation and 1 above-knee amputation) for a major/minor amputation ratio of 0.06. Ambulatory status was preserved or improved in 74% (67 of 91) of patients. The 30-day readmission rate was 11%, which was lower than that observed (21%) in a contemporaneous but all-inclusive population of lower extremity revascularization procedures performed at our institution.

Conclusions.—Multidisciplinary limb salvage teams effectively heal wounds and maintain ambulatory status in patients with limb-threatening neuroischemic wounds. Patient specific factors, such as hindfoot or ankle wounds, can adversely influence the outcome. Even with aggressive care, healing can be prolonged and a substantial proportion of patients can be expected to have a recurrence, making subsequent surveillance mandatory. Our data also suggest that a coordinated amputation prevention program may help to minimize hospital readmissions in this high-risk population (Table 3).

▶ Providers who treat patients with peripheral artery disease (PAD) are invested in avoiding amputations whenever possible. Nonetheless, amputations are a necessary component of the spectrum of treatments necessary to provide comprehensive care to patients with PAD. Surgeons who perform amputations therefore may take offense at the notion that a vascular surgery, vascular medicine, or critical limb ischemia clinic (or service) does not also share the goal of amputation prevention regardless of whether it is directly branded as such. Incorporating amputation prevention into the name of the enterprise, however, serves as both an indicator and reminder of the shared goal all specialists have in mind. The clinic described in this study was codirected by podiatry and vascular surgery specialists who referred to other specialties (presumably not located in the same clinic enterprise) on an as-needed basis. Debridement and toe amputation, both of which are routinely performed by most vascular surgeons, were categorized as podiatry procedures in this analysis. Conversely, some podiatry operations that are not commonly performed by vascular surgeons but may contribute to wound healing and limb salvage (such as tendon release) were conspicuously absent from the list procedural characteristics (Table 3).

TABLE 3.—Procedural Characteristics

			Number	%
Total procedures			248	
Inpatient cases			218	88
Outpatient cases			30	12
Emergent cases			35	14
Multiple procedures on single admission			66	69
	Inpatient	**%**	**Outpatient**	**%**
Procedures				
Podiatry	127	51	24	10
Debridement	37		10	
Drainage procedure	12			
Partial toe amp	6		3	
Complete toe amp	5		1	
Ray amp	16		2	
Multiple digit ray amp	8		2	
TMA	11		1	
Open amputation	7		—	
Delayed primary closure	7		—	
Hammertoe correction	1		1	
Calcanectomy	8		1	
Midfoot amputation	4		—	
Metatarsal head resection	5		—	
Other	—		3	
Plastic surgery	8	3		
Debridement	3			
Skin graft	1			
Rotational flap	2			
Free flap	2			
Vascular Surgery	80	32	6	2
Diagnostic angiogram	23		4	
Angioplasty or stent	28		2	
Femoral endarterectomy	3			
Thrombolysis	1			
Bypass procedure	22			
Aortobifemoral	2			
Axillary-femoral	1			
Iliofemoral	1			
Femoral-popliteal	6			
Femoral-distal	8			
Popliteal-distal/pedal	4			
Major amputations				
BKA	2			
AKA	1			
High:low amputation ratio	0.06			

AKA, above-knee amputation; BKA, below-knee ampuation; DP, dorsalis pedis; PT, posterior tibial; TMA, transmetatarsal amputation.

Reprinted from Vartanian SM, Robinson KD, Ofili K, et al. Outcomes of neuroischemic wounds treated by a multidisciplinary amputation prevention service. *Ann Vasc Surg*. 2015;29:534-542, with permission from Elsevier.

Given the room for improvement that these investigators identified in terms of medical management (the average hemoglobin A1C was 8.3% and only 52% of patients were on statins at the time of initial evaluation), there may be a case for expanding their concept to include in-clinic medical specialists from vascular medicine, endocrinology, and/or internal medicine. Limitation of this multidisciplinary clinic to surgical specialists may reflect the organizational structure and/or financial model of the health system, which sometimes presents barriers to establishing more comprehensive collaborative initiatives due to logistics and/or competition. Vascular providers might do well to borrow a page from other models where medical and surgical specialists routinely collaborate to deliver better care to a focused population such as organ transplantation, cancer, and spinal disease.

The patient population in this study was defined based on new patient referrals to an outpatient clinic. Patients with foot wounds admitted through the hospital emergency department were therefore excluded. Because patients presenting to the emergency department might be expected to have higher amputation rates resulting from issues related to health care access and/or more advanced wounds deemed inappropriate for the slower outpatient referral process. This "referral bias" (mentioned in the discussion) is a form of selection bias that may have contributed to the low rates of major extremity amputation reported. Additionally, outcomes may have been affected by exclusion of patients with venous ulcers and, by extension, patients with mixed disease (ie, PAD plus venous insufficiency) who often have worse outcomes than those with PAD alone.

Construction of a Venn diagram illustrating the overlapping skill sets and specialists required to provide comprehensive care to patients with foot wounds would locate vascular surgeons at its center. Vascular surgeons can provide revascularization (both endovascular and open surgical), wound care, and both major and minor amputations and are often asked to assume patients initially managed by providers with more focused skill sets. Because vascular surgeons are often the final "common pathway" for complex patients who have exhausted more basic treatment options, they therefore often apply a distinct, longer term perspective of the clinical course of PAD. This perspective often influences their attitude about treatment decisions, allowing them to consider how treatments A, B, and C will affect options X, Y, and Z. These comments aside, vascular surgeons should embrace the multidisciplinary approach to amputation prevention that includes unique contributions from other specialties and in many ways are well situated to lead these initiatives. Multidisciplinary care appears to be the way of the future and potentially offers a more patient-centered treatment experience with potential for better outcomes.

M. Corriere, MD, MS

Prospective, randomized, multi-institutional clinical trial of a silver alginate dressing to reduce lower extremity vascular surgery wound complications

Ozaki CK, Hamdan AD, Barshes NR, et al (Brigham and Women's Hosp, Boston, MA; Harvard Med School, Boston, MA; Baylor College of Medicine, Houston, TX)

J Vasc Surg 61:419-427, 2015

Objective.—Wound complications negatively affect outcomes of lower extremity arterial reconstruction. By way of an investigator initiated clinical trial, we tested the hypothesis that a silver-eluting alginate topical surgical dressing would lower wound complication rates in patients undergoing open arterial procedures in the lower extremity.

Methods.—The study block-randomized 500 patients at three institutions to standard gauze or silver alginate dressings placed over incisions after leg arterial surgery. This original operating room dressing remained until gross soiling, clinical need to remove, or postoperative day 3, whichever was first. Subsequent care was at the provider's discretion. The primary end point was 30-day wound complication incidence generally based on National Surgical Quality Improvement Program guidelines. Demographic, clinical, quality of life, and economic end points were also collected. Wound closure was at the surgeon's discretion.

Results.—Participants (72% male) were 84% white, 45% were diabetic, 41% had critical limb ischemia, and 32% had claudication (with aneurysm, bypass revision, other). The overall 30-daywound complication incidence was 30%, with superficial surgical site infection as the most common. In intent-to-treat analysis, silver alginate had no effect on wound complications. Multivariable analysis showed that Coumadin (Bristol-Myers Squibb, Princeton, NJ; odds ratio [OR], 1.72; 95% confidence interval [CI], 1.03-2.87; $P = .03$), higher body mass index (OR, 1.05; 95% CI, 1.01-1.09; $P = .01$), and the use of no conduit/material (OR, 0.12; 95% CI, 0.82-3.59; $P < .001$) were independently associated with wound complications.

Conclusions.—The incidence of wound complications remains high in contemporary open lower extremity arterial surgery. Under the study conditions, a silver-eluting alginate dressing showed no effect on the incidence of wound complications.

▶ Surgical site infections remain an all too common postoperative complication after vascular surgical procedures that result in increased patient morbidity and health care expenditures. Silver pharmacologic compounds and silver-eluting biomaterials have shown efficacy in a variety of clinical applications for infection prophylaxis and therapy. This prospective, randomized, multi-institutional clinical trial of a silver alginate dressing expands on a previously published nonconcurrent, single-institution study that demonstrated a reduction in wound complications with the use of an Acticoat postoperative dressing, compared with a conventional nonsilver dressing after defined lower extremity revascularization (5% vs 14%).[1] The authors theorized that lowering bacterial counts overlying the incisions with a silver alginate dressing might have a durable beneficial effect on postoperative wound infections. The Acticoat Absorbent dressing (Smith & Nephew PLC, London, United Kingdom) is an antimicrobial barrier dressing coated with nanocrystalline silver that delivers a controlled, sustained (up to 3 days) dose of silver while also absorbing moisture to minimize wound maceration.

Although the study failed to demonstrate a significant effect on the incidence of infrainguinal wound complications following elective surgery for both occlusive and aneurysmal peripheral vascular disease, the authors did demonstrate that the incidence of wound complications following open arterial surgery remains high (30%) in a contemporary vascular surgical practice despite increased attention toward perioperative wound prevention measures like timely and appropriate administration of perioperative antibiotics, maintenance of normothermia, and the use of skip incisions for vein harvest. There is tremendous value in this realistic assessment of surgical site infection rates after infrainguinal arterial surgery. The authors also identified preoperative Coumadin (Bristol-Myers Squibb, Princeton, NJ) use, elevated body mass index, and the use of vascular conduit/material as factors independently associated with wound complications by multivariate analysis.

Wound closure technique, incision orientation, tobacco abuse, and identification of redo surgical procedures were not included as covariates. Additionally, wound classification as clean/contaminated was not felt to be reliably captured in this study for appropriate analysis. It may be that a subtype of wound, for example, a clean contaminated wound in patients with infected tissue loss might benefit from this dressing. Moreover, the optimal amount of silver in each dressing and the cost-effectiveness of such dressings may warrant further investigation.

D. Coleman, MD

Reference

1. Childress BB, Berceli SA, Nelson PR, Lee WA, Ozaki CK. Impact of an absorbent silver-eluting dressing system on lower extremity revascularization wound complications. *Ann Vasc Surg*. 2007;21:598-602.

Determinants of survival and major amputation after peripheral endovascular intervention for critical limb ischemia

Vierthaler L, Callas PW, Goodney PP, et al (Univ of Vermont College of Medicine, Burlington; Dartmouth Hitchcock Med Ctr, Lebanon, NH; et al)
J Vasc Surg 62:655-664, 2015

Objective.—Our objective was to analyze periprocedural and 1-year outcomes of peripheral endovascular intervention (PVI) for critical limb ischemia (CLI).

Methods.—We reviewed 1244 patients undergoing 1414 PVIs for CLI (rest pain, 29%; tissue loss, 71%) within the Vascular Study Group of New England (VSGNE) from January 2010 to December 2011. Overall survival (OS), amputation-free survival (AFS), and freedom from major amputation at 1 year were analyzed using the Kaplan-Meier method. Cox proportional hazards models were used to calculate hazard ratios (HRs) and 95% confidence intervals (CIs).

Results.—The number of arteries treated during each procedure were 1 (49%), 2 (35%), 3 (12%), and ≥4 (5%). Target arterial segments and TransAtlantic Inter-Society Consensus classifications were aortoiliac, 27% (A, 48%; B, 28%; C, 12%; and D, 12%); femoral-popliteal, 48%

(A, 29%; B, 34%; C, 20%; and D, 17%); and infrapopliteal, 25% (A, 17%; B, 14%; C, 25%; D, 44%). Technical success was 92%. Complications included access site hematoma (5.0%), occlusion (0.3%), and distal embolization (2.4%). Mortality and major amputation rates were 2.8% and 2.2% at 30 days, respectively. Overall percutaneous or open reintervention rate was 8.0% during the first year. At 1-year, OS, AFS, and freedom from major amputation were 87%, 87%, and 94% for patients with rest pain and 80%, 71%, and 81% for patients with tissue loss. Independent predictors of reduced 1-year OS (C index = .74) included dialysis (HR, 3.8; 95% CI, 2.8-5.1; $P < .01$), emergency procedure (HR, 2.5; 95% CI, 1.0-6.2; $P = .05$), age >80 years (HR, 2.2; 95% CI, 1.7-2.8; $P < .01$), not living at home preoperatively (HR, 2.0; 95% CI, 1.4-2.8; $P < .01$), creatinine >1.8 mg/dL (HR, 1.9; 95% CI, 1.3-2.8; $P < .01$), congestive heart failure (HR, 1.7; 95% CI, 1.3-2.2; $P < .01$), and chronic β-blocker use (HR, 1.4; 95% CI, 1.0-1.9; $P = .03$), whereas independent preoperative ambulation (HR, 0.7; 95% CI, 0.6-0.9; $P = .014$) was protective. Independent predictors of major amputation (C index = .69) at 1 year included dialysis (HR, 2.7; 95% CI, 1.6-4.5; $P < .01$), tissue loss (HR, 2.0; 95% CI, 1.1-3.7; $P = .02$), prior major contralateral amputation (HR, 2.0; 95% CI, 1.1-3.5; $P = .02$), non-Caucasian race (HR, 1.7; 95% CI, 1.0-2.9; $P = .045$), and male gender (HR, 1.6; 95% CI, 1.1-2.6; $P = .03$), whereas smoking (HR, .60; 95% CI, 0.4-1.0; $P = .042$) was protective.

Conclusions.—Survival and major amputation after PVI for CLI are associated with different patient characteristics. Dialysis dependence is a common predictor that portends especially poor outcomes. These data may facilitate efforts to improve patient selection and, after further validation, enable risk-adjusted outcome reporting for CLI patients undergoing PVI (Fig 2, Table 4).

▶ It is important for physicians and patients considering treatment options to establish shared goals and expectations. When considering critical limb ischemia (CLI) survival outcomes, we should remember that death among these patients is usually related to coronary heart disease or stroke rather than leg-specific causes.[1] Along those lines, although it is certainly important to understand the epidemiology of CLI mortality, revascularization is not performed to prolong survival but instead to alleviate rest pain, promote wound healing, and avoid amputation. Successful revascularization therefore accomplishes important patient-centered goals related to palliation, physical function, and quality of life. Patients who sleep through the night, maintain independent living, or preserve their body image through revascularization undoubtedly benefit from the procedure even if it does not extend their survival.

There may be scenarios where the less invasive (and lower risk) procedure might be the best choice, even if it may not be the most durable one. Although the authors mention long-term durability and repeat intervention as important considerations, one could justifiably argue that these issues may be less relevant among CLI patients because of their poor survival. This may be particularly relevant when amputation healing, rather than amputation prevention, is the goal

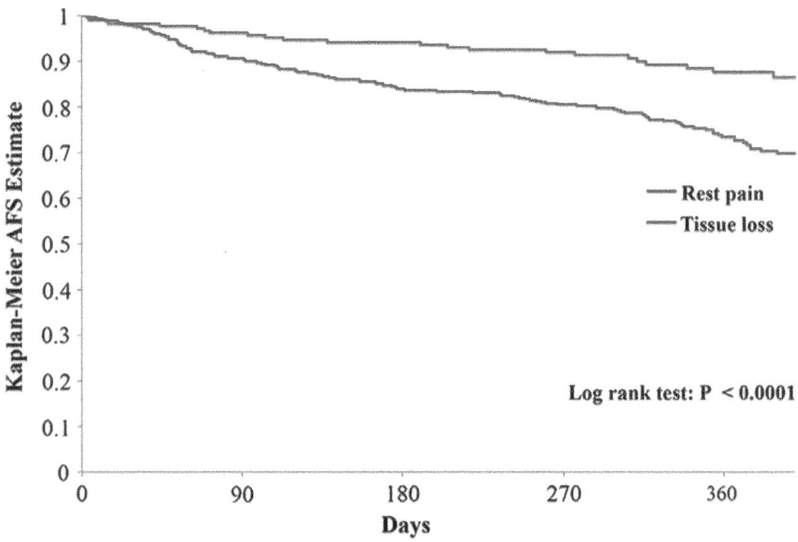

Rest pain					
# at risk	215	191	174	149	104
EST (SE)	-	0.96 (0.013)	0.94 (0.016)	0.92 (0.02)	0.88 (0.025)
Tissue loss					
# at risk	514	437	381	326	186
EST (SE)	-	0.91 (0.013)	0.84 (0.017)	0.80 (0.018)	0.73 (0.022)

FIGURE 2.—Kaplan-Meier curve of amputation-free survival (AFS) after peripheral vascular intervention (PVI) for critical limb ischemia (CLI). *EST*, Estimated survival; *SE*, standard error.. (Reprinted from Vierthaler L, Callas PW, Goodney PP, et al. Determinants of survival and major amputation after peripheral endovascular intervention for critical limb ischemia. *J Vasc Surg*. 2015;62:655-664, with permission from the Society for Vascular Surgery.)

TABLE 4.—Multivariable Cox Proportional Hazards Model of Factors Associated with 1-Year Survival After Peripheral Vascular Intervention (PVI) for Critical Limb Ischemia (CLI)[a]

Preoperative Characteristic	HR	95% CI	*P* Value
Dialysis dependence	3.8	2.8-5.1	<.01
Emergency procedure	2.5	1.0-6.2	.046
Age >80 years	2.2	1.7-2.8	<.01
Not living at home preoperatively	2.0	1.4-2.8	<.01
Creatinine >1.8 mg/dL	1.9	1.3-2.8	<.01
CHF	1.7	1.3-2.2	<.01
Chronic β-blocker use	1.4	1.0-1.9	.03
Independent ambulation preoperatively	0.7	0.6-0.9	.014

CHF, Congestive heart failure; *CI*, confidence interval; *HR*, hazard ratio.
[a]C index = 0.74.
Reprinted from Vierthaler L, Callas PW, Goodney PP, et al. Determinants of survival and major amputation after peripheral endovascular intervention for critical limb ischemia. *J Vasc Surg*. 2015;62:655-664, with permission from the Society for Vascular Surgery.

of the intervention. Conversely, the focus on short-term gains can be taken too far, particularly if endovascular intervention burns bridges for more definitive surgical options without a realistic chance of meaningful symptomatic improvement, even in the setting of technical success. This analysis did not specify whether the percutaneous revascularizations included were primary versus repeat procedures. Repeat intervention is common among patients with CLI (including those whose first intervention was performed for claudication), and failure of a previous endovascular intervention has a demonstrated negative impact on subsequent revascularization options (both endovascular and surgical) as well as their outcomes.

Although causes of death were not included in this analysis, none of the variables associated with decreased survival would surprise anyone who takes care of CLI (Table 4). Overall survival in this study was poor (82%) but better than published data from many series, likely reflecting exclusion of patients not offered a revascularization (perhaps due to extensive gangrene, risk, or lack of target vessels). As mentioned in the discussion, mortality also may have been affected by bias favoring endovascular treatment over lower extremity bypass among higher risk patients. Mortality and major amputation rates at 30 days were 2.8% and 2.0%, respectively, and amputation-free survival was worse among patients who presented with gangrene. Amputation rates occurred at a relatively consistent rate over time, rather than as a precipitous decrease in AFS during the immediate postoperative period (Fig 2). These observations suggest that the endovascular procedures were not futile.

Qualitative research studies have demonstrated that many patients with peripheral artery disease who undergo amputation later wish that amputation had been performed earlier in their treatment course.[2] Although hindsight is often more clear, patients almost never choose amputation over any alternative option the provider is willing to consider with potential (even minimal) for limb salvage. An amputation cannot be undone once it has been performed, but patients ultimately undergoing amputation may gain greater peace of mind knowing that their providers did everything the could to accomplish limb salvage. In the current era in which amputation rates are viewed as a quality indicator and increased attention is given to disparities in revascularization versus amputation as primary therapy,[3,4] providers are often caught in a dilemma between doing everything possible versus everything reasonable to attempt limb salvage. The critical point in the decision process therefore may be identifying when the next revascularization is unlikely to have meaningful impact on quality of life or limb salvage.

M. Corriere, MD, MS

References

1. Norgren L, Hiatt WR, Dormandy JA, Nehler MR, Harris KA, Fowkes FG. Inter-society consensus for the management of peripheral arterial disease (TASC II). *J Vasc Surg*. 2007;45:S5-S67.
2. Suckow BD, Goodney PP, Nolan BW, et al. Domains that determine quality of life in vascular amputees. *Ann Vasc Surg*. 2015;29:722-730.

3. Holman KH, Henke PK, Dimick JB, Birkmeyer JD. Racial disparities in the use of revascularization before leg amputation in Medicare patients. *J Vasc Surg*. 2011; 54:420-426.
4. Goodney PP, Travis LL, Nallamothu BK, et al. Variation in the use of lower extremity vascular procedures for critical limb ischemia. *Circ Cardiovasc Qual Outcomes*. 2012;5:94-102.

Predictors of Lower-Extremity Amputation in Patients With an Infected Diabetic Foot Ulcer

Pickwell K, Siersma V, Kars M, et al (Maastricht Univ Med Centre, the Netherlands; Univ of Copenhagen, Denmark; et al)
Diabetes Care 38:852-857, 2015

Objective.—Infection commonly complicates diabetic foot ulcers and is associated with a poor outcome. In a cohort of individuals with an infected diabetic foot ulcer, we aimed to determine independent predictors of lower-extremity amputation and the predictive value for amputation of the International Working Group on the Diabetic Foot (IWGDF) classification system and to develop a risk score for predicting amputation.

Research Design and Methods.—We prospectively studied 575 patients with an infected diabetic foot ulcer presenting to 1 of 14 diabetic foot clinics in 10 European countries.

Results.—Among these patients, 159 (28%) underwent an amputation. Independent risk factors for amputation were as follows: periwound edema, foul smell, (non) purulent exudate, deep ulcer, positive probe-to-bone test, pretibial edema, fever, and elevated C-reactive protein. Increasing IWGDF severity of infection also independently predicted amputation.We developed a risk score for any amputation and for amputations excluding the lesser toes (including the variables sex, pain on palpation, periwound edema, ulcer size, ulcer depth, and peripheral arterial disease) that predicted amputation better than the IWGDF system (area under the ROC curves 0.80, 0.78, and 0.67, respectively).

Conclusions.—For individuals with an infected diabetic foot ulcer, we identified independent predictors of amputation, validated the prognostic value of the IWGDF classification system, and developed a new risk score for amputation that can be readily used in daily clinical practice. Our risk score may have better prognostic accuracy than the IWGDF system, the only currently available system, but our findings need to be validated in other cohorts.

▶ Diabetic foot ulcers (DFU) are a clinical problem in which peripheral artery disease (PAD) is often a barrier to wound healing that must be addressed. The morbidity and costs associated with DFU (particularly with the rising prevalence of type II diabetes in the United States) are considerable. These authors observed a 1-year amputation rate of 28% among patients following diagnosis of an infected DFU, supporting an aggressive attitude toward revascularization when PAD is also present, even if the most likely primary cause of the ulcer is neuropathy rather than ischemia. In the era of wound-care centers, where vascular specialists may or may not participate in the initial diagnostic evaluation or treatment planning for patients with DFU, valuable time may be lost if the initial focus includes debridement, topical therapy, and medical management without a simultaneous evaluation for PAD and pursuit of revascularization if indicated. Along those lines, it is curious (given the study population and publication from which this article was selected) that no mention of toe pressures, toe brachial index, or digital waveforms was included as part of the definition of PAD in this study's diabetic patient cohort. Given the high prevalence of tibial and small vessel arterial calcification among patients with diabetes, the stated criteria based on ankle brachial index alone may have misclassified some patients with PAD and noncompressible arteries.

It is interesting to compare the amputation risk score from this analysis (Table 3 in the original article) with the Society for Vascular Surgery Wound, Ischemia and foot Infection (WIfI) classification system, which has been validated as a predictor of amputation-free survival in several studies since its initial description.[1] PAD severity, wound size and depth, edema, and tenderness are variables shared by both systems (infection is also included as part of the SVS-WIfI, but all patients in this study had infected ulcers). Although this analysis included patients with or without PAD, it is clear that a central group of amputation risk factors exists that should activate an aggressive management strategy to achieve limb salvage with or without revascularization. As stated rather eloquently by the WIfI authors, "Perfusion is only one determinant of outcome, wound extent and the presence and severity of infection also greatly impact the threat to a limb." Data from the endocrinology literature seem to concur with this sentiment, strengthening the case that a multidisciplinary approach to foot ulcers makes sense to maximize the chance of limb salvage for all patients.

M. Corriere, MD, MS

Reference

1. Mills JL Sr, Conte MS, Armstrong DG, et al. Society for Vascular Surgery Lower Extremity Guidelines Committee. The society for vascular surgery lower extremity threatened limb classification system: risk stratification based on wound, ischemia, and foot infection (WIfI). *J Vasc Surg.* 2014;59:220-234.e1-2.

Rates and predictors of readmission after minor lower extremity amputations

Beaulieu RJ, Grimm JC, Lyu H, et al (Johns Hopkins Hosp, Baltimore, MD)
J Vasc Surg 62:101-105, 2015

Objective.—One goal of the Patient Protection and Affordable Care Act is to reduce hospital readmissions, with financial penalties applied for excessive rates of unplanned readmissions within 30 days among Medicare beneficiaries. Recent data indicate that as many as 24% of Medicare patients require readmission after vascular surgery, although the rate of readmission after limited digital amputations has not been specifically examined. The present study was therefore undertaken to define the rate of unplanned readmission among patients after digital amputations and to identify the factors associated with these readmissions to allow the clinician to implement strategies to reduce readmission rates in the future.

Methods.—The electronic medical and billing records of all patients undergoing minor amputations (defined as toe or transmetatarsal amputations using International Classification of Diseases, Ninth Revision, codes) from January 2000 through July 2012 were retrospectively reviewed. Data were collected for procedure- and hospital-related variables, level of amputation, length of stay, time to readmission, and level of reamputation. Patient demographics included hypertension, diabetes, hyperlipidemia, smoking history, and history of myocardial infarction, congestive heart failure, peripheral arterial disease, chronic obstructive pulmonary disease, and cerebrovascular accident.

Results.—Minor amputations were performed in 717 patients (62.2% male), including toe amputations in 565 (72.8%) and transmetatarsal amputations in 152 (19.5%). Readmission occurred in 100 patients (13.9%), including 28 (3.9%) within 30 days, 28 (3.9%) between 30 and 60 days, and 44 (6.1%) >60 days after the index amputation. Multivariable analysis revealed that elective admission ($P < .001$), peripheral arterial disease ($P < .001$), and chronic renal insufficiency ($P = .001$) were associated with readmission. The reasons for readmission were infection (49%), ischemia (29%), nonhealing wound (19%), and indeterminate (4%). Reamputation occurred in 95 (95%) of the readmitted patients, including limb amputation in 64 (64%) of the patients (below knee in 58, through knee in 2, and above knee in 4).

Conclusions.—Readmission after minor amputation was associated with limb amputation in the majority of cases. This study identified a number of nonmodifiable patient factors that are associated with an increased risk of readmission. Whereas efforts to reduce unplanned hospital readmissions are laudable, payers and regulators should consider these observations in defining unacceptable rates of readmission. Further, although beyond the scope of this study, it is not unreasonable to assume that pressure to reduce readmission rates in the population of patients with extensive comorbidity may induce practitioners to undertake amputation at a higher level initially to minimize the risk of readmission for reamputation and associated financial penalties and thus deprive the patient the chance for limb salvage (Table 2).

► The relative timing of a minor amputation and ipsilateral leg revascularization procedure is a decision that is commonly encountered among patients with critical limb ischemia. Performing a toe amputation first may allow a staged revascularization to be performed with decreased concerns about acute infectious issues or even avoid the need for revascularization if noninvasive studies suggest a reasonable chance for wound healing. Conversely, performing revascularization first may give ulcers a chance to heal and potentially avoid more

TABLE 2.—Univariate and Multivariable Predictors of Readmission

	Univariate Analysis			Multivariable Analysis		
	OR	95% CI	*P* Value	OR	95% CI	*P* Value
Age, years	1.00	0.98-1.01	.70	–	–	–
Male	1.49	0.97-2.28	.07	1.22	0.77-1.92	.40
Nonelective status	2.94	1.92-4.53	<.001	2.78	1.77-4.35	<.001
Hypertension	2.77	1.48-5.19	.002	1.92	0.99-3.74	.06
Diabetes mellitus	1.62	0.94-2.79	.08	–	–	–
Congestive heart failure	1.20	0.66-2.18	.55	–	–	–
Chronic obstructive pulmonary disease	0.83	0.32-2.15	.69	–	–	–
Myocardial infarction	0.77	0.42-1.40	.39	–	–	–
Cerebrovascular accident	1.29	0.68-2.44	.43	–	–	–
Hyperlipidemia	1.52	0.99-2.33	.06	1.23	0.79-1.93	.92
Tobacco abuse	0.94	0.61-1.45	.80	–	–	–
Peripheral vascular disease	4.89	2.41-9.89	<.001			
Previous lower extremity bypass	1.66	1.03-2.67	.04	3.74	1.82-7.71	<.001
Renal insufficiency	2.85	1.85-4.39	<.001	2.19	1.39-3.45	.001
Length of stay, index, days	0.98	0.96-1.01	.24	–	–	–

CI, Confidence interval; *OR*, odds ratio.

Reprinted from Beaulieu RJ, Grimm JC, Lyu H, et al. Rates and predictors of readmission after minor lower extremity amputations. *J Vasc Surg*. 2015;62:101-105, with permission from the Society for Vascular Surgery.

proximal necrosis at the site of the minor amputation wound. Discharging a patient with digital ulcers, gangrene, or a minor amputation wound with borderline healing potential risks readmission if infection or further necrosis occur, making close observation and early-interval follow-up important when these circumstances exist. This analysis therefore provides some criteria useful for anticipating readmission after minor (either toe or transmetatarsal) lower extremity amputation.

Readmission was common after minor amputation in this study, occurring at a rate of 13.9% and was followed by major extremity amputation among more than 60% of readmitted patients. As the authors point out, the Affordable Care Act has created heightened scrutiny related to readmission. Although readmission may be an appropriate outcome for targeted quality initiatives, punitive nonreimbursement in the setting of readmission for critical limb ischemia has several potential negative consequences that warrant thoughtful consideration. Overly aggressive policies directed toward avoidance of readmission may discourage providers from performing minor amputations when the outcome is uncertain, leading to major extremity amputations that were potentially avoidable (a consequence that seems much more difficult to accept than a readmission). For most patients, risk tolerance for wound complications and/or readmission is quite high when then only alternative is major extremity amputation. This attitude seems reasonable from a societal perspective given the lifelong costs of a major extremity amputation (and conversely the lifelong savings associated with limb salvage, even if readmission is necessary to accomplish this goal). Provider risk tolerance is under siege as short-term financial margins increasingly take precedence in the current health care environment however, and a surge in above-knee amputation rates as a consequence of this attitude seems neither desirable nor far-fetched.

Studies like this one demonstrate that it is unreasonable to expect readmission to become a "never" event for patients with critical limb ischemia. The key to deciding between a minor versus major amputation often comes down to where one draws the line between reasonable odds of success and futility. Providers caring for patients with peripheral artery disease must advocate for patient-centered goals that tolerate readmission among a minority of patients with a reasonable chance at the better functional independence, body image, and quality of life gained through limb salvage. As the authors opine, identification of modifiable risk factors for readmission is necessary if we hope to develop evidence-based strategies to avoid this outcome. Along those lines, perhaps appropriate screening before minor extremity amputation would be a better target for quality initiatives than readmission rates. A step in that direction might be routine consideration of the risk factors for readmission identified in this study (Table 2) before proceeding with minor amputation. It would be interesting to know whether all patients undergoing minor amputations were screened with ankle or toe brachial indexes; such a policy would be difficult to argue against among patients with diabetes and/or kidney disease. Hopefully the pendulum won't swing too far toward major amputation by default for the sake of avoiding readmissions because it is unlikely that many patients would accept this trade as higher quality care.

M. Corriere, MD, MS

8 Nonatherosclerotic

Inflammatory disease of the aorta: Patterns and classification of giant cell aortitis, Takayasu arteritis, and nonsyndromic aortitis

Svensson LG, Arafat A, Roselli EE, et al (Cleveland Clinic, OH)

J Thorac Cardiovasc Surg 149:S170-S175, 2015

Objective.—Inflammatory diseases of the aorta, other than those of known infective etiology, are poorly understood. We analyzed a large series of affected patients who had histologic diagnoses with a view to improving the classification of the extent of aortitis to enable a more targeted approach of treatment.

Methods.—Between 1996 and 2012, we operated on 7551 patients with ascending or aortic arch disease, of whom 279 had clinically diagnosed inflammatory disease. Of these, 156 (2%) were found to have aortitis on histologic examination.

Results.—Patients were divided into 4 histologically based groups: giant cell aortitis, 31% (49/156); Takayasu arteritis, 5.1% (8/156); isolated aortitis, 59% (92/156); and other, 4.5% (7/156). Patterns of anatomic extent were also analyzed, and in particular it was noted that giant cell aortitis and isolated aortitis had more extensive disease. In addition, specimen analysis suggested early indications of unrecognized preexistent infections. Death after surgery occurred in 3.2% (5/156), and stroke in 1.9% (3/156). Kaplan-Meier survival at 8 years was 55%. We present a classification for disease extent and management.

Conclusions.—Aortitis continues to be a conundrum; however, good results are achievable with surgery. Intervention should be based on a clearer understanding of the histologic pattern and extent of disease, which helps in subsequent targeted disease management (Fig 2).

► Inflammatory disease of the aorta includes many overlapping forms and etiologies. Dr Svensson and the Cleveland Clinic group have expertly reviewed an extensive volume of patients with ascending aorta or arch disease to improve their original classification of Takayasu arteritis patients as published by Svensson and Crawford in 1997. By evaluating 156 of the 7551 patients with histologic aortitis who underwent surgical repair, they propose a classification of 4 types (Fig 2) with various aortic aneurysm/narrowing as a guide for further treatment. For example, in patients with type 1 disease, they recognize little

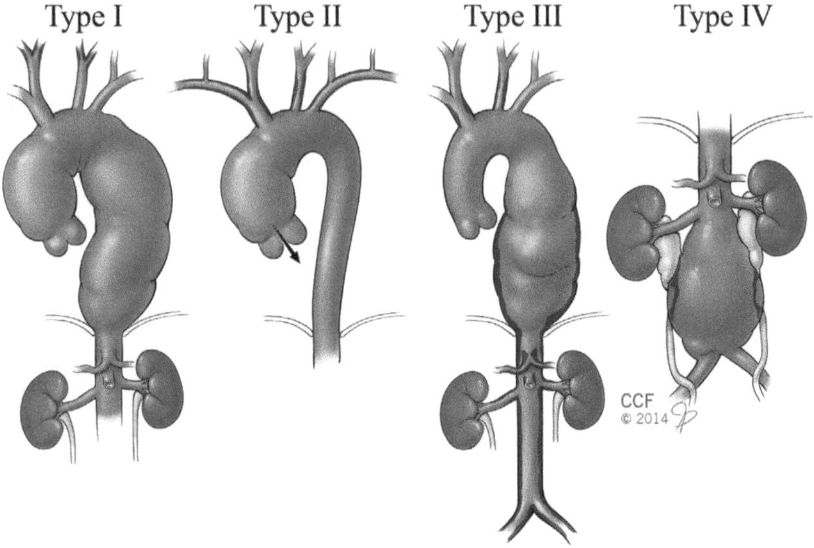

FIGURE 2.—Aortic aneurysm–narrowing classification. (Reprinted from Svensson LG, Arafat A, Roselli EE, et al. Inflammatory disease of the aorta: patterns and classification of giant cell aortitis, Takayasu arteritis, and nonsyndromic aortitis. *J Thorac Cardiovasc Surg*. 2015;149:S170-S175, with permission from The American Association for Thoracic Surgery.)

need for clinical distinction between giant cell aortitis and isolated aortitis. This population, however, should be considered for prophylactic elephant trunk procedure because natural progression will likely necessitate future intervention. Overall, the authors confirmed that histological aortitis is fairly common in patients undergoing ascending or arch aortic repair and occurred at a rate of 2%. New to this study was the presence of rare unrecognized microorganisms in the aortic samples. This subclinical infection may contribute to the etiology of the disease and has already been suggested in tumor biology (Bebek 2012). Infective etiology to aortitis will certainly be a renewed topic of future research thanks to this study.

K. C. Orion, MD

Retrospective Comparison of Open versus Endovascular Procedures for Takayasu Arteritis

Labarca C, Makol A, Crowson CS, et al (Mayo Clinic, Rochester, MN; Univ of California at Los Angeles (UCLA))

J Rheumatol 43:427-432, 2016

Objective.—To compare the outcomes between vascular surgery and endovascular procedures in a cohort of patients with Takayasu arteritis (TA).

Methods.—A retrospective cohort study was conducted of patients with TA who underwent vascular interventions at a tertiary center between 1984 and 2009. The American College of Rheumatology criteria for TA were used to select patients. Disease activity was assessed according to the Kerr criteria. Data are reported using descriptive statistics and Kaplan-Meier methods for complication rates.

Results.—The cohort included 66 patients with TA who underwent 119 vascular procedures (surgery 93; endovascular repair 26). The most frequent indication for vascular surgery and endovascular procedure was arm claudication (surgical group 43%, endovascular repair group 31%). In 59% of the vascular surgical procedures and in 38% of endovascular procedures, the disease was active within 1 month of intervention. The most frequent arterial lesion requiring intervention was the aorta (28%) in the vascular surgery group and the subclavian (35%) in the endovascular repair group. Early complications occurred after 15 surgeries and 4 endovascular repair procedures ($p = 0.93$). Late complications occurred after 34 surgical procedures and 10 endovascular repair procedures (44% vs 66%, respectively; $p = 0.33$). The majority of complications in both groups were restenosis. Hypertension, dyslipidemia, and higher doses of corticosteroids were associated with an increased risk of postprocedural complications and restenosis.

Conclusion.—In patients with TA, both open surgical and endovascular revascularization procedures are associated with high failure rates and frequent operative complications. Traditional cardiovascular risk factors, corticosteroid dose, and active disease are risk factors for restenosis after revascularization procedures (Table 6).

▶ Takayasu arteritis (TA) is a large-vessel vasculitis affecting primarily the aorta and its branches, which can lead to extremity and end-organ ischemia. First-line therapy is typically with corticosteroids; however, patients often develop chronic lesions that are not responsive to medical management. More than half of patients with TA undergo some type of vascular intervention. The authors of this article sought to compare the outcomes of patients undergoing open versus endovascular repair for their disease.

They performed a retrospective study from 1984 to 2009 and identified 126 patients. Of these, 66 patients underwent vascular intervention; 119 procedures were performed: 93 open and 26 endovascular. The most frequent indications for endovascular or surgical intervention were claudication, hypertension, and heart failure. As with other studies, revascularization procedures were associated with high failure rates. Restenosis was the most common procedure-related late complication for both groups, 26 after surgery and 9 after endovascular repair (37% vs 62%, $P = .19$). Several risk factors were correlated with increased complications. These included presence of hypertension ($P = .02$), corticosteroid dose ($P = .004$), and dyslipidemia ($P = .005$) (see Table 6). The increased rate of complication seen with patients on corticosteroids may indicate procedures undertaken during the active phase of the disease, which is frequently associated with higher complication rates.

TABLE 6.—Risk Factors for Postprocedural Complications and Restenosis

Variable	Any Postprocedural Complication, HR (95% CI)	Restenosis, HR (95% CI)
Endovascular repair	1.15 (0.59–2.25)	1.33 (0.58–3.06)
Age at surgery	0.87* (0.67–1.13)	0.70* (0.48–1.01)
Sex male	0.41 (0.12–1.39)	0.43 (0.09–2.07)
Corticosteroid use	1.45 (0.83–2.52)	2.08 (0.96–4.51)
Corticosteroid dose**	**1.15 (1.04–1.26)**	**1.23 (1.05–1.45)**
Immunosuppressant use	1.08 (0.59–1.97)	1.32 (0.59–2.92)
Aorta	1.10 (0.59–2.07)	**0.33 (0.11–0.99)**
Thoracic	1.35 (0.77–2.36)	1.82 (0.86–3.85)
Abdominal	1.33 (0.72–2.45)	0.95 (0.41–2.23)
Emergency procedure	2.53 (0.99–6.48)	**1.41** (0.29–6.81)
Arm claudication	0.83 (0.47–1.47)	1.14 (0.54–2.41)
Leg claudication	0.93 (0.43–1.98)	0.85 (0.29–2.44)
Heart failure	0.73 (0.28–1.90)	0.22 (0.03–1.67)
Myocardial infarction	1.34 (0.49–3.66)	2.49 (0.77–8.12)
Hypertension	**2.40 (1.12–5.16)**	**4.91 (1.42–17.00)**
Dyslipidemia	**2.93 (1.38–6.25)**	**4.25 (1.41–12.79)**
Diabetes mellitus	0.79 (0.09–6.91)	—
Current smoker (vs never)	0.41 (0.18–0.94)	0.37 (0.11–1.24)
Former smoker (vs never)	0.78 (0.41–1.49)	0.93 (0.37–2.32)
NIH criterion 1 (systemic features, fever, musculoskeletal pain)	0.72 (0.22–2.35)	0.89 (0.19–4.09)
NIH criterion 2 (elevated ESR)	2.59 (0.94–7.09)	1.92 (0.33–11.9)
NIH criterion 3 (features of vascular ischemia or inflammation)	1.99 (0.95–4.18)	**3.14 (1.06–9.27)**
NIH criterion 4 (typical angiographic features)	1.8 (0.63–5.16)	1.89 (0.43–8.32)
NIH criteria (2+ vs 0–1)	1.45 (0.80–2.63)	1.75 (0.77–3.99)

*HR reported per 10-year increase (values in bold type are statistically significant).

**Per 10 mg/day increase. NIH: US National Institutes of Health; ESR: erythrocyte sedimentation rate.

Reprinted from Labarca C, Makol A, Crowson CS, et al. Retrospective comparison of open versus endovascular procedures for takayasu arteritis. *J Rheumatol.* 2016;43:427-432, with permission from The Journal of Rheumatology.

Although this is a retrospective study, it has a relatively large cohort of patients with TA. It illustrates the inherent risks and frequent complications associated with vascular interventions in these patients, both endovascular and open.

M. Arnold, MD

Vessel Wall Inflammation of Takayasu Arteritis Detected by Contrast-Enhanced Magnetic Resonance Imaging: Association with Disease Distribution and Activity

Kato Y, Terashima M, Ohigashi H, et al (Tokyo Med and Dental Univ, Japan; Cardiovascular Imaging Clinic, Tokyo, Japan)
PLoS One 10:e0145855, 2015

Aims.—The assessment of the distribution and activity of vessel wall inflammation is clinically important in patients with Takayasu arteritis. Magnetic resonance imaging (MRI) is a useful tool, but the clinical utility of late gadolinium enhancement (LGE) in Takayasu arteritis has yet to be determined. The aim of the present study was to evaluate the utility of LGE in assessing vessel wall inflammation and disease activity in Takayasu arteritis.

Methods and Results.—We enrolled 49 patients with Takayasu arteritis who had undergone 1.5 T MRI. Patients were divided into Active (n = 19) and Inactive disease (n = 30) groups. The distribution of vessel wall inflammation using angiography and LGE was assessed by qualitative analysis. In 79% and 63% of patients in Active and Inactive groups, respectively, greater distribution of vessel wall inflammation was observed with LGE than with conventional angiography. MRI values of pre- and post-contrast signal-to-noise ratios (SNR), SNR increment (post- SNR minus pre-SNR), pre- and post-contrast contrast-to-noise ratios (CNR), and CNR increment (post-CNR minus pre-CNR) were evaluated at arterial wall sites with the highest signal intensity using quantitative analysis of post-contrast LGE images. No statistically significant differences in MRI parameters were observed between Active and Inactive groups. Contrast-enhanced MRI was unable to accurately detect active disease.

Conclusion.—Contrast-enhanced MRI has utility in detecting the distribution of vessel wall inflammation but has less utility in assessing disease activity in Takayasu arteritis (Fig 1).

▶ Takayasu arteritis can have many distributions throughout the aortic arch and aortic branches, as shown in Fig 1. What is equally important to the disease location is whether the disease is active. This is paramount in surgical planning because operating during active inflammation markedly increases the risk. The authors herein have attempted to use late gadolinium enhancement (LGE) to determine whether this can be a useful tool to determine disease activity. Magnetic resonance imaging (MRI) is increasingly being used for this purpose.

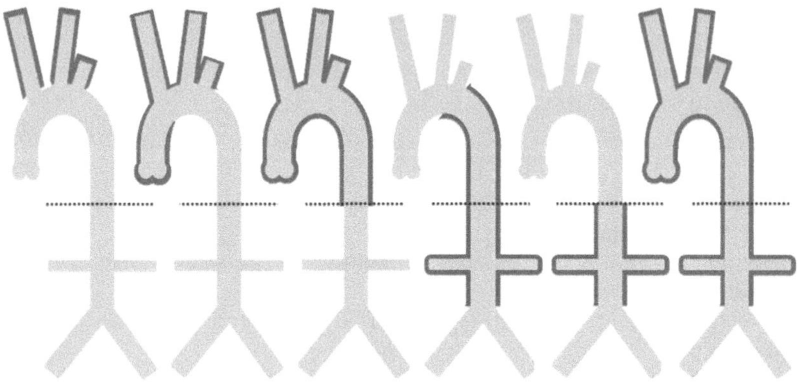

FIGURE 1.—Angiographic classification of Takayasu arteritis. The dotted lines refer to the diaphragms. (Reprinted from Kato Y, Terashima M, Ohigashi H, et al. Vessel wall inflammation of Takayasu arteritis detected by contrast-enhanced magnetic resonance imaging: association with disease distribution and activity. *PLoS One*. 2015;10:e0145855, with permission Kato et al.)

Interestingly, although many patients with Takayasu arteritis are Japanese in heritage, the use of intravascular gadolinium contrast agent, the most commonly used agent in magnetic resonance imaging (MRI), is not currently available in Japan. Therefore, they used gadopentetate dimeglumine, which is widely used clinically. Authors found that LGE was sensitive to detect disease but not able to assess activity versus inactivity even with a well-thought-out subgroup analysis. Many surgeons rely on C-reactive protein (CRP) to guide judgment on disease activity, and these authors also found a significant difference in CRP levels in patients with active disease. Still, because MRI is far more sensitive than CT or traditional angiography to detect vessel wall inflammation, the authors smartly propose further studies with MRI to find a contrast agent more targeted such as elastin, collagen, or macrophages.

K. C. Orion, MD

Surgical Treatment of Middle Aortic Syndrome with Takayasu Arteritis or Midaortic Dysplastic Syndrome

Kim SM, Jung IM, Han A, et al (Seoul Natl Univ College of Medicine, Republic of Korea; et al)

Eur J Vasc Endovasc Surg 50:206-212, 2015

Objective.—Middle aortic syndrome (MAS) is a rare condition characterized by severe stenosis of the distal thoracic or abdominal aorta. The aims of this study are to define the anatomic characteristics of MAS and to review the various surgical methods and their outcomes in terms of long-term durability.

Materials and Methods.—Ten adult patients were diagnosed with MAS caused by Takayasu arteritis (TA) or midaortic dysplastic syndrome and underwent surgical treatment between July 1992 and January 2013.

Result.—The aortic lesions were mostly suprarenal ($n = 7$) and stenoses were commonly found in the celiac axis ($n = 6$), SMA ($n = 7$), and renal artery ($n = 6$). Indications for operation were uncontrolled hypertension in six patients and lower extremity claudication in four. Eight aortic bypasses, one supraceliac aortic interposition graft, and one bilateral aorto-renal bypass were performed. Adjunctive renal bypass with saphenous vein graft ($n = 4$) and IMA reimplantation ($n = 2$) were performed simultaneously. There was no post-operative mortality, and one complication of iliac dissection at the distal anastomosis site was detected and treated by stenting. Hypertension was cured or improved in five of the six patients, and lower extremity claudication improved in all of them. With a median follow up of 60 months (range, 12–263), all the aortic bypasses were patent and one adjunctive renal artery bypass graft with aortic bypass was occluded 29 months post-operatively.

Conclusions.—Aortic bypass for MAS is safe and shows excellent long-term durability. Considering the patients are relatively young with a long life expectancy, aggressive surgical treatment could be beneficial. Lifelong follow up to monitor complications and disease progression is necessary (Fig 2).

▶ Although treatment of coarctation of the thoracic aorta is well described, little is known about the treatment of stenosis of the abdominal aorta due to inflammatory arteritis. Termed "middle aortic syndrome" (MAS), these patients present with uncontrolled hypertension as well as symptoms of lower extremity claudication. Treatment options include thoracoabdominal bypass. The authors of this article did a retrospective review of the evaluation and treatment of 10 patients with middle aortic syndrome.

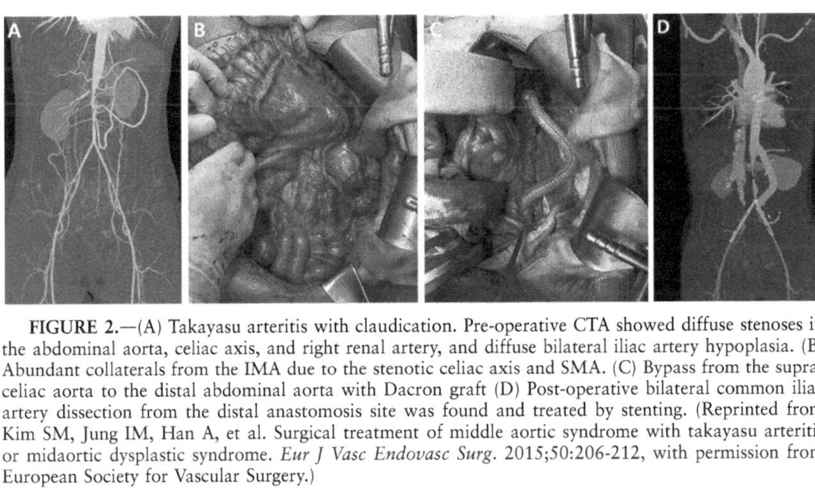

FIGURE 2.—(A) Takayasu arteritis with claudication. Pre-operative CTA showed diffuse stenoses in the abdominal aorta, celiac axis, and right renal artery, and diffuse bilateral iliac artery hypoplasia. (B) Abundant collaterals from the IMA due to the stenotic celiac axis and SMA. (C) Bypass from the supraceliac aorta to the distal abdominal aorta with Dacron graft (D) Post-operative bilateral common iliac artery dissection from the distal anastomosis site was found and treated by stenting. (Reprinted from Kim SM, Jung IM, Han A, et al. Surgical treatment of middle aortic syndrome with takayasu arteritis or midaortic dysplastic syndrome. *Eur J Vasc Endovasc Surg*. 2015;50:206-212, with permission from European Society for Vascular Surgery.)

MAS syndrome was diagnosed by its radiologic features, stenosis or occlusion in the distal thoracic or abdominal aorta. The majority of patients (8 of 10) were treated with aorto-aortic bypass. Seven of 8 of those also underwent a concomitant procedure, either renal bypass or internal mammary artery reimplantation (Fig 2). There were no perioperative mortalities. The 1 reported complication was an iliac artery dissection, likely due to clamp injury, that was treated with stenting. At follow-up, hypertension was cured or improved in 5 of 6 patients in whom that was a presenting symptom, and all patients presenting with claudication had improvement in their symptoms. No progression of aortic stenosis or problems at the anastomotic sites were seen at follow-up.

Of note only 2 of the 10 patients were on steroids or immunosuppression. Although there are no clear-cut markers for active disease, it is recommended that revascularization procedures not be performed during the active phase of the disease.

The authors of this article describe an elegant and effective technique for the treatment of a challenging problem. However, as they acknowledge, their patient group is small, and they were only treated with open repair. A more robust, perhaps multicenter prospective study that also includes endovascular techniques would help further delineate indications, technical challenges, and outcomes for these complex patients.

M. Arnold, MD

Efficacy of Biological-Targeted Treatments in Takayasu Arteritis Multicenter, Retrospective Study of 49 Patients

Mekinian A, for the French Takayasu Network (Hôpital Saint Antoine, Paris, France; et al)

Circulation 132:1693-1700, 2015

Background.—The goal of this work was to assess the safety and efficacy of biologics (ie, tumor necrosis factor-α antagonists and tocilizumab) in patients with Takayasu arteritis.

Methods and Results.—This was a retrospective, multicenter study of the characteristics and outcomes of 49 patients with Takayasu arteritis (80% female; median age, 42 years [20–55 years] treated by tumor necrosis factor-α antagonists [80%] or tocilizumab [20%]) and fulfilling American College of Rheumatology or Ishikawa criteria. Factors associated with complete response were assessed. Eighty-eight percent of patients with Takayasu arteritis were inadequately controlled with or were intolerant to conventional immunosuppressive therapy (median number, 3 [1–5]). Overall response (ie, complete and partial) to biological-targeted treatments at 6 and 12 months was 75% and 83%, respectively. There were significantly lower C-reactive protein levels at the initiation of biological-targeted treatments (22 mg/L [10–46 mg/L] versus 58 mg/L [26–76 mg/L]; $P = 0.006$) and a trend toward fewer immunosuppressants drugs used before biologics ($P = 0.054$) in responders (ie, complete or partial responders) relative to nonresponders to biological-targeted treatments. C-reactive protein levels and daily prednisone dose significantly decreased after 12 months of biological-targeted treatments (30 versus 6 mg/L [$P < 0.05$] and 15 versus 7.5 mg [$P < 0.05$] at baseline and 12 months, respectively). The 3-year relapse-free survival was 90.9% (83.5%–99%) over the biological treatment period compared with 58.7% (43.3%–79.7%; $P = 0.0025$) with disease-modifying anti-rheumatic drugs. No difference in efficacy was found between tumor necrosis factor-α antagonists and tocilizumab. After a median follow-up of 24 months (2–95 months), 21% of patients experienced adverse effects, with biological-targeted treatments discontinued in 6.6% of cases.

Conclusion.—This nationwide study shows a high efficacy of biological-targeted treatments in refractory patients with Takayasu arteritis with an acceptable safety profile.

▶ This article is a review of patients with refractory Takayasu arteritis (TA) and the response to biologic therapy. In general, the results of this article suggest a positive benefit to instituting biologic therapy for patient with refractory TA. Most impressive is the 3-year data indicating high rates of symptomatic relief with a relative safe side effect profile. The article is a retrospective review, and patients were not randomized to different therapies. There would be clear benefit of a long-term prospective randomized trial; however, the disease process is rare, and this study looks specifically at refractory disease. From the review, it appears that biologic therapy has promising results in this selected population and should be remembered for patients suffering from refractory disease.

B. Propper, MD, FACS

Eligibility and Disqualification Recommendations for Competitive Athletes With Cardiovascular Abnormalities: Task Force 7: Aortic Diseases, Including Marfan Syndrome: A Scientific Statement From the American Heart Association and American College of Cardiology

Braverman AC, on behalf of the American Heart Association Electrocardiography and Arrhythmias Committee of the Council on Clinical Cardiology, Council on Cardiovascular Disease in the Young, Council on Cardiovascular and Stroke Nursing, Council on Functional Genomics and Translational Biology, and the American College of Cardiology ()

Circulation 132:e303-e309, 2015

Background.—Both acute aortic dissection and rupture can cause sudden death in athletes with Marfan syndrome or similar aortopathies. These athletes have increases in blood pressure and aortic stress during intense physical exertion, which can lead to aortic catastrophe from dissection or rupture or accelerate the development of an aneurysm. Therefore these athletes should know what levels of exercise are safe for them to participate in from an early age. Marfan syndrome and similar disorders affect multiple organ systems and include cardiovascular features such as mitral valve prolapse, mitral regurgitation, aortic root dilatation, and aortic dissection. Aneurysm formation and dissection are also more likely in the descending aorta.

Patient Evaluation.—Individuals with Marfan syndrome and similar disorders should have their aortic diameters measured serially to determine if they are enlarged or enlarging. However, the various imaging methods used to determine aortic diameter result in different values. Therefore *z* scores that incorporate the individual's height, weight, age, and sex are now preferred over single aortic dimensional determination. A *z* score describes the number of standard deviations over or under a size or age-specific population that a specified measurement falls. The score helps to assess cardiac dimensions in young persons, whose normal values change with growth. Mild, moderate, and severe aortic dilatation is defined by *z* score values of 2 to 3, 3.01 to 4.0, and over 4.0, respectively.

Athletic participation can produce hemodynamic changes that increase aortic wall tension and aortic dimension. In addition, elite athletes have somewhat larger aortas at the Valsalva sinuses than nonathletes. Mild aortic enlargement may be a normal adaptive response to intense training, but larger increases are not normal, most often indicating the presence of an underlying pathologic condition. Exercise training can exacerbate the underlying condition.

Tall athletes may also demonstrate a slightly larger aortic dimension than that considered the upper limit of normal, but it is important to not assume that an enlarged aorta in a tall or large athlete is nonpathologic. For athletes whose aortic *z* scores are above normal for their age, sex, and body surface area (BSA), a knowledgeable specialist or a multidisciplinary team should be engaged to exclude the presence of any underlying disorder associated with aortic dilatation, including Marfan syndrome.

Risk Assessment.—The long-term prognosis for athletes who have unexplained aortic dilatation remains unclear. In addition, no prospective data exist to clarify the risks of competitive athletics for patients who have had surgical correction of aortic dissection or aneurysm. However, persons with Marfan syndrome and similar disorders remain at risk for distal aortic complications for their lifetime.

Conclusions.—For aortic root enlargement of more than 40 mm in adults or more than 2 standard deviations from the mean for BSA in children and adolescents, participation should be limited to low-intensity competitive sports. For patients with mildly dilated aortic diameters (*z* score of 2 to 2.5 or 1 to 2 mm above normal range) and no diagnosis of connective tissue disorder, family history of aortic disease, or pathogenic gene mutation associated with aneurysm, individual choices must be made on a case-by-case basis. Discussions should include the athlete, parents (as appropriate), and coaches/trainers and fully disclose the potential risks of further training and competition. If participation in competitive sports is continued, the athlete should undergo close aortic surveillance (every 6 to 12 months) with echocardiography or magnetic resonance angiography. Frequency of imaging should be determined by the absolute size of the aorta, *z* score, stability of the aorta's size, and intensity of the sport. For patients whose aorta continues to enlarge, disqualification from competition is appropriate. In addition, because mildly dilated aortic roots have required aortic aneurysm surgery in later years, long-term aortic surveillance is recommended even after the athlete's competitive days are past. (Fig 1).

▶ Athletes with aortic disease or a condition associated with aortic disease are at risk for acute aortic dissection or rupture. This includes patients with Marfan syndrome, Loeys-Dietz syndrome, familial thoracic aortic aneurysm and dissection syndrome, and bicuspid aortic valve aortopathy. An important step in counseling these patients is accurate measurement of the aortic root and ascending aorta. Measurements should be taken perpendicular to the axis of blood flow and should include the largest measured aortic diameter (attach figure from paper). In addition to the measurement, clinicians should also consider the *z* score when making recommendations to patients. The *z* score describes how many standard deviations above or below a mean of a specific population a value lies. A *z* score of 2 to 3 signifies mild aortic dilatation, whereas a *z* score >4.0 is suggestive of severe dilation.

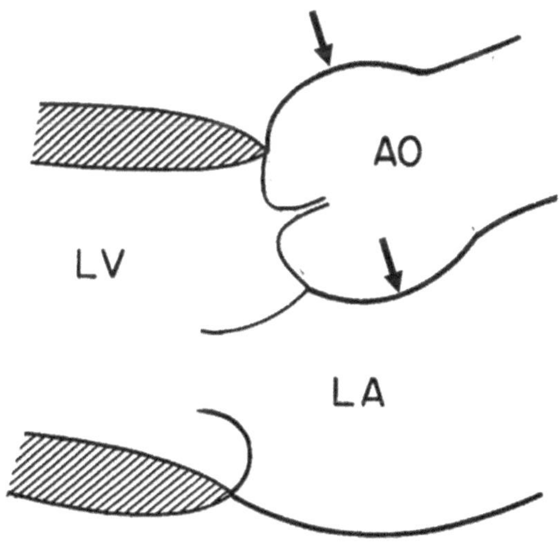

FIGURE 1.—Schematic of the aortic root showing measurement of the aortic root diameter at maximum width parallel to the aortic annular plane by American Society of Echocardiography leading-edge convention (arrows). AO indicates aorta; LA, left atrium; and LV, left ventricle. (Reprinted from Braverman AC, on behalf of the American Heart Association Electrocardiography and Arrhythmias Committee of the Council on Clinical Cardiology, Council on Cardiovascular Disease in the Young, Council on Cardiovascular and Stroke Nursing, Council on Functional Genomics and Translational Biology, and the American College of Cardiology. Eligibility and disqualification recommendations for competitive athletes with cardiovascular abnormalities: task force 7: aortic diseases, including Marfan syndrome: a scientific statement from the American Heart Association and American College of Cardiology. *Circulation.* 2015;132:e303-e309, with permission from the American Heart Association, Inc. and the American College of Cardiology Foundation.)

Of note, elite athletes have slightly larger aortas at the sinuses of Valsalva than control subjects. However a large increase in aortic size is unusual in athletes and should be investigated further. Athletes with aortic *z* scores >2 to 2.5 should be evaluated by a specialist.

There are limited data as to the long-term outcomes of athletes with aortic dilatation. In addition, there is no evidence that beta-blockers, angiotensin receptor blockers, or angiotensin-converting enzyme inhibitors protect athletes from dissection or rupture.

The authors include an extensive updated list of guidelines for managing athletes with aortic pathology. Indeed, these patients need special attention and require long-term follow-up and surveillance even after they have stopped competing in athletic activities at an elite level.

M. Arnold, MD

Visceral Renal

Outcomes of Hypertensive Patients with Renal Fibromuscular Dysplasia Compared with Patients with Concomitant Atherosclerotic Renal Artery Stenosis following Endovascular Therapy

Jenkins TL, Baker MG, Baheti AR, et al (Univ of Virginia School of Medicine, Charlottesville)
J Vasc Interv Radiol 26:625-633, 2015

Purpose.—To examine if the outcomes after endovascular treatment in hypertensive patients with renal artery fibromuscular dysplasia (FMD) and incidental atherosclerotic renal artery stenosis (ARAS) differ from the outcomes in patients with FMD alone.

Materials and Methods.—All cases of patients with renal artery FMD undergoing percutaneous transluminal angioplasty during the period 2002–2012 were reviewed. The patients with complete data before and after the procedure were identified (N = 84). Based on the procedural reports, these patients were separated into two cohorts: patients with isolated FMD (n = 59) and patients with concomitant atherosclerotic renal artery stenosis and FMD (ARAS-FMD) (n = 25). The medical record of each patient was reviewed for baseline blood pressure, antihypertensive medication use, and renal function data and the same data after the procedure. Procedural details including the angiographic findings, the number of stents placed, the average number of revascularization procedures, and the number of patients requiring more than one revascularization procedure were noted.

Results.—The study population included 68 patients (FMD, n = 46; ARAS-FMD, n = 22). Patients in the FMD and ARAS-FMD cohorts experienced comparable significant decreases in systolic and mean arterial pressures after endovascular intervention. There was no change in the number of antihypertensive medications after the procedure within or between groups. Patients in the ARAS-FMD cohort had lower baseline estimated

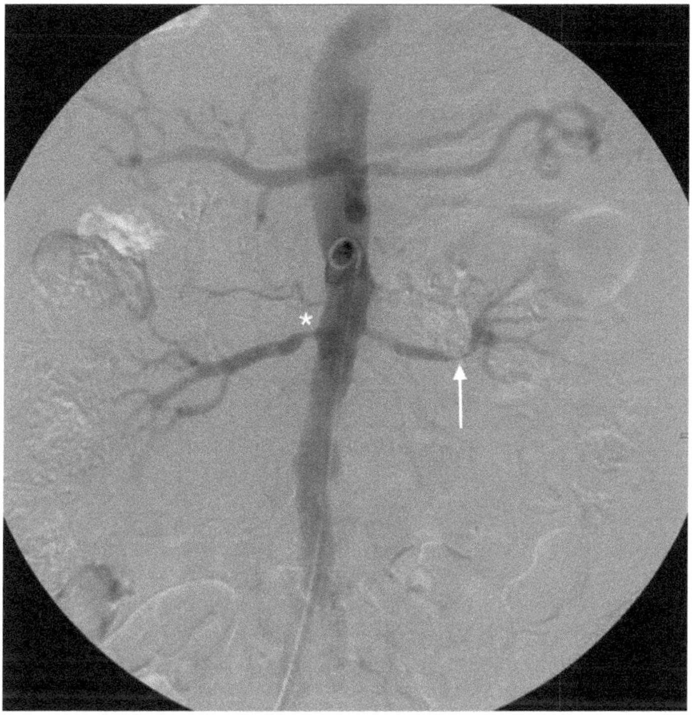

FIGURE 1.—Aortogram reveals a smooth concentric narrowing of the distal left renal artery consistent with focal MD (arrow) and a significant ostial eccentric right renal artery lesion (asterisk) representing ARAS. There is also atherosclerotic disease in the proximal left renal artery. (Reprinted from Jenkins TL, Baker MG, Baheti AR, et al. Outcomes of hypertensive patients with renal fibromuscular dysplasia compared with patients with concomitant atherosclerotic renal artery stenosis following endovascular therapy. *J Vasc Interv Radiol.* 2015;26:625-633, with permission from SIR.)

glomerular filtration rates ($P = .007$); however, renal function stabilized in both groups after endovascular therapy.

Conclusions.—Patients with ARAS-FMD respond to endovascular therapy with outcomes similar to patients with isolated renal artery FMD (Figs 1 and 5).

▶ The authors of this article present a retrospective review comparing patient with fibromuscular dysplasia (FMD) to those with FMD and renal artery stenosis (RAS). The conclusions indicate that both groups respond similar to endovascular therapy. From the review, the authors indicate that a diagnosis of FMD was established based on angiographic imaging. Additionally, a diagnosis of RAS was also based on angiographic imaging. I do not believe that angiographic imaging is appropriate for determining RAS from proximal FMD using angiogram. It is well believed that the majority of RAS stems from extension of aortic disease into the proximal renal vessels. The authors point to Figs 1 and 5 as an example of RAS and FMD. From the images, there is minimal to no aortic disease, and I would propose that the right-sided lesion is truly proximal

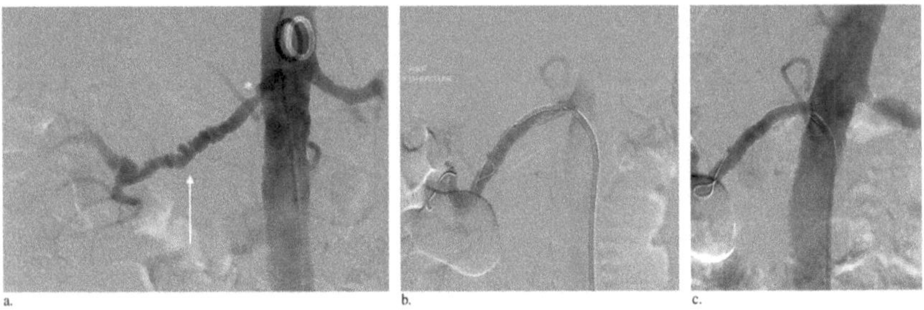

FIGURE 5.—(a) Aortogram revealing multifocal FMD affecting the right renal artery (arrow) and a 70% ostial stenosis (asterisk) representing ARAS. Note atherosclerotic involvement of the infrarenal aorta. (b) Selective right renal angiogram after treatment with balloon percutaneous transluminal angioplasty of FMD lesion. (c) Successful deployment of a stent across the ostial lesion with resolution of the pressure gradient. (Reprinted from Jenkins TL, Baker MG, Baheti AR, et al. Outcomes of hypertensive patients with renal fibromuscular dysplasia compared with patients with concomitant atherosclerotic renal artery stenosis following endovascular therapy. *J Vasc Interv Radiol.* 2015;26:625-633, with permission from SIR.)

FMD and not RAS. Given the difficulty in truly defining FMD versus RAS, I think the results of this study must be examined further. There is a clear age difference between the 2 groups noted by the authors. My suspicion is that many of the RAS patients were patient with proximal FMD in the later stages and who thus do not truly represent a comparison of age-related RAS with FMD. When we examine both populations together, what can be seen is that patients with FMD respond well to angioplasty as the primary treatment modality and that those patients with FMD and systemic manifestation represent a patient population that should be targeted as the response to therapy is far greater than the group analyzed in the 2014 CORAL Trial.

B. Propper, MD, FACS

9 Upper Extremity

Venous Disease

Utilization of venous duplex scanning and postoperative venography in patients with subclavian vein thrombosis

Orlando MS, Likes KC, Lum YW, et al (Johns Hopkins Univ School of Medicine, Baltimore, MD)

J Vasc Surg Venous Lymphat Disord 3:173-177, 2015

Objective.—The purpose of this study was to review preoperative and postoperative duplex scans and postoperative venograms in patients with subclavian vein thrombosis who underwent first rib resection and scalenectomy (FRRS) during 2005 to 2013.

Methods.—Preoperative venous duplex scans revealed no compression (NC), venous compression (VC, ≥50% decrease in velocity on abduction), venous ablation (VA, 0 velocity on abduction), and acute thrombus (AT, 0 velocity on abduction and adduction). Correlation with 2-week postoperative venograms (open, stenosis requiring dilation, or occluded) and postoperative (2- to 4-month, 6- to 8-month, and 12-month) duplex scans was performed.

Results.—Of 215 patients treated with FRRS for effort thrombosis, 140 had an ipsilateral preoperative duplex scan and postoperative venogram. Twenty-nine patients (21%) had VC, 70 (50%) had VA, 8 (5.7%) had AT, and 33 (24%) had NC. Patients with preoperative NC or VC were more likely to have an open vein on venography ($P = .014$). Six to 8 months after FRRS, patients with preoperative VA were more likely to have compression or ablation ($P = .009$); no difference was seen at 1 year. Patency rates at last follow-up were 100% in the preoperative VC and AT groups, 96% in those with VA, and 94% in patients with no preoperative compression. The 128 preoperative scans of the asymptomatic side revealed that 67 patients (52%) had NC, 29 (23%) had VC, 32 (25%) had VA, and 0 had AT. Patients with NC ($P = .027$), VC ($P = .017$), or VA ($P = .008$) were significantly more likely to have the same result on the opposite side.

Conclusions.—Postoperative duplex scans reveal that VC and VA resolve during the year after FRRS, obviating the need for repeated venography or intervention. Patency rates are excellent in all patients when postoperative venography directs intervention. Patients with NC, VC, or VA on preoperative scans often show the same result on the opposite side.

▶ The continued experience of Dr Freischlag et al refines the treatment algorithms for venous thoracic outlet syndrome. The current recommendations of decompression followed by interval venography and potential angioplasty, and the findings of the venography, dictate the duration of continued anticoagulation. Using this protocol, excellent long-term patency of the vein is achieved. The treatment of thoracic outlet syndrome is largely variable based on the presentation of the patient, and most definitive surgical procedures (decompression with first rib resection and scalenectomy) are performed at institutions separate from the initial presenting institution. Hence, protocols such as these are vital. What is curious within this report is that even with appropriate surgical decompression, a significant proportion of the patients are seen on duplex to have at least some venous compression up to a year postoperatively, even if there was none preoperatively. Although this is puzzling and somewhat suggests "inadequate" decompression, patients overwhelmingly experience symptom relief and absence of acute thrombosis, which remain the primary goals of therapy. It is a reminder that patients are treated and not the ultrasounds.

R. J. Feezor, MD, FACS

Thoracic Outlet

Concurrent venography during first rib resection and scalenectomy for venous thoracic outlet syndrome is safe and efficient

Hawkins AT, Schaumeier MJ, Smith AD, et al (Brigham & Women's Hosp, Boston, MA)

J Vasc Surg Venous Lymphat Disord 3:290-294, 2015

Objective.—Surgical treatment of acute axillosubclavian vein thrombosis from venous thoracic outlet syndrome (VTOS) traditionally involves first rib resection and scalenectomy (FRRS) followed by interval venography and balloon angioplasty. This approach can lead to an extended need for anticoagulation and a separate anesthesia session. We present outcomes for FRRS with concurrent venography.

Methods.—Retrospective chart review was performed for consecutive patients undergoing FRRS with concurrent venography for VTOS from February 2007 to April 2014. Venography was performed immediately after FRRS with the arm in neutral and provocative positions. The primary outcomes of this study were primary and primary-assisted patency. Secondary outcomes included whether concurrent venography resulted in modification of the procedure, postoperative anticoagulation use, and postoperative complications.

Results.—Thirty patients underwent first rib resection with venography with a mean follow-up time of 24.4 months. The mean age was 29.5 years (range, 17-52 years), and 17 (56.7%) were female. All were maintained on anticoagulation before the procedure. Concurrent venography resulted in modification of the procedure in 28 patients (93.3%). Of these, 27 patients (96.4%) underwent balloon angioplasty and two patients (7.1%) underwent further rib resection. Twenty patients (66.7%) were discharged after the procedure with no anticoagulation. For those receiving postoperative anticoagulation for persistent minor thrombus, median time for anticoagulation duration was 5.0 months (range, 0.8 and 16.7 months). Two patients (6.7%) had postoperative bleeding requiring thoracentesis or video-assisted thoracoscopic evacuation of hemothorax. One patient (3.3%) suffered rethrombosis and was successfully lysed open, resulting in a 2-year subclavian vein (SCV) primary patency of 96.7% and primary-assisted patency of 100%. No patients required reoperation for VTOS, and all reported improvements in symptoms. Three patients (10.0%) later underwent prophylactic first rib resection on the contralateral side for symptoms and SCV stenosis.

Conclusions.—FRRS with concurrent venography is a safe procedure for VTOS that allows effective intraoperative modification of the surgical plan, resulting in excellent patency of the SCV, early cessation of anticoagulation, and durable relief of symptoms.

▶ Although algorithms for treatment of venous thoracic outlet syndrome (TOS) vary and consensus is unclear, there is growing evidence, as supported by this study, in favor of using concurrent venography at the time of first rib resection. As noted in this study, 93% of the patients had additional modification based on venography, most of which was the addition of balloon angioplasty. The advantage of a completion venogram is underscored by the additional need for venous balloon angioplasty and minimizing the need for additional venous reconstruction. Although the primary patency at 2 years of 96.7% is excellent, other series have reported higher restenosis rates, with need for repeat angioplasty. Still, with the use of repeat angioplasty, results in all series have been excellent. Overall, this study supports my own bias and practice pattern with routine completion venography and angioplasty under direct operative vision of the decompressed thoracic outlet, which I have also found to be efficient and effective.

M. Passman, MD

Hemodialysis Access

Impact of Duplex Ultrasound Surveillance Program on Patency of Prosthetic Arteriovenous Graft for Hemodialysis: A Single-Center Experience

Mauro R, Pini R, Faggioli G, et al (Univ of Bologna, Italy)
Ann Vasc Surg 29:1211-1217, 2015

Background.—Arteriovenous prosthetic graft (AVG) is an alternative hemodialysis vascular access choice; however, its performance is limited by a high rate of thrombosis. The aim of the study was to compare the long-term secondary patency of AVG in patients undergoing a surveillance program and the long-term secondary patency of AVG in patients with clinical assessment of AVG malfunction.

Methods.—From 2009 to 2012, all patients with AVG entered in a duplex ultrasound (DUS) surveillance program (at 3 months and then every 6 months postoperatively) to assess AVG malfunction and/or stenosis (stenosis >50% and blood flow decrease [<600 mL/min]) and eventually treated by endovascular revascularization. AVG long-term patency in the surveillance group was compared with that obtained in a historical control group in which the malfunction was clinically detected. As secondary end point, the central vein catheter (CVC) placement after AVG thrombosis was compared in the 2 groups.

Results.—Sixty patients were included in the study, 33 (55%) in the surveillance program and 27 (45%) in the historical group. The 2 groups had similar clinical characteristics and follow-up (59, interquartile range [IQR]: 45 vs. 56 [IQR, 40 months], $P = 0.32$). Fifteen (45%) AVG malfunctions were detected in the surveillance group and successfully treated (10 [66.6%] angioplasty and 5 [33.4%] angioplasty stenting). No malfunction was detected in the historical control group. By Kaplan–Meier analysis, the 5-year secondary patency was significantly higher in the surveillance group compared with the historical group: 42 ± 13% vs. 9 ± 7%, $P = 0.03$. By Cox analysis, the DUS surveillance was a significantly protective factor for AVG thrombosis, otherwise the use of CVC before the AVG and diabetes mellitus were AVG thrombosis risk factors. The CVC placement was significantly lower in the surveillance group compared with the historical group (14.0% vs. 42.2%, $P = 0.02$).

Conclusions.—The DUS surveillance allows a greater secondary patency compared with a clinical evaluation and reduces CVC placement rate.

▶ Use of arteriovenous (AV) prosthetic grafts for dialysis is performed in the absence of adequate venous conduit; however, resultant high rates of graft failure make this a suboptimal option. The authors hypothesize that a surveillance program to detect early malfunction and to allow early treatment will increase AV graft patency rates as well as decrease subsequent tunneled dialysis catheter placement. This was a single-center observational cohort study comparing 27 patients who underwent routine clinical evaluation consisting of physical examination of the graft with measurements of bleeding time after removal of needle at the completion of dialysis by nephrologists, and a second group of 33 patients enrolled in a duplex ultrasound surveillance program with examination at 3 months and then every 6 subsequent months, with results interpreted by vascular surgeons. The primary end point was graft secondary patency, and a secondary end point was incidence of tunneled dialysis catheter placement after creation of AV graft. Over the time period of the study, no patients in the clinical evaluation group were identified with failing access compared with 15 (45%) patients with detected stenosis by duplex ultrasound in the surveillance group. Of note, 87% of these patients had "normal" functioning grafts. These patients all underwent angioplasty (67%) or stenting (33%). Secondary patency-defined in this study as patency following any procedure to correct graft stenosis or thrombosis, was 42% versus 9% at 5 years in the clinical evaluation versus duplex surveillance group, respectively. Cox analysis confirmed surveillance ultrasound had a significant protective factor in AV graft patency, whereas use of central catheter before AV graft and diabetes mellitus were risk factors for thrombosis. These results are limited by the small number of patients and single-center nature of the design; however, it suggests that routine use of duplex surveillance strategies after AV graft placement may decrease graft failure rates.

M. R. Smeds, MD, FACS

The Necessity for Routine Pre-operative Ultrasound Mapping Before Arteriovenous Fistula Creation: A Meta-analysis

Georgiadis GS, Charalampidis DG, Argyriou C, et al (Democritus Univ Hosp, Alexandroupolis, Greece)

Eur J Vasc Endovasc Surg 49:600-605, 2015

Objective/Background.—Existing guidelines suggest routine use of pre-operative color Doppler ultrasound (DUS) vessel mapping before the creation of arteriovenous fistulae (AVF); however, there is controversy about its benefit over traditional clinical examination or selective ultrasound use.

Methods.—This was a systematic review and meta-analysis of randomized controlled trials (RCTs) comparing routine DUS mapping before the creation of AVF with patients for whom the decision for AVF placement was based on clinical examination and selective ultrasound use. A search of MEDLINE/PubMed, SCOPUS, and the Cochrane Library was carried out in June 2014. The analyzed outcome measures were the immediate failure rate and the early/midterm adequacy of the fistula for hemodialysis. Additionally, assessment of the methodological quality of the included studies was carried out.

Results.—Five studies (574 patients) were analyzed. A random effects model was used to pool the data. The pooled odds ratio (OR) for the immediate failure rate was 0.32 (95% confidence interval [CI] 0.17–0.60; $p < .01$), which was significantly in favor of the DUS mapping group. The pooled OR for the early/midterm adequacy for hemodialysis was 0.66 (95% CI 0.42–1.03; $p = .06$), with a trend in favor of the DUS mapping group; however, subgroup analysis revealed that routine DUS mapping was more beneficial than selective DUS ($p < .05$).

Conclusion.—The available evidence, based mainly on moderate quality RCTs, suggests that the pre-operative clinical examination should always be supplemented with routine DUS mapping before AVF creation. This

policy avoids negative surgical explorations and significantly reduces the immediate AVF failure rate.

▶ Hemodialysis access surgery can be a vexing challenge for surgeons with persistently high rates of failure to mature and primary failure for arteriovenous fistulae (AVF). Although routine use of preoperative duplex ultrasound examination (DUS) of the upper extremities is recommended by current guidelines, including the Disease Outcomes Quality Initiative, consensus Level I evidence of its benefit is unfortunately lacking. It may seem intuitive that DUS would more accurately identify veins suitable for use in constructing an AV fistula, but there is also the question of whether DUS might "convince" the surgeon to attempt AVF with a marginal vein that otherwise is unimpressive on physical examination alone. Evidence from many randomized control trials (RCTs) has been conflicted when comparing routine preoperative DUS with physical examination either alone or with selective DUS. This meta-analysis of 5 RCTs found a statistically significant higher odds ratio of immediate failure rate that favored routine use of DUS compared with physical examination with selective DUS. Although this result will not settle the issue, it lends further support that DUS, at least as a supplement to a careful preoperative physical examination, should be recommended for all patients intending to undergo arteriovenous fistula creation for hemodialysis access.

M. Williams, MD

10 Carotid and Cerebrovascular

Relationship between histologic features and outcomes of carotid revascularization for radiation-induced stenosis

Sano N, Satow T, Maruyama D, et al (Natl Cerebral and Cardiovascular Ctr, Suita, Japan)

J Vasc Surg 62:370-377, 2015

Objective.—This study aimed to elucidate the relationships between preoperative carotid imaging results, histologic characteristics, and surgical treatment outcomes of radiation-induced carotid stenosis (RICS), using control subjects without RICS for comparison.

Methods.—We retrospectively reviewed records of 17 patients who underwent carotid revascularization for 22 instances of RICS, including 10 cases of carotid artery stenting (CAS), 11 cases of carotid endarterectomy (CEA), and 1 case of CEA with retrograde CAS, between July 2004 and April 2013. The controls were 475 patients with no history of radiation therapy who underwent carotid revascularization in a similar period. Preoperative magnetic resonance imaging (MRI), ultrasonography (US), and computed tomography angiography results were correlated with outcomes of histologic analysis of CEA specimens. End points included ipsilateral and contralateral stroke, myocardial infarction, restenosis, instent thrombosis, and target lesion revascularization.

Results.—Vulnerable plaques on carotid MRI (86% vs 64.2%; $P = .010$) and mobile (27% vs 8.0%; $P = .008$) and ulcerative (50% vs 15.8%; $P < .001$) plaques on US were more frequent in the RICS group. All revascularization procedures were successful, and no occlusion occurred. Adverse events in the CAS group, including one minor stroke and one transient ischemic attack within 30 days as well as five ipsilateral neurologic events after 30 days, including three minor strokes and two transient ischemic attacks, were significantly more frequent than in the CEA group. All three cases of late ipsilateral stroke displayed vulnerable plaque on preoperative MRI and late in-stent thrombosis or restenosis on US.

Conclusions.—Our radiologic and histologic analyses revealed that advanced RICS is often accompanied by formation of vulnerable plaque. CEA can prevent undesirable late outcomes in such cases.

► Cervical radiation is highly effective in treating some head and neck cancers, but its use can lead to radiation-induced carotid stenosis (RICS). The mechanism through which radiation causes RICS is considered to be secondary to intimal hyperplasia and accelerated atherosclerosis. During the early stages of carotid artery stenting (CAS), it was felt that patients with RICS would be better served with CAS than carotid endarterectomy (CEA) due to soft tissue changes induced by the radiation, making surgery more risky. Recent evidence has shown that short-term and long-term outcomes are actually better with CEA compared with CAS in the setting of RICS. The purpose of this study was to investigate the relationships among preoperative imaging, specimen histology, and surgical treatment outcomes in patients undergoing revascularization for RICS.

In this study, 22 carotid revascularization procedures were performed in patients with RICS. Specifically, there were 10 cases of CAS, 11 cases of CEA, and 1 case of CEA with retrograde CAS. Characteristics of the RICS cohort were compared with a control group of 475 patients who underwent carotid revascularization without a history of radiation. Carotid duplex was used to characterize mobile plaques and ulcerated plaques. The presence of high signal intensity within plaques on MRI indicated intraplaque hemorrhage with large necrotic cores, a characteristic of a vulnerable plaque. A high proportion of necrotic core to total plaque seen on histology was also indicative of a vulnerable plaque. Results demonstrated that mobile and ulcerated plaques on duplex, vulnerable plaques on MRI, and the proportion of necrotic core on histology were all significantly worse in the RICS group compared with controls. Looking specifically at outcomes in the RICS group, there were no ipsilateral neurological events seen in CEA patients, whereas there were 5 ipsilateral neurological events in the CAS group. Additionally, all of the patients in the CAS group who had clinically silent ischemic events on MRI or early in-stent thrombosis had vulnerable plaques on preoperative MRI. Therefore, in the setting of vulnerable plaques seen with RICS, CEA may be a better option for carotid revascularization compared with CAS, especially when considering the high incidence of late restenosis and neurological events seen in CAS patients.

B. Peterson, MD, FACS

2015 American Heart Association/American Stroke Association Focused Update of the 2013 Guidelines for the Early Management of Patients With Acute Ischemic Stroke Regarding Endovascular Treatment: A Guideline for Healthcare Professionals From the American Heart Association/American Stroke Association

Powers WJ, on behalf of the American Heart Association Stroke Council ()
Stroke 46:3020-3035, 2015

Purpose.—The aim of this guideline is to provide a focused update of the current recommendations for the endovascular treatment of acute ischemic stroke. When there is overlap, the recommendations made here supersede those of previous guidelines.

Methods.—This focused update analyzes results from 8 randomized, clinical trials of endovascular treatment and other relevant data published since 2013. It is not intended to be a complete literature review from the date of the previous guideline publication but rather to include pivotal new evidence that justifies changes in current recommendations. Members of the writing committee were appointed by the American Heart Association/American Stroke Association Stroke Council's Scientific Statement Oversight Committee and the American Heart Association/American Stroke Association Manuscript Oversight Committee. Strict adherence to the American Heart Association conflict of interest policy was maintained throughout the consensus process. Recommendations follow the American Heart Association/American Stroke Association methods of classifying the level of certainty of the treatment effect and the class of evidence. Prerelease review of the draft guideline was performed by 6 expert peer reviewers and by the members of the Stroke Council Scientific Statement Oversight Committee and Stroke Council Leadership Committee.

Results.—Evidence-based guidelines are presented for the selection of patients with acute ischemic stroke for endovascular treatment, for the endovascular procedure, and for systems of care to facilitate endovascular treatment.

Conclusions.—Certain endovascular procedures have been demonstrated to provide clinical benefit in selected patients with acute ischemic stroke. Systems of care should be organized to facilitate the delivery of this care.

▶ Significant new data on the endovascular management of acute stroke have been published, and as such the American Heart Association, together with the American Stroke Association, have released these evidence-based clinical guidelines. The authors stress early (within 4.5 hours of symptoms) administration of intravenous (IV) tissue-type plasminogen activator (r-tPA) as mainstay of acute stroke management. Three randomized controlled trials for endovascular management of acute stroke with intra-arterial fibrinolysis and/or use of mechanical embolectomy devices were reviewed, none of which showed benefit with IV r-TPA for either initial treatment or in those with persistent occlusion after initial systemic thrombolysis. Use of stent retrievers have been studied in 5 randomized clinical trials, all of which have shown improved recanalization rates and outcomes, with better outcomes in those with complete/nearly complete recanalization of large vessel arterial occlusion. Nearly all patients in these trials received r-TPA initially before endovascular therapy, and all required noninvasive arterial imaging (CTA or MRA) before endovascular therapy but after initial r-TPA systemic dosing (because a minority of patients [37%] will clear occlusions of large vessel arteries with systemic therapy alone). The authors then outlined a number of recommendations, with level of evidence grading. Recommendations with the highest grades (Class I, Level of Evidence A) include:

1. Patients eligible for IV r-tPA should receive, even if endovascular therapy is being considered.
2. Patients should receive endovascular therapy with a stent retriever if they meet all the following criteria:

a. Prestroke mRS score 0 to 1

b. Acute ischemic stroke receiving IV r-tPA within 4.5 hours of onset

c. Causative occlusion of the internal carotid artery or proximal middle cerebral artery

d. Age ≥18

e. National Institutes of Health Stroke Scale score ≥6

f. Alberta Stroke Program Early Computed Tomography score (ASPECTS) ≥6

g. Treatment can be initiated (groin puncture) within 6 hours of symptom onset

3. Use of the stent retrievers is preferable to the MERCI device. The use of mechanical thrombectomy devices other than stent retrievers may be reasonable in some circumstances.
4. Emergency imaging of the brain is recommended before any specific treatment for acute stroke is initiated. In most instances, nonenhanced computed tomography will provide necessary information.
5. If endovascular therapy is contemplated, a noninvasive intracranial vascular study is strongly recommended during initial imaging but should not delay r-tPA administration. For those receiving r-tPA, it should be given before this imaging.
6. Patients should be transported rapidly to the closest available certified primary stroke center, or the most appropriate institution that provides emergency stroke care and regional systems of stroke care should be developed.

M. R. Smeds, MD, FACS

Risk of Stroke and Cardiac Events in Medically Treated Asymptomatic Carotid Stenosis

Divya KP, Sandeep N, Sarma S, et al (Sree Chitra Tirunal Inst for Med Sciences and Technology, Thiruvananthapuram, Kerala, India)

J Stroke Cerebrovasc Dis 24:2149-2153, 2015

Background.—The risk of stroke in patients with 50% or more asymptomatic carotid stenosis (ACS) on intensive medical treatment is low. Hence, the optimal treatment of ACS remains controversial at this point of time.

Aim.—We assessed the risk of stroke/transient ischemic attack (TIA) and cardiac events in patients with 50% or more ACS on intensive medical treatment.

Methods.—All patients with TIA/minor stroke (National Institutes of Health Stroke Scale score ≤5) who had undergone vessel imaging as part of their evaluation and patients with coronary artery disease who had undergone vessel imaging before cardiac intervention were screened for the presence of asymptomatic carotid stenosis. The risk of TIA/stroke, cardiac events, and vascular deaths were evaluated.

Results.—Of 1,800 patients, 92 patients (.05%) had ACS having 50% to 99% stenosis; 63 had TIA/minor stroke, and 29 had coronary artery disease, of whom 7 patients had bilateral ACS, thus constituting 99 study units of ACS. The mean follow-up was 34.7 months (range 3-120 months). Two patients developed ischemic events on the side ipsilateral to the ACS and 9 patients developed cardiac events during the follow-up. The average annual event rate for cerebral ischemic events was .93% (95% confidence interval [CI], .11-3.37), 4.21% (95% CI, 1.92-7.98) for cardiac events, and 3.27% (95% CI, 1.31-6.74) for death.

Conclusions.—Although the risk of stroke in patients with ACS is low, acute coronary events and vascular deaths were significant. This highlights the importance of intensive risk factor modification to reduce adverse cardiovascular events in ACS rather than revascularization of the carotid stenosis.

▶ The landmark early 1990s Asymptomatic Carotid Atherosclerosis Study (ACAS)[1] compared carotid endarterectomy with medical therapy for patients with 60% or greater asymptomatic carotid stenosis. The outcomes of aggregate risk of ipsilateral stroke and any perioperative stroke or death at 5 years of 5.1% for endarterectomy patients versus 11.0% for medical therapy patients (aggregate risk reduction of 53% in favor of surgical treatment) led the authors to recommend surgery for good operative candidates for the purpose of improved stroke risk reduction. Medical therapy in the ACAS trial consisted of daily aspirin and adequate management of other medical risk factors, such as hypertension and diabetes. "Best medical therapy" has evolved in the 20+ years since ACAS was published, particularly with the massive increase in the use of statins, making it necessary to reexamine the benefit that surgery has to offer for asymptomatic patients.

This small single-center retrospective study looked at outcomes of modern best medical management in asymptomatic moderate (50%–69%) and severe (70%–99%) carotid stenosis patients over an 8-year period in the Indian population. Only 92 patients were identified for the study, a number that was further reduced after 17 patients were excluded from the analysis for having undergone open or endovascular carotid intervention. The study also suffers from a significant selection bias because more than two-thirds of the patients in the analysis, although asymptomatic from the carotid stenosis identified on imaging, had a symptomatic transient ischemic attack (TIA) or stroke from the contralateral carotid artery or the posterior circulation. At a mean follow-up of 34 months, there were 2 ischemic events (both TIAs with 70%–99% stenosis) attributed to the carotid stenosis being studied, reported as a low average annual risk of 0.93% with wide confidence intervals due to the small sample size. The study of surgical intervention for asymptomatic carotid stenosis versus modern best medical therapy is an immensely important topic that will not be settled in the near future. CREST 2 (Carotid Revascularization for Primary Prevention of Stroke), which will reexamine this topic in a randomized prospective trial, will be eagerly anticipated by all physicians with an interest in the treatment of carotid artery disease.

M. Williams, MD

Reference

1. Endarterectomy for asymptomatic carotid artery stenosis. Executive Committee for the Asymptomatic Carotid Atherosclerosis Study. *JAMA*. 1995;273: 1421-1428.

Summary of Evidence on Early Carotid Intervention for Recently Symptomatic Stenosis Based on Meta-Analysis of Current Risks

De Rango P, Brown MM, Chaturvedi S, et al (Hosp S.M. Misericordia, Perugia, Italy; Univ College London, UK; Univ of Miami Miller School of Medicine, FL; et al)

Stroke 46:3423-3436, 2015

Background and Purpose.—This study aimed to assess the evidence on the periprocedural (<30 days) risks of carotid intervention in relation to timing of procedure in patients with recently symptomatic carotid stenosis.

Methods.—A systematic literature review of studies published in the past 8 years reporting periprocedural stroke/death after carotid endarterectomy (CEA) and carotid stenting (CAS) related to the time between qualifying neurological symptoms and intervention was performed. Pooled estimates of periprocedural risk for patients treated within 0 to 48 hours, 0 to 7 days, and 0 to 15 days were derived with proportional meta-analyses and reported separately for patients with stroke and transient ischemic attack as index events.

Results.—Of 47 studies included, 35 were on CEA, 7 on CAS, and 5 included both procedures. The pooled risk of periprocedural stroke was 3.4% (95% confidence interval [CI], 2.6–4.3) after CEA and 4.8% (95% CI, 2.5–7.8) after CAS performed <15 days; stroke/death rates were 3.8% and 6.9% after CEA and CAS, respectively. Pooled periprocedural stroke risk was 3.3% (95% CI, 2.1–4.6) after CEA and 4.8% (95% CI, 2.5–7.8) after CAS when performed within 0 to 7 days. In hyperacute surgery (<48 hours), periprocedural stroke risk after CEA was 5.3% (95% CI, 2.8–8.4) but with relevant risk differences among patients treated after transient ischemic attack (2.7%; 95% CI, 0.5–6.9) or stroke (8.0%; 95% CI, 4.6–12.2) as index.

Conclusions.—CEA within 15 days from stroke/transient ischemic attack can be performed with periprocedural stroke risk <3.5%. CAS within the same period may carry a stroke risk of 4.8%. Similar periprocedural risks occur after CEA and CAS performed earlier, within 0 to 7 days. Carotid revascularization can be safely performed within the first week (0–7 days) after symptom onset.

▶ Consensus regarding the timing of carotid revascularization following transient ischemic attack (TIA) or stroke is lacking in the current literature. Traditionally, surgeons would wait 4 to 6 weeks after the initial onset of symptoms to allow for recovery and to reduce the theoretical risk of reperfusion injury. Unfortunately, patients were developing recurrent events while waiting to undergo revascularization. Along these lines, more recent guidelines are suggesting intervention less than 2 weeks after the onset of nondisabling stroke or TIA. Here, the authors review the current literature related to early carotid intervention for recently symptomatic stenoses.

After sifting through the available literature, the authors identified 47 studies that satisfied their search criteria. Three distinct time courses were evaluated. The times were from the onset of symptoms to revascularization and were set up as follows: intervention within 15 days, 7 days, or 48 hours. For the intervention within 15 days group, the pooled risk of stroke within 30 days of intervention was 3.4% for carotid endarterectomy (CEA) and 4.8% for carotid artery stenting (CAS). For the intervention within 7 days group, risk of stroke was 3.3% following CEA and 4.8% for CAS. Outcomes were worse if the interventions followed stroke compared with interventions after TIA. In the less than 48 hours group, stroke risk was 5.3% after CEA and 2.1% after CAS (although this analysis was limited to 5 studies). From these results, the authors concluded that carotid revascularization can be performed safely within the first week of symptoms. Limitations of this meta-analysis are largely due to the lack of randomized controlled trials on this topic, limiting this review to case series and registries. Additionally, the severity of symptoms patients were experiencing preoperatively cannot be elucidated. Nevertheless, these findings support early carotid revascularization in patients with symptomatic carotid stenoses, although caution should still be practiced in patients with larger, more disabling strokes.

B. Peterson, MD, FACS

Systematic Review of Guidelines for the Management of Asymptomatic and Symptomatic Carotid Stenosis

Abbott AL, Paraskevas KI, Kakkos SK, et al (Monash Univ, Melbourne, Victoria, Australia; St George's Hosp, London, UK; Univ of Patras, Greece; et al)
Stroke 46:3288-3301, 2015

Background and Purpose.—We systematically compared and appraised contemporary guidelines on management of asymptomatic and symptomatic carotid artery stenosis.

Methods.—We systematically searched for guideline recommendations on carotid endarterectomy (CEA) or carotid angioplasty/stenting (CAS) published in any language between January 1, 2008, and January 28, 2015. Only the latest guideline per writing group was selected. Each guideline was analyzed independently by 2 to 6 authors to determine clinical scenarios covered, recommendations given, and scientific evidence used.

Results.—Thirty-four eligible guidelines were identified from 23 different regions/countries in 6 languages. Of 28 guidelines with asymptomatic carotid artery stenosis procedural recommendations, 24 (86%) endorsed CEA (recommended it should or may be provided) for ≈50% to 99% average-surgical-risk asymptomatic carotid artery stenosis, 17 (61%) endorsed CAS, 8 (29%) opposed CAS, and 1 (4%) endorsed medical treatment alone. For asymptomatic carotid artery stenosis patients considered high-CEA-risk because of comorbidities, vascular anatomy, or undefined reasons, CAS was endorsed in 13 guidelines (46%). Thirty-one of 33 guidelines (94%) with symptomatic carotid artery stenosis procedural recommendations endorsed CEA for patients with ≈50% to 99% average-CEA-risk symptomatic carotid artery stenosis, 19 (58%) endorsed CAS and 9 (27%) opposed CAS. For high-CEA-risk symptomatic carotid artery stenosis because of comorbidities, vascular anatomy, or undefined reasons, CAS was endorsed in 27 guidelines (82%). Guideline procedural recommendations were based only on results of trials in which patients were randomized 12 to 34 years ago, rarely reflected medical treatment improvements and often understated potential CAS hazards. Qualifying terminology summarizing recommendations or evidence lacked standardization, impeding guideline interpretation, and comparison.

Conclusions.—This systematic review has identified many opportunities to modernize and otherwise improve carotid stenosis management guidelines.

▶ Although you may lose focus reading this article from beginning to end, this article truly is a "Systematic Review of Guidelines for the Management of Asymptomatic and Symptomatic Carotid Stenosis," as the title states. With its 114 references, I could not think of any deficiencies in terms of citing the most important articles in publication over the past 7 years associated with the management of patients with carotid artery disease.

Thirty-four guidelines published in the literature from January 2008 to 2015 met the authors' inclusion criteria. In the guidelines addressing asymptomatic carotid disease, 86% recommended carotid endarterectomy (CEA) for average risk patients with 50% to 99% stenoses. In the guidelines addressing symptomatic carotid disease, 94% recommended CEA for average risk patients with 50% to 99% stenoses. In symptomatic, high-risk patients, CAS was endorsed in 82% of the guidelines. The authors recognize one of the major flaws of current guidelines in the literature: they fail to recognize the advancement in the best medical therapy for the treatment of carotid artery disease. Nevertheless, if you are looking for an exhaustive list of guidelines from the past 8 years regarding the treatment of carotid artery disease, look no further than the bibliography from this article.

B. Peterson, MD, FACS

Urgent carotid intervention is safe after thrombolysis for minor to moderate acute ischemic stroke

Bazan HA, Zea N, Jennings B, et al (Ochsner Clinic, New Orleans, LA)

J Vasc Surg 62:1529-1538, 2015

Objective.—Carotid intervention shortly after an acute neurologic ischemic event is being performed more frequently in stroke centers to reduce the risk of recurrent stroke. Thrombolysis with recombinant tissue plasminogen activator (tPA) is offered to select patients with ischemic stroke symptoms who present within 4.5 hours. However, there is a paucity of data as to whether tPA followed by urgent carotid endarterectomy (CEA) or carotid artery stenting (CAS) has an increased risk of complications, particularly intracerebral hemorrhage (ICH). We sought to determine the periprocedural complications of urgently performed CEA or CAS following tPA.

Methods.—From January 2009 to January 2015, 762 patients underwent carotid interventions (CEA, n = 440; CAS, n = 322) at a tertiary referral center and 165 patients (21.6%) underwent an urgent CEA or CAS during the index hospitalization for an acute transient ischemic attack or stroke. We compared the effect of intravenous tPA on 30-day complications, including ICH. The χ^2 and Fisher exact tests were used to determine significance between groups.

Results.—During the 6-year period, 165 patients underwent urgent carotid interventions (CEA, n = 135; CAS, n = 30) for acute neurologic symptoms. Of these, 19% (31 patients [CEA, n = 25; CAS, n = 6]) had tPA for an acute stroke; the remaining (134 patients [CEA, n = 110; CAS, n = 24]) fell outside of the tPA time window. Most strokes were minor or moderate with a mean National Institutes of Health Stroke Scale (NIHSS) score of 6.6 (range, 0-19). The mean time to intervention for both groups was 2.4 days (0-15 days). The 30-day stroke, death, and myocardial infarction rates were 9.7% (3 of 31) for the tPA group compared with 4.5% (6 of 134) for the no-tPA group (P =.37). Including bleeding complications in these 30-day outcomes, there was no difference between the tPA (3 of 31) and the no-tPA cohorts (8 of 134; $P = .43$). In the tPA group, there were one ICH, one neck hematoma/death, and an additional death; in the no-tPA group, there were one ICH, two neck hematomas, one stroke, two myocardial infarctions, one ICH/death, and one additional death. No significant increased rates of bleeding were noted within the tPA group (2 of 31) compared with the no-tPA group (4 of 134; $P = .32$). Moreover, in the tPA cohort, more than half of the patients (17 of 31) underwent revascularization within 72 hours (CEA = 13; CAS = 4) with outcomes similar to those who underwent revascularization after 72 hours.

Conclusions.—Thrombolysis followed by urgent CEA or CAS is not associated with an increased risk of complications in select patients who present with acute neurologic symptoms. Selection of patients is important; there was no ICH and only one death in each group for patients with minor to moderate ischemic stroke (NIHSS score <10).

▶ The latest trend in the treatment of symptomatic carotid artery disease is early intervention, and this trend is supported by a meta-analysis of the large randomized carotid trials that demonstrated carotid endarterectomy (CEA) has the greatest benefit when performed within 2 weeks of symptom onset.[1] Thrombolysis with recombinant tissue plasminogen activator (tPA) has been shown to be beneficial if given within a short time from the onset of symptoms, and the advent of stroke centers and telestroke networks will likely increase the use of tPA. There are few data to suggest that carotid intervention shortly after the administration of tPA is accompanied by more bleeding complications. The authors sought to determine the effect of tPA administration on complications in patients undergoing urgent CEA or carotid artery stenting.

In this retrospective review, 165 patients underwent urgent carotid interventions, with 19% of these patients having received tPA. Most strokes were mild to moderate, with the tPA group having a mean National Institutes of Health Stroke Scale (NIHSS) score of 6.6 and the no-tPA group having a mean NIHSS score of 6.1. There were early carotid interventions in both groups with a mean time to carotid intervention of 2.4 days in the tPA group and 2.2 days in the no-tPA group. There was no difference in 30-day complications between groups, testing for any bleeding, including intracranial hemorrhage (ICH) and access site bleeding, stroke, death, and myocardial infarction. An overriding theme from these results is the importance of patient selection and reserving early carotid revascularization for patients with mild to moderate strokes (ie, NIHSS score <10). There was no incidence of ICH in either group when NIHSS scores were <10, and all 3 patients who developed ICH had NIHSS scores >10. This study gives further credence to early carotid revascularization after an acute ischemic event, even in the setting of tPA administration, so long as the stroke is deemed mild to moderate, there is evidence of clinical recovery, and there is no evidence of bleeding on brain imaging.

B. Peterson, MD, FACS

Reference

1. Rothwell PM, Eliasziw M, Gutnikov SA, Warlow CP, Barnett HJ. Carotid Endarterectomy Trialists Collaboration. Endarterectomy for symptomatic carotid stenosis in relation to clinical subgroups and timing of surgery. *Lancet*. 2004;363: 915-924.

Extracranial Internal Carotid Artery Dissection Treated with Self-expandable Stents: A Single-Centre Experience

Juszkat R, Liebert W, Stanisławska K, et al (Poznań Univ of Med Sciences, Poland)

Cardiovasc Intervent Radiol 38:1451-1457, 2015

Purpose.—Treatment of choice for the internal carotid artery dissection (ICAD) is anticoagulation for three to 6 months. Endovascular procedures may be a promising alternative for patients (pts) with haemodynamic impairment, recurrent ischaemic symptoms or symptomatic pseudoaneurysms. Thus, the purpose of this study was to evaluate the efficacy and safety of carotid artery stenting in treatment of selected pts with extracranial ICAD.

Methods.—This study involved 18 symptomatic pts with the mean age of 44.6 ± 10.4 years with ICAD treated with the use of self-expandable stents. Six months after primary procedures, pts were readmitted to hospital and physical examination followed by cerebral angiography was performed. In the late follow-up period, clinical evaluations completed by duplex Doppler ultrasonography were carried out every 6 months and at the end of the follow-up period.

Results.—Nobody died and no life-threatening adverse events were observed during either the in-hospital stay or post-discharge follow-up period (median 21 months). Stent deployment immediately restored flow in the true lumen of ICA in all cases. However, residual blood flow through the false lumen was observed in one pt. Complete resolution of clinical symptoms was observed in 14 pts (78%), partial improvement in 2 (11%) and persistence of neurological deficit in 2 (11%).

Conclusions.—Implantation of self-expandable stents in treatment of selected extracranial ICAD cases is safe. This method may enable us to restore immediately and usually permanently proper arterial blood flow in the ICA and in consequence lead to significant clinical improvement in the late follow-up period.

▶ Recommendations for the treatment of uncomplicated extracranial carotid artery dissection (CAD), regardless of etiology, typically call for medical treatment alone either with anticoagulation or antiplatelet therapy. Cases of symptomatic (complicated) CAD may benefit from endovascular or open surgical intervention over medical therapy alone. The authors of this single-center series of 18 cases report their experience in treating complicated CAD (all patients either had a stroke, transient ischemic attack, or symptomatic pseudoaneurysm) with self-expanding nitinol stents. Overall the patients did well with no adverse events and the majority had an improvement in preprocedure neurologic symptoms, allowing the authors to recommend that the procedure is safe and effective for treatment of complicated extracranial CAD.

There are several limitations of this study. Spontaneous and posttraumatic dissections were both included, although they may respond differently to treatment and could be better studied separately. The etiology of neurologic symptoms in these patients, either from thromboembolism or impaired hemodynamics from reduced flow in the true lumen, is uncertain. In patients with symptomatic thromboembolic disease, carotid artery stenting may be safe and effective but may be of no benefit over medical treatment alone. Additionally, the selective use of distal embolic protection in some but not all patients in the study, while recognizing that risk of distal embolization is not the same in this pathology compared with atherosclerotic embolic disease, is still controversial.

M. Williams, MD

Periprocedural Myocardial Infarction After Carotid Endarterectomy and Stenting: Systematic Review and Meta-Analysis

Boulanger M, Camelière L, Felgueiras R, et al (Université de Caen Basse Normandie, Caen, France; Hosp Santo António, Porto, Portugal; et al)

Stroke 46:2843-2848, 2015

Background and Purpose.—Carotid angioplasty and stenting (CAS) is associated with higher risk of periprocedural stroke and death when compared with carotid endarterectomy (CEA). By contrast, the risk of myocardial infarction (MI) was higher after CEA than after CAS in randomized trials. However, numbers were small, and risk factors are unknown.

Methods.—We performed a systematic review and a meta-analysis of studies published from January 1980 to June 2014 and collected unpublished data. We extracted data on 9 predefined risk factors (age, contralateral carotid occlusion, coronary artery disease, diabetes mellitus, sex, hypertension, peripheral artery disease, type stenosis, and clinical presentation). We selected studies with data available on MI in at least 1 subgroup, calculated absolute and relative risks, and identified differential effects on risks of MI.

Results.—The 30-day absolute risk of MI was 0.87% (95% confidence interval, 0.69–1.07) after CEA and 0.70% (95% confidence interval, 0.54–0.88) after CAS ($P_{\text{int}} = 0.38$). After CAS, patients with symptomatic stenosis and restenosis were at higher risk of MI, whereas men were at lower risk. After CEA, age, history of coronary artery disease, peripheral artery disease, and restenosis increased the risk of MI. Only the effect of sex differed between CAS and CEA with men being at lower risk of MI than women after CAS, whereas there was no difference between after CEA ($P_{\text{int}} = 0.01$).

Conclusions.—The risk of MI after CEA and CAS did not significantly differ. Risk factors for MI are overall similar in both techniques except that men are at lower risk of MI after CAS but not after CEA.

▶ Multiple studies have demonstrated increased risk of myocardial infarction (MI) after carotid endarterectomy (CEA) compared with carotid stenting (CAS); however, these overall risks are low, and factors associated with risk have not been fully elucidated. The authors sought to determine absolute risk of perioperative MI and identify risk factors associated with this outcome using a meta-analysis of 52 independent studies of CEA, 68 independent studies of CAS, and 1609 patients from the authors' own retrospective review of their patients treated from 2000 to 2013 at a single center. Publications used in the meta-analysis had to have MI and death data that could be extracted for any subgroup among 9 predefined risks factors (age, contralateral carotid occlusion, coronary artery disease, diabetes, sex, hypertension, peripheral arterial disease, type of stenosis, or clinical presentation). There was no difference in 30-day absolute risk of MI between CEA and CAS (0.87% vs 0.7%). Risk factors identified in both included increased age, history of coronary artery disease, peripheral arterial disease, symptomatic stenosis, and restenosis. Males were more likely to have MI following CEA but not CAS, and the main risk factor identified was history of coronary artery disease. This study is limited by its design, with meta-analysis only as good as the studies used for comparison. Validity and similarity of the individual studies used and selection criteria entertained is not determinable and biases from these studies may be amplified in the analysis. However, these data suggest that periprocedural MI may not be as prevalent in CEA patients compared with CAS patients as initially thought.

M. R. Smeds, MD, FACS

Carotid Artery Revascularization: What's the Best Strategy?

Hussain MA, Verma S, Gupta N, et al (Li Ka Shing Knowledge Inst of St. Michael's Hosp, Toronto, Ontario, Canada; Ottawa Hosp, Ontario, Canada; et al)

Circulation 131:2226-2231, 2015

Background.—Stroke is the acute development of a focal neurological deficit caused by disruption of the blood flow to the brain and can be either ischemic or hemorrhagic in etiology. Over 80% are ischemic, and between 15% and 20% of these are caused by atherosclerosis of the extracranial carotid arteries. After an ischemic stroke, patients are at increased risk for death and for recurrent stroke. Narrowing or stenosis of the carotid bulb and internal carotid artery (ICA) caused by atherosclerosis can produce plaque embolization or hypoperfusion, leading to stroke. Patients who smoke; those who have hypertension, hyperlipidemia, coronary artery disease (CAD), diabetes mellitus, peripheral arterial disease, or abdominal aortic aneurysm; and those of the Native American or white race are at increased risk of ICA stenosis. Treatment options include medical therapy, carotid endarterectomy (CEA), and carotid artery stenting (CAS). The best treatment for a patient with stroke is determined by considering factors related to the patient, the disease, and available resources.

Patient Factors.—Among the patient factors to be considered are age, sex, comorbid conditions, operative risk, life expectancy, functional status, and patient preferences. Patients age 70 years or older have an increased risk of complications with CAS compared to CEA. Women tend to experience less benefit from CEA than men, but the evidence does not indicate female sex is a high-risk factor for CAS. CEA has a higher risk of periprocedural myocardial infarction than CAS, so the patient's cardiac status should be carefully assessed before determining which procedure is best. Life expectancy is important, with symptomatic patients having a significant reduction in stroke rate with CEA after 2 to 3 years. Asymptomatic patients show minimal benefit for CEA over medical therapy after 5 years. Patients who have dense hemispheric neurological deficits, significant dementia, or severally limited functional status tend not to benefit from any of the carotid revascularization procedures, but the family, physician, and patient should be consulted before a final decision is made. Patients should be given a complete picture of the benefits and risks associated with each procedure.

Disease Factors.—With respect to disease status, the choice of treatment should consider whether the patient is symptomatic, the degree of stenosis present, the characteristics of any plaque, and if contralateral disease is also present. Anatomically, patients should be assessed for challenging neck anatomy, difficult carotid artery presentations, and the configuration, tortuosity, and extent of calcification of the aortic arch.

Resources.—CAS is technically demanding and should only be performed by experienced operators in specialized centers to achieve the highest chance of success and the lowest possibility of complications. If CAS is considered, patients should be referred to the best operator and center available.

CEA should be selected for asymptomatic patients after a careful assessment of their life expectancy, comorbid conditions, surgeon/institution stroke and death rate, and patient preferences. It is the gold standard for symptomatic patients with ICA stenosis. CAS has undergone significant changes since its initial introduction, and several contemporary RCTs find that its outcomes are comparable to those with CEA, making it an increasingly attractive option. The increased risk of periprocedural stroke or death is 1.5- to 2-fold for CAS compared to normal patients, but it has about half as much risk for myocardial infarction as CEA. CEA has a higher risk for damage to cranial nerves, but patients age 70 years or older have better outcomes with CEA than CAS.

Guidelines.—CEA is generally superior for symptomatic patients who have significant ICA stenosis, even if they are older than 70 years. CAS is an alternative for symptomatic patients at high operative risk, even if their anatomy is challenging or they have significant comorbid conditions.

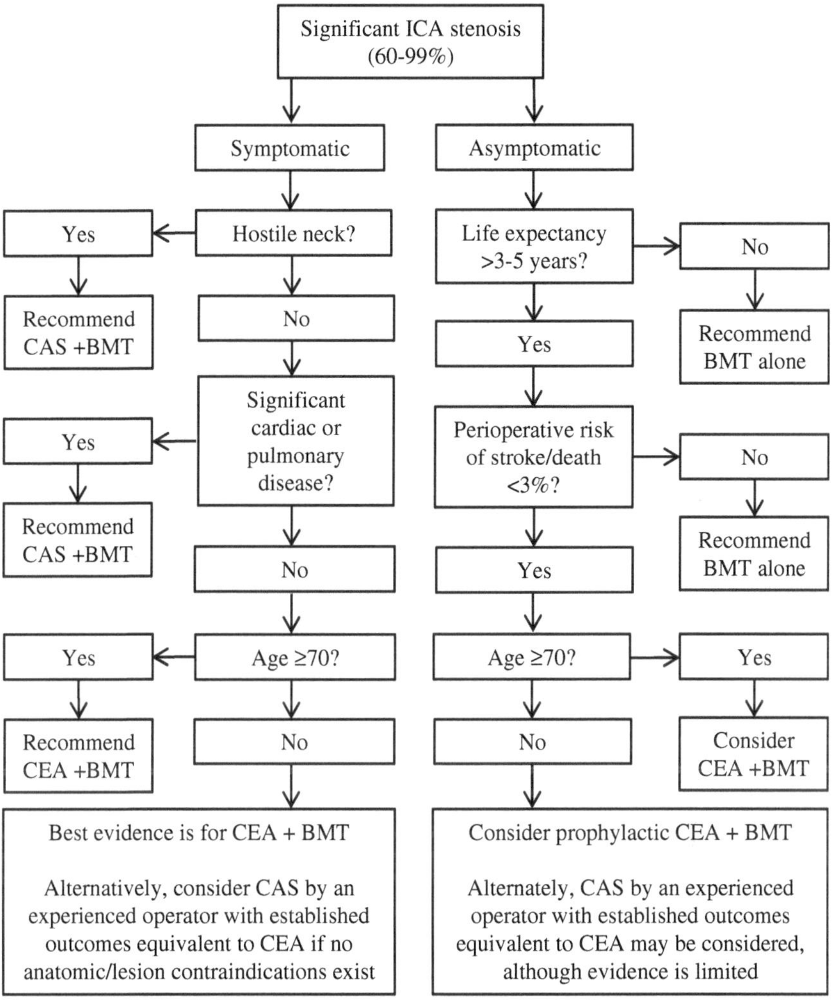

FIGURE 2.—Algorithm for carotid revascularization decision making. BMT indicates best medical therapy; CAS, carotid artery stenting; CEA, carotid endarterectomy; and ICA, internal carotid artery. (Reprinted from Hussain MA, Verma S, Gupta N, et al. Carotid artery revascularization: what's the best strategy? *Circulation*. 2015;131:2226-2231, with permission from American Heart Association, Inc.)

For asymptomatic patients, CEA should be done for patients who have significant ICA stenosis with a life expectancy of at least 3 to 5 years and a low risk of perioperative stroke or death (less than 3%). CAS may be appropriate for asymptomatic patients who are carefully selected and treated at high-volume centers by experienced operators who have achieved low stroke and death rates (Fig 2).

▶ Starting with a case scenario that will sound familiar to all physicians who take care of patients with carotid artery disease, the authors present a clear, concise summary of the current state of carotid artery revascularization. Although best medical therapy is something of an afterthought in this review, the authors succeed in presenting the key points of the recent major trials and meta-analyses comparing carotid endarterectomy (CEA) to carotid artery stenting (CAS).

I wanted to highlight several points from this article. First, it is relatively clear from a subanalysis of CREST and a Cochrane meta-analysis that patients 70 years of age and older have increased periprocedural risk with CAS compared with CEA. Next, symptomatic patients realize benefit from CEA in terms of stroke risk reduction almost immediately, whereas asymptomatic patients need to have a life expectancy of 3 to 5 years to have significant benefit from carotid revascularization. Third, symptomatic patients without characteristics that would make them high risk for surgery should be treated with CEA, and ideally within the first week of symptoms. Next, most randomized controlled trials have failed to show noninferiority of CAS to CEA. CAS patients have a 1.5- to 2-fold higher risk of periprocedural stroke and death, but half the risk of myocardial infarction compared with CEA patients. Finally, the authors provide us with an outstanding algorithm for carotid revascularization decision making based on the evidence currently available (Fig 2). All in all, this is an easy-to-read synopsis of the current state of carotid revascularization.

B. Peterson, MD, FACS

Characteristics that define high risk in carotid endarterectomy from the Vascular Study Group of New England

Gates L, Botta R, Schlosser F, et al (Yale Univ School of Medicine, New Haven, CT; et al)

J Vasc Surg 62:929-936, 2015

Objective.—The Stenting with Angioplasty and Protection in Patients at High Risk for Endarterectomy (SAPPHIRE) trial compared carotid endarterectomy (CEA) to carotid artery stenting (CAS) among high-risk patients using a model of risk that has not been validated by previous publications. The objective of our study was to determine the accuracy of this high-risk model and to determine the true risk factors that result in patients being at high risk for CEA.

Methods.—Prospectively collected data for 3098 CEAs between 2003 and 2011 at 20 Vascular Surgery Group of New England (VSGNE) centers were used. SAPPHIRE general inclusion criteria and primary outcomes were assessed. Factors that were associated with the primary outcome by analysis of variance ($P < .10$) and not linearly dependent, as determined by a Pearson correlation analysis, were further assessed for an independent association by multivariate logistic regression. A risk index model was developed for these significant predictors to accurately define high-risk CEA.

Results.—The average patient age was 69.9 ± 9.5 years, 60% were male, and 45.7% were asymptomatic. The 1-year composite outcome event rate, defined as postoperative myocardial infarction and stroke or death, was 14.2%. Multivariate analysis ($P < .05$) found the following independently significant risk factors: age in years (95% confidence interval [CI], 1.0-1.1; $P < .001$), preadmission living in a nursing home (95% CI, 1.2-6.6; $P = .020$), congestive heart failure (95% CI, 1.4-2.8; $P < .001$), diabetes mellitus (DM; 95% CI, 1.1-1.3; $P < .001$), chronic obstructive pulmonary disease (95% CI, 1.2-1.5; $P < .001$), any previous cerebrovascular disease (95% CI, 1.1-1.9; $P = .003$), and contralateral internal carotid artery stenosis (95% CI, 1.0-1.2; $P = .001$). Three of the SAPPHIRE high-risk criteria—abnormal stress test, recurrent stenosis after CEA, and previous radiotherapy to the neck—were not independently associated with an adverse outcome. Independently significant risk factors not included in the SAPPHIRE criteria are inclusion of ages <80 years, preadmission living in a nursing home, DM, contralateral carotid stenosis, and any previous cerebrovascular accident. The risk index predictors are age in years (40-49: 0 points; 50-59: 2 points; 60-69: 4 points; 70-79: 6 points; 80-89: 8 points), living in a nursing home (4 points), any cardiovascular disease (2 points), congestive heart failure (5 points), chronic obstructive pulmonary disease (3 points), DM (2 points), degree of contralateral stenosis (<50%: 0 points; 50%-69%: 1 point; 70%-near occlusion: 2 points; occlusion: 3 points). High-risk CEA is defined as >13 points, representing adverse outcome rate of 22.5%.

Conclusions.—SAPPHIRE and other previously reported high-risk CAS inclusion criteria do not include all of the factors found to be independently associated with outcomes. Further studies are required to determine whether CAS is inferior to CEA in high-risk patients using a validated model of risk. In addition, this preoperative assessment includes novel criteria that can be used to stratify risks.

▶ Carotid artery stenting (CAS) continues to be an important and effective alternative to carotid endarterectomy (CEA), particularly in patients who are identified to be "high risk" based on cardiopulmonary comorbidities or challenging anatomic considerations. This was validated by the Stenting and Angioplasty with Protection in Patients at High-Risk for Endarterectomy (SAPPHIRE) trial, which concluded that CAS with embolic protection was not inferior to CEA in high-risk patients. The authors of this study address one of the main criticisms of SAPPHIRE: that the "high-risk" criteria definitions were subjectively chosen at the investigator's discretion and not validated by evidence. The SAPPHIRE high-risk criteria remain the standard utilized by the Centers for Medicare & Medicaid Services for the Medicare National Coverage Determinations.

In this large multicenter retrospective review, the authors evaluated data from 3098 CEA patients over 9 years with end points nearly identical to SAPPHIRE (missing study data necessitated a slight adjustment) to identify evidence-based variables associated with the primary outcome of myocardial infarction, stroke, or death. Although some of the variables identified are in accordance with those designated by SAPPHIRE, others such as diabetes and living in a nursing home before admission (seemingly a surrogate variable for patient performance status) are not accounted for by the SAPPHIRE criteria. Although the authors took this a step further and developed a risk index model that calculates a percentage risk estimated by a given patient's preoperative characteristics, the accuracy of this model has not been prospectively studied.

M. Williams, MD

Does the Technique of Carotid Endarterectomy Determine Postoperative Hypertension?

Ben Ahmed S, Daniel G, Benezit M, et al (CHU Clermont-Ferrand, France; et al)

Ann Vasc Surg 29:1272-1280, 2015

Background.—Hypertension (HT) after carotid endarterectomy (CEA) is a risk factor for postoperative myocardial infarction, stroke, and neck hematoma. We compared the incidence of postoperative HT within the week after eversion CEA (e-CEA) and patch closure CEA (p-CEA). Postoperative HT was defined as a systolic blood pressure (sBP) ≥ 160 mm Hg and/or the need for postoperative vasodilatators. The aim of our study was to determine if the technique of CEA had an effect on postoperative HT.

Methods.—Between January 2010 and June 2011, we prospectively reviewed 560 consecutive endarterectomies (340 p-CEAs and 220 e-CEAs) performed in 443 patients under general anesthesia. All had >70% stenoses, 119 were symptomatic, and 441 asymptomatic. We compared preoperative, peroperative, and postoperative sBP and diastolic blood pressure, carotid sinus nerve block, postoperative intravenous and oral antihypertensive medications, neurologic and cardiac complications, and mortality.

Results.—The e-CEA group had a higher incidence of women (36.4% vs. 21.8%, $P = 0.0002$) and HT (85.0% vs. 78.2%, $P = 0.04$). The e-CEAs had a significantly higher incidence of carotid sinus nerve block (93.6% vs. 15.6%, $P < 0.0001$). The incidence of postoperative HT was not significantly different between the 2 groups (75.9% in the e-CEA group versus 68.5% in the p-CEA group, $P = 0.06$). The average postoperative sBP between postoperative hour (H) 2 and H12 was significantly higher in the e-CEA group but <160 mm Hg. The sBP dropped between H2 and H6, and this decrease was greater in the p-CEA group (30% vs. 15% in the e-CEA group). The need for postoperative antihypertensive medication was not different between the 2 groups. One independent risk factor of postoperative HT was identified: history of HT. The rate of postoperative complications was not significantly different between the 2 groups.

Conclusions.—The e-CEA technique is not a risk factor and does not have an effect on postoperative HT. The postoperative sBP was more stable in this group. Eversion carotid endarterectomy has been considered, in the literature, as a risk factor of postoperative hypertension. We conducted a large prospective and comparative study of the endarterectomy technique by eversion and with conventional patch closure. The primary end point was the blood pressure value and the administration of antihypertensive treatment. Our study shows that postoperative hypertension after carotid endarterectomy is not related to the surgical technique. Changes in blood pressure after carotid endarterectomy by eversion are lower than those observed after conventional endarterectomy with patch closure. This technique prevents the occurrence of possible hypotension occurrence, which can be the cause of perioperative complications.

► Postoperative hypertension after carotid endarterectomy is associated with myocardial infarction, stroke, and neck hematoma. Mehta et al previously suggested that eversion carotid endarterectomy was associated with a significantly higher incidence of postoperative hypertension.[1] Here, the authors sought to compare the effects of technique of carotid endarterectomy-eversion (e-CEA) or patch (p-CEA), on postoperative hypertension. In comparing 220 e-CEAs to 340 p-CEAs and using a primary end point of systolic blood pressure greater than 160 mm Hg and/or the need for a vasodilator agent after blood pressure measurement within the first 24 hours after surgery, the authors state that there is no significant difference in blood pressure between groups. However, even though these groups were not statistically different with regard to the primary endpoint, these groups were different in three aspects. First, for the first 12 hours after surgery, e-CEA patients had statistically higher blood pressures than the patch group (analogous to the patients in the Mehta study), but the pressures remained below the 160 mm Hg end point. Second, p-CEA patients experienced more hypotensive events. Finally, the e-CEA patients experienced less variability in their postoperative blood pressures. These findings demonstrate that patients undergoing carotid endarterectomy, regardless of the technique, can experience significant variability in postoperative blood pressure in the first 12 to 24 hours after surgery, thus mandating close hemodynamic monitoring in the initial postoperative period.

B. Peterson, MD, FACS

Reference

1. Mehta M, Rahmani O, Dietzek AM, et al. Eversion technique increases the risk of post-carotid endarterectomy hypertension. *J Vasc Surg*. 2001;34:839-845.

Dual Antiplatelet Therapy Prior to Expedited Carotid Surgery Reduces Recurrent Events Prior to Surgery without Significantly Increasing Perioperative Bleeding Complications

Batchelder A, Hunter J, Cairns V, et al (Leicester Royal Infirmary, UK)

Eur J Vasc Endovasc Surg 50:412-419, 2015

Objective.—A daily Rapid-Access TIA Clinic was introduced in 2008, where symptomatic patients were started on 75 mg aspirin + 40 mg simvastatin by the referring doctor, before attending the clinic. Following clinic assessment, patients with 50–99% stenoses were transferred to the vascular unit for carotid endarterectomy (CEA). In two audits ($n = 212$ patients), the median delay from transfer to the vascular unit to undergoing CEA was 3 days, during which time 28 patients (13%) suffered recurrent neurological events. It was hypothesized that early introduction of dual antiplatelet therapy (by adding clopidogrel 75 mg once parenchymal haemorrhage was excluded in the TIA clinic) might significantly reduce recurrent events between transfer to the surgical unit and undergoing CEA.

Methods.—Prospective audit in 100 consecutive, recently symptomatic patients receiving dual antiplatelet therapy. Endpoints were: prevalence of recurrent events between transfer from the TIA clinic and undergoing CEA; rates of spontaneous embolization prior to undergoing CEA; and prevalence of haemorrhagic complications

Results.—The median delay from symptom to CEA was 8 days (IQR 5–15). The median delay between transfer from the TIA clinic to CEA was 3 days (IQR 2–5), during which time three patients (3%) suffered recurrent TIAs. This represents a fivefold reduction compared with previous audit data (OR 4.9, 95% CI 1.5–16.6, $p = .01$) and was matched by a fourfold reduction in the prevalence of spontaneous embolization from 39/189 (21%) previously to 5/83 (5%) in the current audit (OR 4.1, 95% CI 1.5–10.7, $p = .0047$). The 30-day death/stroke rate was 1%. There were three haemorrhagic complications: stroke caused by haemorrhagic transformation of an infarct; exploration for neck haematoma; and debridement and skin grafting for spontaneous shin haematoma.

Conclusion.—Early introduction of dual antiplatelet therapy was associated with a significant reduction in recurrent neurological events and spontaneous embolization prior to CEA, without incurring a significant increase in major peri-operative bleeding complications.

▶ There has been a recent trend toward performing carotid endarterectomy as soon and as safely possible after the onset of cerebral symptoms secondary to the high rate of recurrent symptoms in the intervening time period (up to 25% at 14 days). The authors hypothesize that institution of early dual antiplatelet therapy with aspirin and clopidogrel before surgical therapy will reduce rates of recurrent stroke and transient ischemic attack (TIA). This is based on the observation that recurrent embolization results from unstable plaques with the highest rates in the early time period after onset of symptoms. Patients' outcomes from a "rapid-access TIA" clinic were compared between an initial group treated with aspirin alone (and a single dose of Plavix the night before the procedure) with a median time frame of 3 days from clinic evaluation and carotid endarterectomy, and a contemporary group treated with aspirin and Plavix preoperatively treated over a median time frame of 3 days. There was an overall reduction in recurrent TIA/stroke from 13% to 3% and a 5-fold reduction in spontaneous embolization from 21% to 5% (determined by transcranial Doppler examination the afternoon before surgery) between these 2 groups. Three patients (3%) in the dual antiplatelet cohort suffered hemorrhagic complications in the perioperative period: 1 with hemorrhagic stroke, 1 with neck hematoma, and 1 with spontaneous shin hematoma. This is compared with 7 patients (3%) in the previous group treated with only aspirin.

During this time frame, the authors also began using bovine pericardium as a patch rather than polyester patches. To differentiate perioperative bleeding complications from prosthetic path, 3 comparison groups were made consisting of those with prosthetic patch and aspirin, those with prosthetic patch and dual antiplatelet medications, and those with bovine pericardium and dual antiplatelet medications. Time from restoration of flow to removal of drapes was used as surrogate for achieving hemostasis. While there was a significant decrease in this time when switched to bovine pericardium, dual antiplatelet medication did not statistically increase the hemostasis time. These results suggest that early dual antiplatelet therapy is associated with a reduction in recurrent neurologic events before carotid endarterectomy without a significant increase in bleeding complications.

This article is limited by its retrospective nature as well as single-center design. Most centers do not have a rapid-access TIA clinic. However, more aggressive antiplatelet therapy may be indicated during this vulnerable time period.

M. R. Smeds, MD, FACS

Effect of Patching on Reducing Restenosis in the Carotid Revascularization Endarterectomy Versus Stenting Trial

Malas M, Glebova NO, Hughes SE, et al (Johns Hopkins Univ, Baltimore, MD; Univ of Colorado Denver, Aurora; Rutgers Univ, Newark, NJ; et al)

Stroke 46:757-761, 2015

Background and Purpose.—The purpose is to determine whether patching during carotid endarterectomy (CEA) affects the perioperative and long-term risks of restenosis, stroke, death, and myocardial infarction as compared with primary closure.

Methods.—We identified all patients who were randomized and underwent CEA in Carotid Revascularization Endarterectomy versus Stenting Trial. CEA patients who received a patch were compared with patients who underwent CEA with primary closure without a patch. We compared periprocedural and 4-year event rates, 2-year restenosis rates, and rates of reoperation between the 2 groups. We further analyzed results by surgeon specialty.

Results.—There were 1151 patients who underwent CEA (753 [65%] with patch and 329 [29%] with primary closure). We excluded 44 patients who underwent eversion CEA and 25 patients missing CEA data (5%). Patch use differed by surgeon specialty: 89% of vascular surgeons, 6% of neurosurgeons, and 76% of thoracic surgeons patched. Comparing patients who received a patch versus those who did not, there was a significant reduction in the 2-year risk of restenosis, and this persisted after adjustment by surgeon specialty (hazard ratio, 0.35; 95% confidence interval, 0.16–0.74; $P = 0.006$). There were no significant differences in the rates of periprocedural stroke and death (hazard ratio, 1.58; 95% confidence interval, 0.33–7.58; $P = 0.57$), in immediate reoperation (hazard ratio, 0.6; 95% confidence interval, 0.16–2.27; $P = 0.45$), or in the 4-year risk of ipsilateral stroke (hazard ratio, 1.23; 95% confidence interval, 0.42–3.63; $P = 0.71$).

Conclusions.—Patch closure in CEA is associated with reduction in restenosis although it is not associated with improved clinical outcomes. Thus, more widespread use of patching should be considered to improve long-term durability.

Clinical Trial Registration.—URL: http://www.clinicaltrials.gov. Unique identifier: NCT00004732.

▶ Previous trials have suggested that patching during carotid endarterectomy (CEA) leads to better results than primary closure of the arteriotomy; however, results from these trials have been somewhat variable and consist of small numbers of patients. In this study, the authors use a robust data set from the Carotid Revascularization Endarterectomy versus Stenting Trial (CREST), to assess the superiority of patching over primary closure in CEA patients. The authors analyzed 1082 patients from CREST, 70% of whom underwent patch closure during CEA and 30% of whom underwent primary closure. Interestingly, the utilization of patching by physicians varied by board specialty. Specifically, vascular surgeons and thoracic surgeons were more likely to patch (89% and 76%, respectively), and neurosurgeons were less likely to patch (only 6%). The authors demonstrated that 2-year restenosis rates were significantly lower in the patching group compared with the primary closure group, and after adjusting for specialty, patching was associated with a 65% reduction in the 2-year risk of restenosis. Although clinical outcomes of periprocedural stroke and death, need for immediate reoperation, and 4-year risk of ipsilateral stroke did not differ between groups when adjusting for surgical specialty, the aforementioned results strongly support the more widespread use of patching during CEA in an effort to provide a durable repair with low risk of restenosis.

B. Peterson, MD, FACS

Examination of regional anesthesia for carotid endarterectomy

Pasin L, Nardelli P, Landoni G, et al (IRCCS San Raffaele Scientific Inst, Milan, Italy; et al)

J Vasc Surg 62:631-634, 2015

Objective.—Carotid endarterectomy is the most effective treatment for reducing the risk of stroke in patients with significant carotid stenosis. Few studies have focused on the failure rate of regional anesthesia.

Methods.—Data of all patients undergoing carotid endarterectomy (June 2009 to December 2014) in a single center were collected. Combined deep and superficial cervical plexus block or superficial plexus block alone was used according to the attending anesthesiologist's choice and the patient's characteristics (eg, dual antiplatelet or anticoagulation therapy). Intraoperative remifentanil (0.025-0.05 μg/kg/min) was administered to maintain an adequate level of comfort, responsiveness, and cooperation. General anesthesia was planned only in the case of major contraindications or the patient's refusal of locoregional anesthesia. The primary end point of our study was the incidence of intraoperative conversion from locoregional to general anesthesia.

Results.—A total of 2463 carotid endarterectomies were included in the analysis. Regional anesthesia was initially chosen in 2439 patients, whereas 24 patients received planned general anesthesia. In seven cases, regional anesthesia was converted to general anesthesia because of severe agitation of the patient (before clamping in four cases, after carotid clamping in two cases, and after declamping in one case). A shunt was used in 302 patients (12.3%) because of neurologic deterioration at the carotid clamping test. Intraoperative complications were emergent repeated surgical procedures in 13 cases (0.53%) because of acute neurologic deterioration, 1 intraoperative acute myocardial infarction (0.04%), and 3 cases (0.04%) of hemodynamically relevant supraventricular tachyarrhythmia. No intraoperative death occurred. In-hospital mortality was 0.12% (three patients). Major stroke occurred in 23 patients (0.93%); minor stroke occurred in 16 patients (0.65%). The combined stroke and death rate was 1.62% (40 patients).

Conclusions.—In our practice, carotid endarterectomy under regional anesthesia is safe and associated with a very low rate of conversion to general anesthesia.

▶ The use of locoregional anesthesia in carotid endarterectomy is common, but few studies have examined failure rates (conversion to general anesthesia) of this technique. The authors hypothesize that locoregional anesthesia with superficial or deep cervical plexus block and continuous low-dose remifentanil is safe with a low rate of failure. Secondary outcomes entertained included incidence of major in-hospital cardiovascular and neurologic events as well as mortality. A retrospective review was performed on all patients undergoing carotid endarterectomy at a single center by 6 surgeons over a 5-year period (n = 2463). Of these, the majority (n = 2439; 99%) received planned locoregional anesthesia with only 7 (0.28%) requiring conversion to general anesthesia, mostly secondary to severe agitation due to block failure or claustrophobia. There were no differences in demographic or preoperative factors between those requiring conversion to general anesthesia and those who did not. Shunts were placed in 12% of patients treated with locoregional anesthesia, but only 5 of the patients who were treated with a shunt required conversion to general anesthesia. Perioperative complications were low with only 13 patients (0.5%) returning to the operating room and an in-house mortality rate of 0.1%. These results were obtained in a high-volume carotid center with an established locoregional anesthesia protocol; therefore, they may not be applicable to lower volume centers in which locoregional anesthesia is not routinely performed.

M. R. Smeds, MD, FACS

Impact of Cognitive Dysfunction on Survival in Patients With and Without Statin Use Following Carotid Endarterectomy

Heyer EJ, Mergeche JL, Wang S, et al (Columbia Univ, NY; et al)
Neurosurgery 77:880-887, 2015

Background.—Early cognitive dysfunction (eCD) is a subtle form of neurological injury observed in ~25% of carotid endarterectomy (CEA) patients. Statin use is associated with a lower incidence of eCD in asymptomatic patients having CEA.

Objective.—To determine whether eCD status is associated with worse long-term survival in patients taking and not taking statins.

Methods.—This is a post hoc analysis of a prospective observational study of 585 CEA patients. Patients were evaluated with a battery of neuropsychometric tests before and after surgery. Survival was compared for patients with and without eCD stratifying by statin use. At enrollment, 366 patients were on statins and 219 were not. Survival was assessed by using Kaplan-Meier methods and multivariable Cox proportional hazards models.

Results.—Age ≥75 years ($P = .003$), diabetes mellitus ($P < .001$), cardiac disease ($P = .02$), and statin use ($P = .014$) are significantly associated with survival univariately ($P < .05$) by use of the log-rank test. By Cox proportional hazards model, eCD status and survival adjusting for univariate factors within statin and nonstatin use groups suggested a significant effect by association of eCD on survival within patients not taking statin (hazard ratio, 1.61; 95% confidence interval, 1.09-2.40; $P = .018$), and no significant effect of eCD on survival within patients taking statin (hazard ratio, 0.98; 95% confidence interval, 0.59-1.66; $P = .95$).

Conclusion.—eCD is associated with shorter survival in patients not taking statins. This finding validates eCD as an important neurological outcome and suggests that eCD is a surrogate measure for overall health, comorbidity, and vulnerability to neurological insult.

▶ Carotid endarterectomy (CEA) can be complicated by a subtle form of neurological injury termed "early cognitive dysfunction" (eCD) in up to 25% of patients. Statin use has been shown to decrease the incidence of eCD following CEA and has been shown to increase survival after CEA. Here, the authors sought to determine whether eCD status is associated with worse long-term survival and whether this association differs between statin users and non—statin users in patients undergoing CEA.

In this post hoc analysis of an observation study, 585 CEA patients made up the study population, including 366 patients (62.6%) on statins and 219 patients (37.4%) who were not. All patients underwent rigorous neuropsychometric evaluations preoperatively and within 24 hours postoperatively to test for eCD. One hundred forty-five patients (24.8%) tested positive for eCD following CEA (eCD present in 30.1% of patients not on statins and in 21.6% of patients on statins). Interestingly, the authors found that in patients not taking a statin, having eCD led to a higher risk of dying (odds ratio [OR] 2.21), whereas those on statin therapy, having eCD or not, did not lead to a higher mortality risk (OR 1.03) post-CEA. Although the patient cohort is small for a survival analysis, this is the first study to show that eCD after CEA is associated with shorter survival in patients not taking statins, and it provides further evidence that statins are beneficial regardless of lipid levels in patients with carotid artery disease.

B. Peterson, MD, FACS

Long-Term Clinical Outcomes and Cardiovascular Events after Carotid Endarterectomy

Go C, Avgerinos ED, Chaer RA, et al (Univ of Pittsburgh Med Ctr, PA)
Ann Vasc Surg 29:1265-1271, 2015

Background.—Long-term atherosclerotic adverse events are anticipated in patients undergoing carotid endarterectomy (CEA); however, their incidence and risk predictors remain unknown.

Methods.—A consecutive cohort of CEAs between 1/1/2000—12/31/2007 was analyzed. End points were any stroke, coronary event (myocardial infarction, coronary bypass, or stenting), vascular interventions for critical limb ischemia, aortic aneurysm or carotid disease, and death. Survival analysis and Cox regression models were used to identify clinical predictors.

Results.—A total of 1,136 CEAs (bilateral, 89; mean age, 71.2 ± 9.2 years; 56.5% male; 36.3% symptomatic, and 3.9% combined with coronary bypass) were performed during the study period with a mean clinical follow-up of 60 months (0—155 months). The postoperative combined stroke and/or death rate was 2.7% and 1.9% for asymptomatic and 4.1% for symptomatic patients. Five and 10-year risks of the end points were 7.2% and 16.1% for stroke, 18.4% and 31.5% for coronary interventions, 20.6% and 28.5% for major vascular interventions, and 25.8% and 50.1% for death. Statins conferred a significant protective effect for stroke (hazard ratio [HR], 0.53; $P = 0.016$) and death (HR, 0.66; $P < 0.0001$). Baseline vascular disease predicted future vascular interventions: aortic aneurysm (HR, 1.90; $P = 0.003$), peripheral arterial disease (HR, 2.03; $P < 0.0001$), and contralateral internal carotid artery (ICA) stenosis ≥50% (HR, 4.61; $P < 0.0001$). Renal insufficiency predicted worse outcomes for all other end points (HR, 2.21; $P = 0.023$ for stroke; HR, 1.62; $P = 0.008$ for coronary events; HR, 2.38; $P < 0.0001$ for death).

Conclusions.—Patients undergoing CEA continue to derive long-term low stroke rate benefit but still sustain major coronary events and require vascular interventions, indicating a need for more intensive medical treatment and rigorous follow-up.

► Patients who undergo carotid endarterectomy for extracranial carotid occlusive disease are clearly at risk for other systemic manifestations of atherosclerosis. A large retrospective chart review of more than 1000 CEA patients over the span of 8 years by the authors of this study, with 5- and 10-year outcomes reported, provides a more specific view of the severity of the problem. The patients in the study had early postoperative adverse outcomes (stroke, myocardial infarction, death) at rates comparable to data available from other recent studies, including data available from the National Surgical Quality Improvement Program. The long-term outcomes for these patients are sobering, but not surprising. Ten-year risks of stroke, coronary interventions, major vascular interventions, and death were reported at 16.1%, 31.5%, 28.5%, and 50.1%, respectively.

One promising aspect of this study is that over the course of the 8 years that were reviewed, a larger percentage of the patients were treated with statins postoperatively, and in fact, statin use conferred a significant long-term protective effect for stroke and death. This should strongly emphasize that surgeons should consider themselves responsible for medically treating their patients' underlying disease process and not just 1 manifestation of their atherosclerosis. In terms of carotid stenosis, it is not as simple as an either/or choice between surgical intervention and best medical therapy. All operative patients should be treated with best medical therapy in addition to their carotid intervention with the hope of preventing further adverse effects of their atherosclerosis in the future.

M. Williams, MD

Patient and observer scar assessment scores favour the late appearance of a transverse cervical incision over a vertical incision in patients undergoing carotid endarterectomy for stroke risk reduction

Deck M, Kopriva D (Univ of Saskatchewan College of Medicine, Canada; Univ of Saskatchewan, Saskatoon, Canada)

Can J Surg 58:245-249, 2015

Background.—Carotid endarterectomy (CEA) is a very common operation, but there is no agreement on the appropriate orientation of the surgical incision.

Methods.—We retrospectively reviewed the charts of patients who had undergone CEA between Jul. 1, 2010, and Dec. 31, 2013. We contacted patients identified in the review to solicit participation in a clinical follow-up examination, during which the esthetic outcome of the scar was evaluated using the Patient and Observer Scar Assessment Scale (POSAS).

Results.—During the study period 237 CEAs were performed. Nine patients refused the use of their personal health information in this study. There were no significant differences in the neurologic outcomes of patients based on the incision orientation (perioperative stroke and death 1.4% with transverse incision v. 0% with a vertical incision, $p = 0.44$). Fifty-two patients presented for follow-up examination. Thirty-three had a transverse incision and 19 had a vertical incision. Results of the POSAS significantly favoured the transverse incision ($p = 0.03$). Vertical incisions were more often associated with persistent, mild marginal mandibular nerve dysfunction ($p = 0.04$).

Conclusion.—Carotid endarterectomy performed through a transverse skin incision compared with a vertically oriented skin incision is associated with improved esthetic outcome, as measured by the POSAS, without an observed statistically significant difference in the risk of perioperative stroke or death between the 2 techniques.

▶ Carotid endarterectomy (CEA) is one of the most common procedures performed by vascular surgeons, but there is no consensus regarding the orientation of the incision. Traditionally, vertical incisions were made, but now many surgeons perform transverse incisions, often using a skin crease, to produce a less obvious scar. It seems intuitive that a transverse incision oriented along Langer's lines would produce a better cosmetic outcome, but despite this principle, many surgeons continue to make a vertical incision.

In this study, 52 patients underwent CEA: 33 patients through a transverse incision and 19 patients through a vertical incision. The aesthetic outcome of the scar was evaluated by using the Patient and Observer Scar Assessment Scale. This previously validated scale consists of a patient questionnaire portion and an observer portion. All patients were examined by the same observer. There was no difference between groups with regard to the neurological outcomes of patients. The "observer" assessment favored the appearance of the transverse incision, but this did not reach statistical significance. The observer detected mild marginal mandibular nerve dysfunction in 15.7% of patients in the vertical incision group and none in the transverse incision group ($P = .044$). The patient assessment scores showed a significant difference in favor of the transverse incision. Although CEA can be performed with equal efficacy through either a vertical or transverse incision, patients seem to favor the appearance of the transverse incision over the vertical incision in this relatively small patient cohort.

B. Peterson, MD, FACS

Risk factors for cranial nerve injury after carotid endarterectomy

Bennett KM, Scarborough JE, Shortell CK (Duke Univ Med Ctr, Durham, NC)

J Vasc Surg 62:363-369, 2015

Background.—Although numerous studies have described the incidence of postoperative cranial nerve injury (CNI) after carotid endarterectomy (CEA), there have been few attempts to identify risk factors for this complication.

Methods.—The 2012 CEA-targeted American College of Surgeons National Surgical Quality Improvement Program database was used to determine the incidence of CNI after CEA. Multivariate logistic regression analysis was performed to identify independent predictors of CNI after CEA, using a comprehensive array of patient-, carotid disease-, and procedure-related factors as potential predictor variables.

Results.—Of the 3762 CEA patients who were included in our analysis, 84 (2.2%) were noted to have sustained CNI in the first 30 days after their operation. Independent predictors of this complication included age ≥80 years (reference group, <70 years; adjusted odds ratio [AOR] for CNI, 1.74; 95% confidence interval [CI], 1.00-3.03; $P = .05$), presence of a preoperative bleeding disorder (including patients in whom preoperative nonaspirin anticoagulation therapy was not stopped before CEA; AOR, 1.66; 95% CI, 1.03-2.68; $P = .04$), duration of operation (AOR, 1.15 for each 30-minute interval beyond an operative time of 90 minutes; 95% CI, 1.06-1.25; $P = .001$), and need for reoperation (AOR, 2.65; 95% CI, 1.03-6.80; $P = .04$).

Conclusions.—Our study demonstrates clinically evident CNI to be a relatively uncommon event after CEA at institutions that participate in the CEA-targeted American College of Surgeons National Surgical Quality Improvement Program and identifies four separate factors that are independently associated with an increased risk of CNI.

▶ The incidence of cranial nerve injury (CNI) in the setting of patients undergoing carotid endarterectomy (CEA) is quite variable in the literature. For patients (especially asymptomatic patients) to receive benefit from undergoing CEA, the procedure has to be safe and accompanied by few complications. Using a relatively new database, or rather a newly focused long-standing database, the 2012 CEA-targeted American College of Surgeons National Quality Improvement Project (ACS NSQIP), this study attempts to identify factors that are independently associated with increased risk of developing CNI after CEA.

The cohort included 3762 patients, and CNI was detected in 84 patients (2.2%). Roughly one-third of these injuries were diagnosed on the day of surgery, one-third diagnosed the day after surgery, and one-third diagnosed more than 1 day after surgery. Using multivariate analysis, the authors detected 4 risk factors that were independently associated with the development of CNI after CEA: age greater than or equal to 80, the presence of a preoperative bleeding disorder (defined by NSQIP as patients in whom nonaspirin anticoagulation was not stopped), duration of operation (beyond 90 minutes), and the need for reoperation. Interestingly, the "high-risk" anatomical characteristics cited in most CEA and carotid artery stenting studies (ie, prior CEA, neck dissection, or history of radiation) did not preclude patients to CNI.

The major limitation of this study lies in the fact that these are data abstracted from a large database, and the ability to identify patients with CNI relies solely on what is documented in the chart. Prospective, postoperative examination of CEA patients by independent physicians looking for CNI is not possible in this type of review; nevertheless, this study does draw attention to certain clinical scenarios that may lead to increased risk of CNI. Perhaps the findings will heighten surgeons' attention to detail during CEA in these scenarios and lead to a reduced incidence of CNI.

B. Peterson, MD, FACS

Stress Management in Patients Undergoing Carotid Endarterectomy for Carotid Artery Stenosis: A Pilot Randomized Controlled Trial

Vasdekis SN, Roussopoulou A, Lazaris A, et al (Athens Univ Med School, Greece; Univ of Athens Med School, Greece; et al)

Ann Vasc Surg 29:1400-1407, 2015

Background.—Psychological stress is common to patients submitted to cardiovascular operations. The purpose of this pilot, single-center, open-label, randomized controlled trial was to investigate the effects of a stress management program (SMP) on patients undergoing carotid endarterectomy (CEA).

Methods.—A sample of 24 patients with significant (>70%) carotid stenosis was finally randomized to SMP (intervention group; $n = 12$) or no-stress management intervention (control group; $n = 12$) before CEA. SMP consisted of 2 relaxation techniques (relaxation-breathing and guided imagery) before and 8 weeks after CEA. Measurements included Perceived Stress Scale (PSS), Hospital Anxiety and Depression Scale (HADS), Health Locus of Control Scale (HLC), and blood pressure and heart rate.

Results.—The 2 groups did not differ in terms of demographic characteristics, vascular risk factors, and baseline psychometric measurements. No delay on the time of surgery was caused by the practice of the relaxation techniques. Both perceived stress and anxiety improved within the intervention group at the end of the program ($P = 0.005$ and $P = 0.007$, respectively). No improvement in PSS-14, HLC, and HADS scores were documented in control group at the end of the 8-week follow-up period. The intervention group had lower PSS-14 scores at 8 weeks after CEA (median PSS-14 score, 20 points; range, 10–28) compared with control group (median PSS, 25 points; range, 11–47; $P = 0.026$). No significant effect of SMP was found for blood pressure and heart rate measurements.

Conclusions.—Our results indicate that relaxation techniques appear to be beneficial in terms of stress and anxiety reduction in patients undergoing CEA. These findings require independent confirmation in the setting of a larger, double-blind randomized controlled trial.

▶ Unarguably, surgery is stressful for patients. Stress management programs have been shown to have a positive impact on outcomes in pediatrics, obstetrics, orthopedics, and general and cardiac surgery patients. This has never been investigated in patients undergoing carotid endarterectomy (CEA), and therefore, in this open-label, randomized controlled trial, the authors sought to investigate the efficacy of 2 relaxation techniques in improving stress, anxiety, and the feeling of self-control in patients after CEA.

Twenty-four patients were randomized to a stress management program (SMP; n = 12) or no SMP (control; n = 12). The program consisted of a relaxed breathing technique, essentially deep breaths followed by prolonged expirations; and guided imagery-visualization by patients of a relaxed beach setting with themselves as part of it. Patients in the SMP group were taught these methods of relaxation and instructed to practice them 3 times a day before surgery and twice a day after CEA for 8 weeks. Using various proven scoring systems, after 8 weeks, the SMP group members were found to have significant improvement in their perceived stress and anxiety compared with the control group. Although there was no significant difference between groups in terms of blood pressure and heart rate, and despite a small sample size, these simple, inexpensive relaxation techniques should be offered to patients who are about to be subjected to the stress of surgery.

B. Peterson, MD, FACS

Surgeon Case Volume and 30-Day Mortality After Carotid Endarterectomy Among Contemporary Medicare Beneficiaries: Before and After National Coverage Determination for Carotid Artery Stenting

Kumamaru H, Jalbert JJ, Nguyen LL, et al (Harvard Med School, Boston, MA; et al)

Stroke 46:1288-1294, 2015

Background and Purpose.—After the 2005 National Coverage Determination to reimburse carotid artery stenting (CAS) for Medicare beneficiaries, the number of CAS procedures increased and carotid endarterectomy (CEA) decreased. We evaluated trends in surgeons' past-year CEA case-volume and 30-day mortality after CEA, and their association before and after the National Coverage Determination.

Methods.—In a retrospective cohort study of patients undergoing CEA (2001–2008) and CAS (2005–2008) using Medicare data, we described yearly trends of CEA and CAS rates, patient characteristics, and 30-day mortality after CEA. We used logistic regression adjusting for patient- and surgeon-level factors to assess the effect of surgeon case volume on 30-day mortality after CEA.

Results.—We identified 454 717 CEA and 27 943 CAS patients. Patients undergoing CEA in recent years were older and had more comorbidities than earlier years. CEA rates per 10 000 beneficiaries declined from 18.1 in 2002 to 12.7 in 2008, whereas median surgeon past-year case-volume declined from 27 to 21. The CAS rates peaked at 2.3 per 10 000 beneficiaries in 2006 but declined to 1.8 in 2008, resulting in declining overall revascularization procedure rates during 2005 to 2008. Thirty day post-CEA mortality was 1.40% (95% confidence interval, 1.34–1.47) in 2001 to 2002 and 1.17% (1.10–1.24) in 2007 to 2008. Surgeon's past-year case-volume of <10 was associated with higher 30-day mortality consistently during 2001 to 2008.

Conclusions.—The rate of CEA procedures decreased substantially during 2001 to 2008, as did surgeon past-year case-volume. The postprocedural mortality in Medicare beneficiaries was high compared with trial patients but somewhat improved over time. Those operated by lower past-year case-volume surgeons had increased mortality.

▶ Increasing use of carotid artery stenting (CAS) after Medicare began reimbursing this procedure in 2005 has resulted in a decrease in carotid endarterectomy (CEA). Additionally, with improvements in medical management of carotid artery disease, the benefit of CEA has decreased. The authors hypothesize that because of this decrease in case volume as well as decrease in benefit, periprocedural outcomes will be worse compared with years before 2005. Medicare data was analyzed from 2001 to 2008. Over this period, CEA per 10 000 beneficiaries decreased from peak of 18.1 in 2002 to 12.7 in 2008, whereas CAS rates initially increased after 2005 but plateaued at around 1.8. CEA patients became older with more comorbidities over the study, and surgeon's median case volumes decreased from 27 to 21. Perioperative mortality actually decreased from 1.4% to 1.17%, and surgeons who performed fewer than 10 cases per year had a significantly higher rate consistently over the time period. Although the authors confirmed that CEA rates are decreasing, this decrease was not completely explained by a corresponding increase in CAS, and there has not been a corresponding increase in mortality, despite patients being older with higher numbers of comorbidities. This may reflect better medical management of carotid artery stenosis with antiplatelet medications and statins, as well as better patient selection. This study is limited by its database design, which is unable to determine postoperative stroke or indications for initial procedure (stenting vs endarterectomy).

M. R. Smeds, MD, FACS

Ultrasound-guided regional anesthesia for carotid endarterectomy induces early hemodynamic and stress hormone changes

Hoefer J, Pierer E, Rantner B, et al (Med Univ of Innsbruck, Austria)
J Vasc Surg 62:57-67, 2015

Objective.—Locoregional anesthesia is an effective method for evaluating cerebral function during carotid endarterectomy (CEA). Landmark-guided regional anesthesia (RA) is currently used for CEA and can provoke substantial perioperative hypertension. Ultrasound-guided RA (US-RA) is a new method for performing RA in CEA; however, the effect on sympathetic activity and blood pressure is uncertain. This study assessed early sympathetic activity during CEA in US-RA compared with general anesthesia (GA).

Methods.—Patients were prospectively randomized to receive US-RA (n = 32) or GA (n = 28) for CEA. The primary end point was the change in systolic arterial blood pressure after induction of anesthesia (just before starting surgery) comparing US-RA with GA. We also recorded heart rate and analyzed concentrations of plasma blood hormones, including cortisol, metanephrine, and normetanephrine at five different times. Creatinine kinase, troponin I, and N-terminal pro-B-type natriuretic peptide were analyzed to detect potential changes in cardiac biomarkers during the procedure.

Results.—Systolic arterial blood pressure (mean ± standard deviation) increased significantly in US-RA patients compared with GA patients even before surgery was initiated (180 ± 26 mm Hg vs 109 ± 24 mm Hg; $P < .001$), then remained elevated during the entire surgery and returned to baseline values 1 hour after admission to the postoperative anesthesia care unit. Heart rate (US-RA: 78 ± 16 beats/min, GA: 52 ± 12 beats/min; $P < .001$) and cortisol levels (US-RA: 155 ± 97 μg/L, GA: 99 ± 43 μg/L; $P = .006$) were also significantly higher in the US-RA group after induction of anesthesia. Other values did not differ.

Conclusions.—The US-RA technique for CEA induces temporary intraoperative hypertension and an increase in stress hormone levels. Nevertheless, US-RA is a feasible, effective, and safe form of locoregional for CEA that enables targeted placement of low volumes of local anesthesia under direct visualization.

▶ While carotid endarterectomy (CEA) can effectively be performed under regional anesthesia (RA) or general anesthesia (GA), RA has been associated with significant perioperative hypertension. A newer technique of RA uses ultrasound guidance rather than just landmarks in an effort to produce more effective results with perhaps less local anesthetic. This study is designed to compare the early sympathetic response in CEA patients receiving GA with patients receiving ultrasound-guided RA (US-RA). The effect that these different types of anesthesia had on blood pressure and stress hormone levels was evaluated.

In this prospectively randomized study, 32 patients undergoing CEA received US-RA, and 28 patients received GA. Hemodynamic measurements and blood samples were taken immediately after placement of an arterial line, and this measurement served as the "baseline." The next measurement occurred after induction of anesthesia and before skin incision, and other measurements occurred at specific points throughout surgery, leading to the final measurement in the recovery room 1 hour after surgery. Despite using less local anesthetic than landmark-based RA, patients in the US-RA group experienced a similar hypertensive response immediately after induction of anesthesia. Systolic blood pressures were significantly higher in the US-RA group compared with the GA group at the first time point, and this persisted throughout surgery, and eventually normalized 1 hour after surgery. Likewise, cortisol levels varied in a similar fashion, with higher levels seen in the US-RA group at all time points. Although US-RA is effective for patients undergoing CEA, this hemodynamic and hormonal change needs to be anticipated, and this response may need to be avoided in certain patients.

B. Peterson, MD, FACS

Surgical Outcomes for Cervical Carotid Artery Stenosis: Treatment Strategy for Bilateral Cervical Carotid Artery Stenosis

Hokari M, Nakayama N, Kazumata K, et al (Hokkaido Univ Graduate School of Medicine, Sapporo, Japan; et al)

J Stroke Cerebrovasc Dis 24:1768-1774, 2015

Background.—Carotid endarterectomy (CEA) and carotid stenting (CAS) are beneficial procedures for patients with high-grade cervical carotid stenosis. However, it is sometimes difficult to manage patients with bilateral carotid stenosis. To decide the treatment strategy, one of the most important questions is whether contralateral stenosis increases the risk of patients undergoing CEA.

Methods.—This retrospective study included 201 patients with carotid stenosis who underwent a total of 219 consecutive procedures (CEA 189/CAS 30). We retrospectively analyzed outcomes in patients with carotid stenosis who were treated with either CEA or CAS and evaluated whether or not contralateral lesions increases the risk of patients undergoing CEA or CAS. Furthermore, we retrospectively verified our treatment strategy for bilateral carotid stenosis.

Results.—The incidences of perioperative complications were 5.3% in the CEA patients and 6.7% in the CAS patients, respectively. There was no significant difference between these 2 groups. The existences of contralateral occlusion and/or contralateral stenosis were not associated with perioperative complications in both the groups. There were 32 patients with bilateral severe carotid stenosis (>50%). Of those, 13 patients underwent bilateral revascularizations; CEA followed by CEA in 8, CEA followed by CAS in 3, CAS followed by CEA 1 coronary artery bypass grafting in 1, and CAS followed by CAS in 1.

Conclusions.—Our date showed that the existence of contralateral carotid lesion was not associated with perioperative complications, and most of our cases with bilateral carotid stenosis initially underwent CEA.

▶ Patients who require intervention for carotid stenosis often have significant contralateral carotid stenosis or occlusions. The best treatment strategy for these patients is uncertain. It has long been suggested that significant contralateral carotid disease might predispose carotid endarterectomy patients to higher risk for postoperative complications. The Stenting and Angioplasty with Protection in Patients at High Risk for Endarterectomy (SAPPHIRE) trial considered contralateral carotid occlusion as a high risk for surgery.[1] This retrospective study out of Japan looked at 219 consecutive carotid interventions (endarterectomy or stent) in 201 patients over a 7-year span. Thirteen of the patients had contralateral carotid occlusion and 32 had 50% to 99% stenosis. About half of the patients studied were symptomatic. One hundred and eighty-nine patients underwent endarterectomy, and 30 received a stent. All endarterectomy patients were routinely shunted intraoperatively, and all underwent primary arteriotomy repair with running suture without patch angioplasty. All stent patients received routine distal embolic protection. Thirteen of the 32 patients with contralateral greater than 50% stenosis went on to have staged intervention on the other carotid artery (8 endarterectomies and 5 stents). The results showed that patients with contralateral stenosis or occlusion were not associated with higher postoperative complications and those treated with endarterectomy and stenting had equivalent outcomes. The authors concluded that endarterectomy for patients with contralateral carotid disease is safe and effective, but prospective studies with a larger sample size are needed.

M. Williams, MD

Reference

1. Yadav JS, Wholey MH, Kuntz RE, et al. Protected carotid artery stenting versus endarterectomy in high-risk patients. *N Engl J Med*. 2004;351:1493-1501.

11 Vascular Trauma

A Pulseless Limb Poorly Predicts an Arterial Injury in Combat Trauma

Quail JF, McDonald VS, Carter KK, et al (Naval Med Ctr San Diego, CA)
Ann Vasc Surg 29:1097-1104, 2015

Background.—A pulseless limb is considered a hard sign of an arterial injury after penetrating trauma in the civilian population. However, the reliability of this finding has never been examined in combat trauma. The purpose of this study was to examine the reliability of the pulseless limb in the combat trauma population. Reasons for false positive physical examination findings were also identified.

Methods.—The Joint Theater Trauma Registry identified all patients who presented to a military treatment facility (MTF) in Kandahar, Afghanistan, with a penetrating extremity injury over a 2-year period. Patients found to have a pulse deficit on initial physical examination were followed, and the results of the subsequent computed tomographic angiogram or arteriogram recorded. Patient demographics, injury patterns, and physiological data were examined. Standard statistical analysis was performed.

Results.—From 2011 to 2012, 644 patients were treated at a single MTF for lower extremity penetrating injuries. The most common mechanisms of injury were explosions (62%) and gunshot wounds (20%). Of the 577 patients with complete medical records, 448 patients (78%) presented with palpable pulses, 115 patients (20%) presented with a pulseless limb, and 14 (2%) presented with hard signs of vascular injury. Of those with a pulseless limb and abnormal ankle-brachial index (ABI) or no ABI obtained who underwent further radiologic imaging, 38 patients (77%) had no arterial injury identified. Compared with those with a palpable pulse, patients with a pulseless limb without an arterial injury were more likely to have a higher Injury Severity Score (ISS), lower hematocrit, lower pH, greater base deficit, higher heart rate, more frequent use of tranexamic acid, and received greater volumes of packed red blood cells, plasma, and crystalloids.

Conclusions.—Our results demonstrate that a pulseless limb is a poor predictor of arterial injury and should not be considered a hard sign of vascular injury in the combat population. Variables including a high ISS, anemia, acidosis, and need for resuscitation products, each a surrogate for injury severity, may contribute to the decreased accuracy of the physical examination in our troops. This may translate into unnecessary immediate exploration or other interventions in patients who present with more significant injuries from the battlefield. Future studies must continue to focus on improved algorithms for diagnostic accuracy of extremity vascular injuries in this population.

▶ A pulseless limb is often considered a "hard sign" of vascular injury, necessitating exploration or further imaging. Although extremity injuries are increasingly encountered in the Global War on Terrorism, access to higher level imaging is not readily available, and as such, inaccurate pulse exams may lead to unnecessary exploration and delays in transfer to definitive care. The authors sought to determine the reliability of the pulse exam in predicting arterial injury by examining all patients presenting with penetrating trauma to a "Role III facility" (level 1 trauma center equivalent) in Afghanistan using a retrospective review of an administrative database. Over a 2-year period (2011–2012), 644 patients presented with penetrating lower extremity trauma, of which 95 had abnormal or no ankle-brachial index (ABI) recorded. Imaging was performed in 49 patients, of whom only 11 (22%) had arterial injury. Comparing patients with pulseless exam and no arterial injury on imaging with those who had normal pulses/ABI showed the former had higher ISS, lower hematocrit and pH, greater base deficit, higher heart rate, and greater volumes of resuscitation (red blood cells, plasma, crystalloids, and tranexamic acid), suggesting that physiologic stresses may result in inaccurate examination. The authors recommend that pulselessness should not be a hard sign of vascular injury in the combat arena. However, only 22% of patients presenting with a pulseless exam underwent ABI, and had this been performed at a higher rate, ischemia may have been excluded more easily. Additional limitations to the study include the use of a database and the study population, which consisted of mostly younger and healthy men, as well as mechanism of injury that was frequently explosion or high-velocity gunshot wounds. These results are likely not applicable to the civilian arena.

M. R. Smeds, MD, FACS

Editor's Choice – Durability of Endovascular Repair in Blunt Traumatic Thoracic Aortic Injury: Long-Term Outcome from Four Tertiary Referral Centers

Steuer J, Björck M, Sonesson B, et al (Uppsala Univ, Sweden; Univ Hosp, Malmö, Sweden; et al)

Eur J Vasc Endovasc Surg 50:460-465, 2015

Objectives.—To analyze the early and long-term survival and reintervention rate in patients undergoing TEVAR for blunt traumatic thoracic aortic injury.

TABLE 2.—Characteristics of Patients Who Underwent Re-intervention After TEVAR

Sex	Age	Trauma Mechanism	Aortic Injury Type[a]	Stent Graft	Indication for Re-intervention	Time to Re-intervention (Weeks)	Operation
M	56	Car crash	IV	Gore TAG 28 × 100	Hemodynamically unstable, proximal endoleak	0.1	Gore TAG 31 × 150
M	24	Car crash	III	Gore TAG 28 × 100	Infolding	1	Palmaz stent
M	60	Snowmobile accident	II	Gore TAG 34 × 150	Proximal endoleak	1	Gore TAG 34 × 150
M	39	Motor cycle accident	III	Gore TAG 31 × 150	Left arm ischemia	1	Bypass LCCA-LSA
M	44	Fallen 16 m	III	Gore TAG 28 × 100	Infolding	2.5	Gore TAG 34 × 150 + bypass LCCA-LSA
M	17	Car crash Passenger	III	Gore TAG 28 × 150	Stent graft collapse	3	Palmaz stent
M	43	Motorcycle accident	IV	Gore TAG 28 × 100	Retrograde endoleak through LSA	6	Coiling LSA
M	27	Terrain vehicle accident	III	Gore TAG 28 × 150	Stent graft collapse, claudication	14	Sinus-XL stent + Palmaz stent
M	69	One car accident	III	Gore TAG 37 × ?	Proximal endoleak	17	Proximal re-lining
F	31	Car crash Passenger	III	Gore TAG 26 × 100	Malalignment, claudication	22	Surgical explantation
M	27	Pedestrian hit by car	III	Gore TAG 28 × 150	Left arm ischemia	42	Bypass LCCA-LSA
M	62	One car accident	III	Gore TAG 34 × 200	Proximal endoleak	43	Palmaz stent
M	23	Motor cycle accident	III	Medtronic Valiant 24 × 112	Fibrous hyperplasia, claudication	58	Surgical explantation

LCCA = left common carotid artery; LSA = left subclavian artery.
Editor's Note: Please refer to original journal article for full references.
[a]Taken from reference.[1]
Reprinted from Steuer J, Björck M, Sonesson B, et al. Editor's choice – durability of endovascular repair in blunt traumatic thoracic aortic injury: long-term outcome from four tertiary referral centers. *Eur J Vasc Endovasc Surg*. 2015;50:460-465, with permission from European Society for Vascular Surgery.

Methods.—This was a consecutive case series. Between the years 2001 and 2010, a total of 74 patients underwent TEVAR for blunt traumatic thoracic aortic injury at four tertiary referral centers, three in Sweden and one in Switzerland. The median age of the patients was 41 years, and 16% were women. Demographic, procedural, and outcome data were collected and reviewed retrospectively. The patients were followed up during 2013–2014.

Results.—Early (30 day) mortality was 9% (7 patients), with only two cases directly related to the aortic injury; in hospital mortality was 14% as three patients died during the primary hospital admission within the first 6 months. Most patients had sustained severe injuries to other organ systems, and among all in hospital deaths brain injury was the predominant cause. Five year survival in the whole group was 81%. Reintervention was needed in 16% (12 patients) during the first year, half of them within the first month. Only one patient underwent reintervention more than 1 year after the initial procedure. Infolding and partial stentgraft collapse was the reason for the secondary procedure in five of the 13 patients; in three it occurred within 3 weeks of the acute TEVAR.

Conclusion.—TEVAR allows rapid and effective therapy in trauma patients with blunt aortic injury. The outcome is dependent on the severity of the concomitant injuries. The treatment is durable during the first decade after the procedure, but even longer follow up is needed to determine the impact of TEVAR in young patients on the degenerative changes that take place in the aging aorta (Table 2).

▶ The authors sought to describe the long-term thoracic endovascular aneurysm repair (TEVAR) device-related complications and device integrity in the aging aorta when used for blunt thoracic aortic injury. This is a retrospective review of 74 TEVAR case performed for blunt thoracic aortic injury at 4 centers between 2001 and 2010. Grades of injury were: grade I (n = 1), grade II (n = 10, 14%), grade III (n = 55, 74%), and grade IV (n = 8, 11%). Among those, 69 patients were available for follow-up. The left subclavian artery (LSA) was covered in 37 patients (50%), and in 4 (5%) the left common carotid artery (LCCA) also had to be covered, which in 2 cases was managed by placing a stent graft into the LCCA as a chimney graft and in 2 by way of a right to left carotid-carotid bypass. Reinterventions were required in 13 (17.5%) patients as detailed in Table 2. The principal reasons for reintervention were endoleak (n = 5), infolding of the stent graft (n = 5), left arm ischemia (n = 2), and fibrous hyperplasia (n = 1). Five-year survival was 81% + 5%; half of the patients were followed for 5 years or more. Lessons learned during the early experiences are to avoid stent graft oversizing to prevent subsequent stent enfolding or collapse. The experience also reminds us of the importance for long-term follow-up, but most importantly in the first year post repair.[1-3]

S. Shalhub, MD, MPH, FACS

References

1. Rabin J, Harris DG, Crews GA, et al. Early aortic repair worsens concurrent traumatic brain injury. *Ann Thorac Surg*. 2014;98:46-51.
2. Azizzadeh A, Keyhani K, Miller CC 3rd, Coogan SM, Safi HJ, Estrera AL. Blunt traumatic aortic injury: initial experience with endovascular repair. *J Vasc Surg*. 2009;49:1403-1408.
3. Starnes BW, Lundgren RS, Gunn M, et al. A new classification scheme for treating blunt aortic injury. *J Vasc Surg*. 2012;55:47-54.

Endovascular repair for blunt thoracic aortic injury using the Zenith Alpha low-profile device

Starnes BW, Dwivedi AJ, Giglia JS, et al (Univ of Washington, Seattle; Univ of Louisville, KY; Univ of Cincinnati, OH; et al)

J Vasc Surg 62:1495-1503, 2015

Objective.—The objective of this study was to report 30-day results from a prospective, nonrandomized, multicenter trial that evaluated the safety and effectiveness of the Zenith Alpha thoracic endovascular graft (Cook Medical, Bloomington, Ind) for treatment of blunt thoracic aortic injuries (BTAIs).

Methods.—Eligible patients with BTAIs (grade II to grade IV) in the descending thoracic aorta were treated with the Zenith Alpha device, which is available in smaller graft diameters (starting at 18 mm) and lower profile delivery systems (starting at 16F) than currently available thoracic endografts. The device (nitinol stents and polyester graft material) accommodates a tighter aortic curvature (radius of 20 mm) than the predicate Zenith TX2 Pro-Form. Follow-up clinical and imaging evaluations were performed at 30 days, at 6 and 12 months, and annually thereafter through 5 years. The primary end point was 30-day mortality.

Results.—Between January 2013 and May 2014, 50 patients (44 men; mean age, 43 ± 19 years; range, 18-89 years) were treated with the Zenith Alpha device at 17 U.S. sites. The mean Injury Severity Score was 31 ± 14 (range, 3-66). Technical success was achieved in 100% of patients, with 0% intraoperative mortality. Device access was entirely percutaneous in 22 patients (44%). Smaller size grafts (18-24 mm) were used in 15 patients (30%). The mean procedure time was 85 ± 44 minutes (range, 34-278 minutes), and mean blood loss was 103 ± 145 mL (range, 0-1000 mL). The 30-day mortality rate was 2%; one patient died 24 days after the procedure of respiratory failure related to associated injuries and not to the device or procedure as adjudicated by an independent Clinical Events Committee (CEC). One patient experienced a stroke 7 days after the procedure (cause undetermined by the CEC), and one patient underwent reintervention for a site-reported proximal type I endoleak (core laboratory reported unknown endoleak type) at 30 days after the procedure. There have been no conversions to open surgical repair, paraplegia, or aortic rupture within 30 days.

Conclusions.—Short-term results indicate that the Zenith Alpha thoracic endovascular graft appears safe and effective for the treatment of BTAIs. This low-profile device enables complete percutaneous repair in a large percentage of patients and can achieve high rates of technical success and very low rates of aortic injury-related mortality within 30 days (Fig 3, Tables 4 and 7).

▶ This study reports the short-term results of the prospective, nonrandomized, multicenter trial (TRANSFIX trial) of the low-profile Zenith Alpha thoracic endovascular graft for treatment of blunt thoracic aortic injuries (BTAIs). The primary end point was 30-day mortality. The primary effectiveness end point was device success at 30 days with the absence of device collapse, type I or type III endoleak requiring intervention, or conversion to open surgical repair at 30 days. The device was developed in response to the unique needs of the trauma population that differ from patients with degenerative aneurysms. The device design addresses the following specific needs: smaller iliac access vessels, smaller thoracic aortas, and narrower aortic arch curvatures. The study population included 50 patients with BTAI grade II to grade IV enrolled at 17 US sites between January 2013 and May 2014. Table 4 summarizes the anatomic characteristics. Fig 3 illustrates preoperative assessment and subsequent repair. Technical success was achieved in 100% of the cases. The left subclavian artery was covered in 21 patients (47%), without subsequent revascularization and no adverse outcomes on follow-up. One patient died within 30 days. Other complications included stroke (2%), renal failure requiring dialysis (2%), and wound complication requiring operative intervention (2%). No aortic ruptures or conversions to open surgical repair were observed within 30 days. Table 7 summarizes 30-day imaging analysis for 42 of 50 patients (84%). Four late deaths were observed beyond 30 days; of those 1 was related to a pseudoaneurysm at the proximal extent of the stent graft due to presumed graft infection

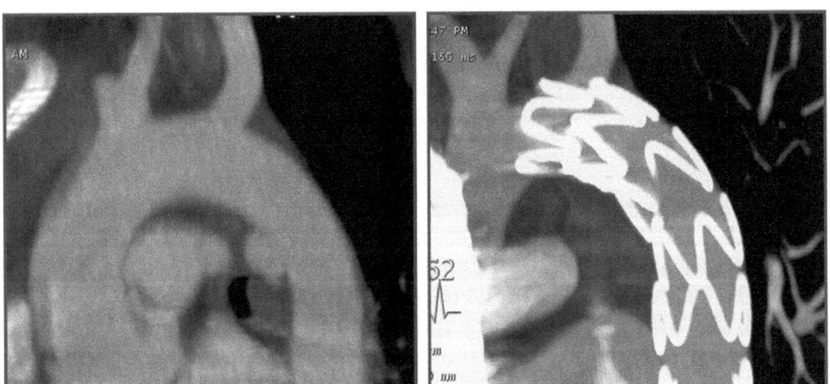

FIGURE 3.—Preassessment aortic injury (*left*) and postprocedure injury healing (*right*). (Reprinted from Starnes BW, Dwivedi AJ, Giglia JS, et al. Endovascular repair for blunt thoracic aortic injury using the Zenith Alpha low-profile device. *J Vasc Surg*. 2015;62:1495-1503, with permission from the Society for Vascular Surgery.)

TABLE 4.—Anatomic Characteristics (Core Laboratory Reported)

Characteristic	% (n/N)
Aortic injury grade[a]	
Grade I: intimal tear	0 (0/49)
Grade II: Intramural hematoma or large intimal flap	8 (4/49)
Grade III: Pseudoaneurysm	86 (42/49)
Grade IV: Free rupture	6 (3/49)
Aortic injury	Mean ± SD (N, range)
Length of aortic injury, mm	32 ± 18 (48, 10-119)
Maximum diameter over the extent of injury, mm	32 ± 6 (46, 21-48)
Aortic arch radius, mm	22 ± 5 (49, 12-35)
Length of LCC to proximal extent of aortic injury, mm	28 ± 13 (47, 0.1-73)
Length of celiac artery to distal aortic injury, mm	186 ± 29 (40, 104-253)

LCC, Left common carotid artery; SD, standard deviation.

[a]The preprocedure computed tomography (CT) scan for one patient (1200059) was not reviewed by the core laboratory at the time of the data lock.

Reprinted from Starnes BW, Dwivedi AJ, Giglia JS, et al. Endovascular repair for blunt thoracic aortic injury using the Zenith Alpha low-profile device. *J Vasc Surg*. 2015;62:1495-1503, with permission from the Society for Vascular Surgery.

TABLE 7.—Thirty-day Core Laboratory Imaging Analysis

Measure	% (n/N)
Injury healing	
Aortic injury no longer visible	76 (32/42)
Injury diameter increase >5 mm compared with before the procedure	0 (0/8)[a]
Endoleak	
Type I[b]	0 (0/41)
Type II	2.4 (1/41)
Type III	0 (0/41)
Type IV	0 (0/41)
Unknown	4.9 (2/41)
Patency	100 (41/41)
Device integrity	
Graft kink	0 (0/42)
Device compression[c]	2.5 (1/42)
Device infolding	0 (0/42)
Barb separation	0 (0/42)
Stent fracture	0 (0/42)

[a]Result based on eight patients with residual injury, and maximum diameter was not assessed in two patients.

[b]One patient was diagnosed from the site as having a proximal type I endoleak; alternatively, the core laboratory evaluated the endoleak as unknown type.

[c]Compression observed in the proximal section of a second main body stent graft.

Reprinted from Starnes BW, Dwivedi AJ, Giglia JS, et al. Endovascular repair for blunt thoracic aortic injury using the Zenith Alpha low-profile device. *J Vasc Surg*. 2015;62:1495-1503, with permission from the Society for Vascular Surgery.

that ultimately resulted in death from exsanguination due to an esophageal-aortic fistula. There were 2 adverse events attributed to significant device undersizing; 1 required a second larger device at the index procedure, and 1 required delayed open repair. The device represents a significant advancement for the management of patients with BTAI. We look forward to improving the results of repair for patients with BTAI as the technology continues to improve.[1,2]

S. Shalhub, MD, MPH, FACS

References

1. Demetriades D, Velmahos GC, Scalea TM, et al. Blunt traumatic thoracic aortic injuries: early or delayed repair results of an American Association for the Surgery of Trauma prospective study. *J Trauma*. 2009;66:967-973.
2. Farber MA, Giglia JS, Starnes BW, et al. Evaluation of the redesigned conformable GORE TAG thoracic endoprosthesis for traumatic aortic transection. *J Vasc Surg*. 2013;58:651-658.

Management and outcome of pediatric vascular injuries

Wahlgren C-M, Kragsterman B (Karolinska Univ Hosp, Stockholm, Sweden; Uppsala Univ, Sweden)

J Trauma Acute Care Surg 79:563-567, 2015

Background.—Vascular injuries in children are relatively uncommon. The objective of this population-based study was to investigate the epidemiology, management, and early outcomes of pediatric vascular injuries.

Methods.—A nationwide survey of prospectively collected data on pediatric vascular injuries in children 15 years or younger between 1987 and 2013 was conducted. Data were retrieved from the National Vascular Surgery registry (Swedvasc) and cross-matched with the National Population Register for mortality data. Demographics, operative techniques, and outcomes were analyzed.

Results.—There were 222 children (boys, n = 148; girls, n = 74) included in this study, with a mean (SD) age of 9.6 (4.1) years (range, 0.5–15 years; <6 years, 18 %; 6–10 years, 39%; >10 years, 42%). Blunt trauma mechanism (n = 146, 66%) was dominant, followed by penetrating (n = 51, 23%) and iatrogenic trauma (n = 21, 9%). Anatomic locations of vascular injuries were primarily upper extremities (n = 134, 60%) and lower extremities (n = 65, 29%), followed by the abdomen (n = 16, 7.2%). Upper extremity injuries were most common in the age group of 10 years or younger (78%, 100 of 128), and lower extremity injuries were most common in the age group of 11 years to 15 years (48%, 45 of 94). Major repair techniques included interposition graft (n = 54, 24%), patch (n = 43, 19%), primary repair (lateral suture/direct anastomosis) (n = 27, 12%), bypass (n = 21, 9.5%), and endovascular techniques (n = 8, 3.7%). Exploration or release of artery was performed in 51 cases (23%). Vein (n = 110) was the dominant graft material, and synthetic grafts (polytetrafluoroethylene/dacron) were only used in four open cases. The most common postoperative complication was arterial occlusion/thrombosis (n = 12). At 30-day follow-up, there was one above-knee and two below-knee amputations as well as one death. No more deaths at 1-year follow-up did occur.

Conclusion.—This nationwide population-based study shows that traumatic vascular injuries in children are associated with high limb salvage rates and low mortality. Blunt trauma mechanism is dominant, and injuries are primarily located to the upper and lower extremities. The preferred repair techniques are venous patch angioplasty and interposition graft, and the frequency of endovascular repair is still low.

Level of Evidence.—Epidemiologic study, level III.

▶ Vascular trauma in pediatric patients is much less common than in adults. The approach to treating vascular injuries in children must account for a few key differences. First, and most obvious, is the relatively small size of the injured vessel. Second, in most cases, pediatric trauma patients will have much longer life expectancy than adults, which makes long-term patency even more of a critical determinant when choosing how to reconstruct the injured vessel. Finally, the expected future vessel growth is a concern when placing a fixed foreign body into a child, such as a synthetic graft or stent graft. In this retrospective review of pediatric (15 years old and younger) vascular trauma patients gathered from a national registry, the authors examined 222 cases from 1987 to 2013. The majority of patients suffered blunt trauma, followed by penetrating and iatrogenic trauma. Extremities were much more commonly injured than the torso. Not surprisingly, given the concerns for long-term patency and future vessel growth, the majority of repairs were vein graft bypasses, patches, and primary repair. Synthetic grafts (PTFE and Dacron) were used in only 4 of 222 patients. Four endovascular stent grafts were placed, 1 of which was for thoracic aortic injury, and all of which were performed from 2009 and onward, presumably because of increasing surgeon comfort in treating adult trauma patients endovascularly. The patients in this review did quite well in early follow-up (30 days and 1 year), with only 1 death (in an extracorporeal membrane oxygenation patient who succumbed to his underlying disease and not his vascular injury), 3 limb amputations, and 12 graft thromboses. Long-term outcomes, which are of bigger concern in successfully treated pediatric vascular trauma, were not addressed by this study.

M. Williams, MD

Proximal humerus fracture with injury to the axillary artery: A population-based study

Menendez ME, Ring D, Heng M (Harvard Med School, Boston, MA)

Injury 46:1367-1371, 2015

Background.—The available evidence regarding axillary artery injury as a result of proximal humerus fracture consists of individual case reports or small series. This study used nationally representative data to determine the prevalence and predictors of axillary artery injury secondary to proximal humerus fracture, and to characterise its influence on inpatient mortality, length of stay, cost and discharge disposition.

Methods.—An estimated 388,676 inpatients with a proximal humerus fracture were identified in the Nationwide Inpatient Sample between 2002 and 2011, 331 with concomitant axillary artery injury (8.5 per 10,000). Multivariable regression modelling was used to identify independent predictors of axillary artery injury and to assess its relationship with inpatient outcomes.

Results.—Factors associated with axillary artery injury were male sex (odds ratio (OR): 1.6, 95% confidence interval (CI): 1.2–2.0), atherosclerosis (OR: 3.7, 95% CI: 2.5–5.4), open fracture (OR: 2.9, 95% CI: 1.9–4.5) and the presence of concomitant injuries, including brachial plexus injury (OR: 109, 95% CI: 79–151), shoulder dislocation (OR: 3.4, 95% CI: 2.0–5.8), scapula fracture (OR: 3.4, 95% CI: 2.1–5.4) and rib fracture (OR: 2.5, 95% CI: 1.6–4.0). Axillary artery injury was associated with increased length of stay, costs and mortality, but it did not affect discharge disposition.

Conclusion.—Our study provides important baseline information regarding the epidemiology of axillary artery injury secondary to proximal humerus fracture. Prompt identification of at-risk patients upon admission might lead to improved diagnosis and management of this vascular injury.

Level of Evidence.—Prognostic level II.

▶ Axillary artery injury has been shown to be associated with the much more common proximal humerus fracture, but because of its low incidence the association has largely been reported in case reports and small case series. In the setting of trauma, axillary artery injuries are oftentimes overlooked because of more pressing concomitant injuries, normal pulse examinations despite injury due to excellent collateral circulation around the shoulder, or patients presenting in shock. Failure to recognize the presence of an axillary artery injury could lead to poor outcomes and increased hospital costs.

Because of its low incidence, the authors used a massive database, the Nationwide Inpatient Sample (NIS), to determine the prevalence and predictive factors of axillary artery injury in the setting of proximal humerus fracture over a 10-year period. They also investigated the effect that axillary artery injury in this setting had on outcomes—specifically, length of stay, cost, inpatient mortality, and discharge disposition. Among the 388 676 patients in the NIS with a proximal humerus fracture, 331 (0.09%) had concomitant axillary artery injuries and

65% of these underwent surgical repair. Multivariate analysis identified the following as risk factors for having an axillary artery injury in the setting of a proximal humerus fracture: male sex, peripheral artery disease, open fracture (3 times more like than closed), and the presence of concomitant injuries (brachial plexus injury, shoulder dislocation, scapula fracture, rib fracture, or other fracture). In fact, brachial plexus injuries occurred in nearly 20% of axillary artery injuries. Axillary artery injury was found to be associated with poorer outcomes in terms of higher inpatient mortality, longer length of stay, and increased hospital costs, but there was no affect on discharge disposition. Overall, despite the low incidence of axillary artery injury in the setting of proximal humerus fracture, the presence of these risk factors and concomitant injuries should raise the physician's index of suspicion and allow for more prompt intervention that could potentially improve outcomes.

B. Peterson, MD, FACS

12 Venous Thrombosis

Association between inflammation biomarkers, anatomic extent of deep venous thrombosis, and venous symptoms after deep venous thrombosis

Rabinovich A, for the BioSOX Investigators (Jewish General Hosp, Montreal, Quebec, Canada; et al)

J Vasc Surg Venous Lymphat Disord 3:347-353, 2015

Objective.—Inflammation may play a role in pathogenesis of venous thromboembolism, but the nature of this relationship is not yet understood. The objective of this study was to assess whether inflammation marker levels measured at diagnosis of deep venous thrombosis (DVT) and change in levels during the first month after DVT are associated with anatomic extent of DVT and severity of venous signs and symptoms at baseline and 1 month.

Methods.—The BioSOX study is a biomarker substudy of the Compression Stockings to Prevent the Post-Thrombotic Syndrome (SOX) trial, a multicenter, randomized controlled trial that included patients with a first, acute, symptomatic, proximal DVT. Blood samples were collected from participants at baseline and 1 month, and C-reactive protein (CRP), intercellular adhesion molecule 1, interleukin (IL)-6, and IL-10 were measured by established assays. Linear regression was used to assess the association between continuous log-transformed baseline biomarker levels and anatomic extent of DVT, classified as iliac or common femoral DVT vs femoral or popliteal DVT (reference). Proportional odds ordinal logistic regression models were used to analyze the association between biomarker level and Villalta score (as a measure of severity of venous signs and symptoms) at baseline and 1 month.

Results.—Among 717 patients, 60.2% were male, and the mean age was 55.2 years. There was a significant association between more extensive DVT (common femoral or iliac) and levels of CRP and IL-6 at DVT diagnosis. Median (interquartile range) CRP level was 11.6 mg/L (3.84-39.5) in patients with common femoral or iliac DVT vs 6.86 mg/L (3.11-22) in patients with popliteal or femoral DVT, and median IL-6 level was 6.36 pg/mL (1.09-14.37) vs 4.40 pg/mL (2.35-8.27), respectively. These differences were statistically significant in linear regression analyses. In addition, compared with those in the lowest quartile, each higher quartile of baseline CRP concentration was associated with an odds ratio of 2.89 (1.93-4.33) for having a more severe Villalta category at baseline and 1.98 (1.28-3.08) for having a more severe Villalta category 1 month after DVT. Higher baseline levels of IL-6 were associated with Villalta severity category at baseline (odds ratio, 2.40 [1.61-3.59]). Change in biomarker levels during the first month after DVT was not strongly associated with the 1-month Villalta score.

Conclusions.—Levels of CRP and IL-6 at DVT diagnosis were associated with thrombotic disease burden, as measured by DVT extent, and severity of DVT symptoms and signs. Further studies are required to more fully elucidate the role of inflammation in DVT and its clinical course.

▶ Evidence regarding the inflammatory response associated with venous thrombosis has been expanding. As a substudy of the Compression Stockings to Prevent the Post-Thrombotic Syndrome (SOX) trial,[1] BioSOX evaluates inflammatory biomarker data collected as part of SOX, showing that levels of C-reactive protein and interleukin (IL)-6 were elevated at the time of deep vein thrombosis (DVT) diagnosis and were associated with clot burden, severity of symptoms, and baseline Villalta score. However, this study is limited in measuring only 4 inflammatory biomarkers after thrombotic event, plus as a secondary end point as part of a subtrial by numerous other confounding factors. Although this study adds to the evidence supporting an association of DVT and inflammation, whether inflammation is a cause or effect of venous thrombosis is not within the scope of this subtrial and remains unclear.

M. Passman, MD

Reference

1. Kahn SR, Shapiro S, Wells PS, et al. Compression stockings to prevent post-thrombotic syndrome: a randomised placebo-controlled trial. *Lancet.* 2014;383: 880-888.

The natural history and treatment outcomes of symptomatic ovarian vein thrombosis

Labropoulos N, Malgor RD, Comito M, et al (Stony Brook Univ Med Ctr, NY; et al)

J Vasc Surg Venous Lymphat Disord 3:42-47, 2015

Background.—Information on ovarian vein thrombosis (OVT) is limited to some retrospective studies. The purpose of this prospective study was to evaluate the natural history and treatment outcomes of OVT.

Methods.—Patients with documented symptomatic OVT who were treated with anticoagulation and had at least 3 months of follow-up were included. Outcomes of interest were recanalization rates, pain resolution, pelvic congestion syndrome, recurrent deep venous thrombosis

(DVT), and mortality. All patients underwent clinical examination and duplex ultrasound; computed tomography venography was selectively performed.

Results.—There were 23 women with a mean age of 44 years (range, 23-68 years). Fifteen (65%) right, 5 (22%) left, and 3 (23%) bilateral OVTs were detected. The median follow-up was 27 months (range, 3 months-7 years). The most common presentation was abdominal pain in nine patients (39%), followed by flank pain in six (26%). Two patients (9%) presented with dyspnea due to pulmonary embolism. The most prevalent condition was the puerperium (n = 9; 39%). Complete recanalization occurred in 16 veins (61%), partial recanalization in four veins (15%), and occlusion in six veins (24%) while patients were receiving anticoagulation. Four patients (17%) had lower extremity DVT during follow-up after the interruption of anticoagulation. Three patients (13%) developed pelvic congestion syndrome. All four deaths (17%) were due to cancer-related complications.

Conclusions.—Symptomatic OVT is rare. Patients fare well with anticoagulation; complete recanalization occurs in about two thirds of the patients. Recurrent DVT is found in lower extremity veins after the interruption of anticoagulation in 17% of patients; mortality was seen only in cancer patients.

▶ Natural history studies are important because they define a disease process and its progression or resolution over time. Symptomatic ovarian vein thrombosis is a rare disease process that mainly affects women during pregnancy, but it can also be seen in women with pelvic malignant disease, pelvic surgery, surgical and nonsurgical trauma, and inflammatory bowel disease. This is an interesting study because it evaluated the natural history of ovarian vein thrombosis and clinical outcomes. In this prospective study, 23 patients were identified with symptomatic ovarian vein thrombosis (all treated with anticoagulation), with a variety of etiologies including postpartum, trauma, cancer, inflammatory bowel disease, and hypercoagulable. The right ovarian vein was affected in 65% of patients. Two patients (8.7%) presented with pulmonary embolism. 17% of patient had propagation of the thrombus in the renal veins or inferior vena cava. Complete recanalization occurred in 62% of patients. On long-term follow-up, deep venous thrombosis (DVT) occurred in 17% of patients. Pelvic venous congestion syndrome occurred in 3 patients, all of whom were postpartum. Four deaths occurred; all were patients who presented with ovarian vein thrombosis and cancer. In summary, patients presenting with symptomatic ovarian vein thrombosis do well with anticoagulation; complete recanalization occurs in about two-thirds of veins involved. Recurrent DVT is found in the lower extremity veins after the interruption of anticoagulation in 17% of patients. Postpartum patients were more likely to experience a recurrent DVT than were patients with other causes of ovarian vein thrombosis. Postpartum patients with ovarian vein thrombosis are at risk for developing pelvic venous congestion syndrome. This important study provides information that would help guide the identification, management, and expected outcomes of patients presenting with symptomatic ovarian vein thrombosis.

J. D. Raffetto, MD, FACS, FSVM

Subsequent arterial ischemic events in patients receiving anticoagulant therapy for venous thromboembolism

Madridano O, on behalf of the RIETE Investigators (Hosp Universitario Infanta Sofía, Madrid, Spain)

J Vasc Surg Venous Lymphat Disord 3:135-141.e1, 2015

Objective.—Patients with acute venous thromboembolism (VTE) are at increased risk for the development of subsequent arterial ischemic events unrelated to the diagnosis of VTE. Accurate identification of VTE patients at increased risk for ischemic events during the course of anticoagulation may help to select those who would potentially benefit from concomitant therapy with anticoagulants and antiplatelets.

Methods.—We used the Registro Informatizado de Enfermedad TromboEmbólica (RIETE) Registry to assess the rate and severity of subsequent ischemic events (ie, stroke, myocardial infarction, lower limb amputation, or mesenteric ischemia) appearing during the course of anticoagulant therapy and tried to identify risk factors for these events.

Results.—From February 2009 to March 2014, 23,370 patients were recruited: 12,397 initially presenting with pulmonary embolism (PE) and 10,973 with deep venous thrombosis. During the course of anticoagulation (mean, 9.2 months), 597 patients developed recurrent VTE, 652 bled, 162 had ischemic events (stroke, 86; myocardial infarction, 53; limb amputation, 13; mesenteric ischemia, 11), and 2063 died. Of these, 29 patients died of recurrent PE, 83 of bleeding, and 53 of the ischemic events. On multivariable analysis, cancer (hazard ratio [HR], 1.77; 95% confidence interval [CI], 1.21-2.61), chronic lung disease (HR, 1.54; 95% CI, 1.05-2.26), renal insufficiency (HR, 1.72; 95% CI, 1.25-2.36), anemia (HR, 1.54; 95% CI, 1.11-2.14), prior artery disease (HR, 1.84; 95% CI, 1.29-2.64), and diabetes (HR, 1.58; 95% CI, 1.10-2.27) independently predicted the risk for ischemic events. Most of these variables also predicted major bleeding (cancer, chronic lung disease, renal insufficiency, anemia, and prior artery disease) or recurrent PE (cancer, chronic lung disease, anemia, and prior artery disease).

Conclusions.—In patients receiving anticoagulation for VTE, the mortality due to PE recurrences was lower than the mortality due to ischemic events. Most independent predictors for ischemic events were also predictors for major bleeding and for recurrent PE.

▶ The management of patients with venous thromboembolism, whether deep vein thrombosis (DVT) or pulmonary embolism (PE), is multilayered. The initial therapy is aimed at prevention of immediate sequelae of the event as well as diminishing the risk of progression. However, the underlying pathologic state of the patient must also be considered. In this review of more than 20 000 patients with DVT or PE, there was a significant risk of recurrent venous thromboembolism (VTE) and major bleeding complications. A smaller risk of arterial ischemic events was identified, but when they occurred, the mortality was nearly 3-fold greater than VTE or bleeding events. Hence, it is imperative for physicians not only to treat the initial pathology but to thoroughly review a patient's history for arterial ischemic risk factors.

R. J. Feezor, MD, FACS

Sulodexide for the Prevention of Recurrent Venous Thromboembolism: The Sulodexide in Secondary Prevention of Recurrent Deep Vein Thrombosis (SURVET) Study: A Multicenter, Randomized, Double-Blind, Placebo-Controlled Trial

Andreozzi GM, on behalf of the SURVET Study Investigators (Univ Hosp, Padua, Italy)

Circulation 132:1891-1897, 2015

Background.—Patients with a first episode of unprovoked venous thromboembolism have a high risk of recurrence after discontinuation of anticoagulant therapy. Extending anticoagulation reduces the risk of recurrence but is associated with increased bleeding. Sulodexide, a glycosaminoglycan, exerts antithrombotic and profibrinolytic actions with a low bleeding risk when administered orally, but its benefit for preventing recurrent venous thromboembolism is not well known.

Methods and Results.—In this multicenter, double-blind study, 615 patients with first-ever unprovoked venous thromboembolism who had completed 3 to 12 months of oral anticoagulant treatment were randomly assigned to sulodexide 500 lipasemic units twice daily or placebo for 2 years, in addition to elastic stockings. The primary efficacy outcome was recurrence of venous thromboembolism. Major or clinically relevant bleeding was the primary safety outcome. Venous thromboembolism recurred in 15 of the 307 patients who received sulodexide and in 30 of the 308 patients who received placebo (hazard ratio, 0.49; 95% confidence interval [CI], 0.27–0.92; $P = 0.02$). The analysis in which lost to follow-up was assigned to failure yielded a risk ratio among treated versus control subjects of 0.54 (95% confidence interval, 0.35–0.85; $P = 0.009$). No major bleeding episodes occurred; 2 patients in each treatment group had a clinically relevant bleeding episode. Adverse events were similar in the 2 groups.

Conclusion.—Sulodexide given after discontinuation of anticoagulant treatment reduced the risk of recurrence in patients with unprovoked venous thromboembolism, with no apparent increase of bleeding risk.

Clinical Trial Registration.—URL: https://www.clinicaltrialsregister.eu/. Identifier: EudraCT number 2009-016923-77.

▶ Risk of recurrence of venous thromboembolism (VTE) after discontinuation of anticoagulation is variable and can persist for several years. For patient with first-time unprovoked VTE, sulodexide and compression stockings initiated after discontinuation of anticoagulation decreased risk of recurrent VTE and no increased risk of bleeding out to 2 years. These findings are similar to the WARFASA trial[1] and ASPIRE trial,[2] which were previously published while SURVET was ongoing and similarly showed the benefit of extended aspirin on decreased VTE recurrence. The generalizability of these results along with these other studies supports the need to extend protection after anticoagulation is discontinued, although it is important to note that sulodexide availability in the United States is limited by no Food and Drug Administration approval.

M. Passman, MD

References

1. Becattini C, Agnelli G, Schenone A, et al. Aspirin for preventing the recurrence of venous thromboembolism. *N Engl J Med.* 2012;366:1959-1967.
2. Brighton TA, Eikelboom JW, Mann K, et al. Low dose aspirin for preventing recurrent venous thromboembolism. *N Engl J Med.* 2012;367:1979-1987.

Impact of Institutional Volume on Outcomes of Catheter Directed Thrombolysis in the Treatment of Acute Proximal Deep Vein Thrombosis: A 6-Year US Experience (2005–2010)

Jarrett H, Zack CJ, Aggarwal V, et al (Temple Univ School of Medicine, Philadelphia, PA; Mayo Clinic, Rochester, MN; et al)
Circulation 132:1127-1135, 2015

Background.—The use of catheter-directed thrombolysis (CDT) in the treatment of acute proximal lower-extremity deep vein thrombosis is increasing in the United States and has been linked to higher bleeding rates. Whether this relationship is interrelated with institution volume of CDT is unknown.

Methods and Results.—The Nationwide Inpatient Sample database was used to identify all patients admitted with a principal diagnosis of proximal or inferior vena caval deep vein thrombosis and treated with CDT from 2005 to 2010. Institutions were divided into high-volume (≥6 procedures a year) and low-volume (<6 procedures a year) centers. Propensity score matching was used to create 2 matched groups for comparative analysis. A total of 90 618 patients were hospitalized for proximal lower-extremity deep vein thrombosis, and 3649 patients (4.1%) underwent CDT. In-hospital mortality was significantly lower at high-volume centers (0.6% versus 1.5%; $P = 0.04$) with a trend toward lower intracranial hemorrhage rates compared with low-volume centers (0.4% versus 1%; $P = 0.07$). No significant difference was seen with blood transfusion (10.4% versus 10.8%; $P = 0.70$), gastrointestinal bleeding (1.4% versus 1.8%; $P = 0.35$), or pulmonary embolism rates (18.4% versus 17.9%; $P = 0.72$). Median length of stay was similar (6 days) and hospital charges were higher ($65 500 versus $75 870) at high-volume centers.

Conclusions.—In this observational study, we found that an increase in institutional volume of CDT was associated with lower in-hospital mortality and lower intracranial hemorrhage rates. Further studies are needed to assess whether standardization of CDT protocols across all institutions in the United States improves outcomes.

▶ This study supports procedure volume as a marker for lower in-hospital mortality and intracranial hemorrhage rates with catheter-directed thrombolysis, and this intuitively makes sense. However, the analysis uses an adjusted cut-point analysis to determine a volume cutoff of <6 procedures per year but does not account for higher potential variance in low-volume centers, which may exaggerate the difference in outcomes. Also, using Nationwide Inpatient Sampling has inherent coding data issues, part of which makes it difficult to differentiate additional pharmaco-mechanical and catheter techniques that may have been used. Although general inverse volume—outcome relationships are observed for many procedures, the cutoff used in this study is not absolute.

M. Passman, MD

Outcomes and predictors of failure of thrombolysis for iliofemoral deep venous thrombosis

Avgerinos ED, Hager ES, Naddaf A, et al (Univ of Pittsburgh Med Ctr, PA)
J Vasc Surg Venous Lymphat Disord 3:35-41, 2015

Background.—Catheter-directed thrombolysis (CDT) with adjunctive mechanical techniques, when successful, is reported to alleviate symptoms of acute iliofemoral deep venous thrombosis (IFDVT) and to lower the occurrence of the post-thrombotic syndrome (PTS). This study aimed to determine longer term outcomes of catheter-based interventions for IFDVT and to identify predictors of immediate and mid-long-term failures that would guide optimal patient selection.

Methods.—Consecutive patients who underwent CDT or pharmacomechanical thrombolysis for IFDVT between May 2007 and March 2013 were identified from a prospectively maintained database. Assessment of predictors of immediate periprocedural failure was based on the degree of clot lysis (≤50% vs >50%) and 30-day recurrence of DVT. Long-term anatomic and clinical failures and outcomes were assessed by ultrasound imaging of the lysed segments and Villalta score (≥5 vs <5). Survival analysis was used to assess primary patency and PTS morbidity.

Multivariate binary logistic and Cox regression models were used to determine predictors of anatomic and clinical failures.

Results.—During the study period, 93 patients (118 limbs; mean age, 49.4 ± 16.2 years; 47 women) with symptoms averaging 11.1 ± 9.6 days in duration were treated with various combinations of CDT or pharmacomechanical thrombolysis; in 52 (56%), at least one ilio-caval stent was deployed. Immediate treatment failure was seen in 11 patients (12%) predicted by the preoperative indication "phlegmasia" (odds ratio, 3.12; $P = .042$) and recent surgery (odds ratio, 19.6; $P = .018$). At a mean ultrasonographic follow-up of 16 ± 14 months (range, 1-65 months), six more patients sustained a rethrombosis, accounting for an overall 3-year primary patency of 72.1%. In the long-term model, loss of primary patency was associated with recent surgery (hazard ratio [HR], 4.04; $P = .023$), malignant disease (HR, 6.75; $P = .016$), and incomplete thrombolysis (≤50%) (HR, 5.83; $P < .001$). By stratification of PTS on the basis of postprocedure failures, at 2 years PTS occurred in 50.6% of patients and in 16.3% of patients without failure ($P < .001$).

Conclusions.—Thrombolysis for symptomatic IFDVT can achieve high rates of thrombus resolution and reduce long-term PTS morbidity on careful patient selection. Improved anatomic and clinical outcomes are associated with the completeness of thrombolysis.

▶ Acute iliofemoral deep vein thrombosis (DVT) can be treated with anticoagulation or anticoagulation with pharmacomechanical and catheter-directed thrombolysis. Recently, the CAVENT trial demonstrated a reduction in postthrombotic syndrome with catheter-directed thrombolysis with an absolute risk reduction of 14.4%. The 5-year follow-up resulted in 43% having post-thrombotic syndrome (PTS) in the catheter-directed thrombolysis and 71% in the anticoagulation group ($P < .0001$); however, there was no difference in quality of life measured by the EU-5D and VEINES-QOL/Sym. Despite limited data from randomized controlled trials and disparate recommendations from society guidelines (ACCP, SIR, SVS/AVF), many institutions and practices treat acute iliofemoral DVT with catheter-directed thrombolysis. Of importance would be an ability to predict which patient would benefit significantly from catheter-directed thrombolysis and pharmacomechanical thrombolysis, to increase the valued outcome. This study is important in determining factors associated with favorable outcomes after treatment of acute iliofemoral DVT. The study consisted of 93 patients and 118 limbs treated. Perioperative failures were significantly affected by recent surgery and phlegmasia. These likely are reflected in the inability to use higher doses of thrombolysis in the former and advanced extensive disease associated with malignancy and hypercoagulable state in the latter. On long-term follow-up, predictors of recurrent thrombosis were recent surgery, malignant disease, and incomplete lysis at baseline. By stratification of PTS on the basis of the postoperative failures at 2 years, PTS was seen in 16.3% of the nonfailures versus 50.6% of failures ($P < .001$). The findings from this study can be used to better select patients for intervention or anticoagulation alone, to guide informed patient consent, and to set treatment expectations. Future studies especially the ATTRACT trial will be important to help guide therapy in patients with acute iliofemoral and femoral-popliteal DVT.[1,2]

J. D. Raffetto, MD, FACS, FSVM

References

1. Enden T, Haig Y, Kløw NE, et al. CaVenT Study Group. Long-term outcome after additional catheter-directed thrombolysis versus standard treatment for acute iliofemoral deep vein thrombosis (the CaVenT study): a randomised controlled trial. *Lancet.* 2012;379:31-38.
2. Haig Y, Enden T, Grøtta O, et al. CaVenT Study Group. Post-thrombotic syndrome after catheter-directed thrombolysis for deep vein thrombosis (CaVenT): 5-year follow-up results of an open-label, randomised controlled trial. *Lancet Haematol.* 2016;3:e64-e71.

Safety and efficacy of ultrasound-accelerated catheter-directed lytic therapy in acute pulmonary embolism with and without hemodynamic instability

Nykamp M, VandenHull A, Remund T, et al (Sanford Res, Sioux Falls, SD; et al)
J Vasc Surg Venous Lymphat Disord 3:251-257, 2015

Objective.—The objective of this study was to evaluate the safety and effectiveness of ultrasound-accelerated thrombolysis in acute pulmonary embolism.

Methods.—A retrospective study of 45 patients was performed to evaluate treatment of acute pulmonary embolism at a single center from January 2011 to December 2013. All patients were diagnosed with computed tomography or ventilation-perfusion scan and had hemodynamic instability (systolic blood pressure <100 mm Hg) or right-sided heart strain evidenced by right ventricular dilation, septal deviation, or hypokinesis by echocardiography or computed tomography. EkoSonic catheters (EKOS Corporation, Bothell, Wash) were placed into the affected pulmonary arteries, and recombinant tissue plasminogen activator was infused through the catheters at 0.5 to 1.0 mg/h per catheter.

Results.—Hypotension (systolic blood pressure <100 mm Hg) was present in 12 patients, with 100% resolution by treatment completion. Tachycardia (heart rate >100 beats/minute) was present in 26 patients and resolved in 92% by treatment completion; the average heart rate for all patients decreased from 109 to 77 beats/minute during the treatment period. Direct pulmonary artery pressure measurement showed average decrease of 21.5 mm Hg, representing a 40.2% reduction. Postprocedure echocardiography demonstrated complete resolution of cardiac dysfunction in 64%. Patients received a total dose of 30.5 mg (range, 14-66 mg) recombinant tissue plasminogen activator during an infusion time of

14.2 hours (range, 8-21 hours). There were no deaths through 90 days of follow-up and no major periprocedural bleeding events.

Conclusions.—This retrospective study demonstrates the safety and efficacy of current ultrasound-accelerated thrombolysis methods to treat acute pulmonary embolism.

▶ This retrospective case-control review of ultrasound-accelerated catheter-directed thrombolysis offers clinical evidence that aggressive treatment of pulmonary emboli in patients with hemodynamic embarrassment due to the presence of the emboli is safe and can potentially reduce mortality. The clinical safety naturally hinges on the patient selection, as with all forms of lytic therapy. However, what is well documented here is the reduction in pulmonary artery pressures, relief of heart strain, and resolution of tachycardia. Although not clear why the control group was not offered lytic therapy, the long-term follow-up showing a reduction in mortality is impressive. It is a reminder that chronic right heart strain brought on by pulmonary embolism is associated with significant mortality, and efforts to relieve strain should be endorsed. Especially with the fluctuating availability of catheter-directed lysis adjuncts on the market, ultrasound enhancement offers significant promise. Given the extremely positive safety profile, it seems unlikely that a randomized trial would improve the clinical recommendations.

R. J. Feezor, MD, FACS

Effect of a Retrievable Inferior Vena Cava Filter Plus Anticoagulation vs Anticoagulation Alone on Risk of Recurrent Pulmonary Embolism: A Randomized Clinical Trial

Mismetti P, for the PREPIC2 Study Group (Centre Hospitalier Universitaire de Saint-Etienne, France; et al)

JAMA 313:1627-1635, 2015

Importance.—Although retrievable inferior vena cava filters are frequently used in addition to anticoagulation in patients with acute venous thromboembolism, their benefit-risk ratio is unclear.

Objective.—To evaluate the efficacy and safety of retrievable vena cava filters plus anticoagulation vs anticoagulation alone for preventing pulmonary embolism recurrence in patients presenting with acute pulmonary embolism and a high risk of recurrence.

Design, Setting, and Participants.—Randomized, open-label, blinded end point trial (PREPIC2) with 6-month follow-up conducted from August 2006 to January 2013. Hospitalized patients with acute, symptomatic pulmonary embolism associated with lower-limb vein thrombosis and at least 1 criterion for severity were assigned to retrievable inferior vena cava filter implantation plus anticoagulation (filter group; n = 200) or anticoagulation alone with no filter implantation (control group;

n = 199). Initial hospitalization with ambulatory follow-up occurred in 17 French centers.

Interventions.—Full-dose anticoagulation for at least 6 months in all patients. Insertion of a retrievable inferior vena cava filter in patients randomized to the filter group. Filter retrieval was planned at 3 months from placement.

Main Outcomes and Measures.—Primary efficacy outcome was symptomatic recurrent pulmonary embolism at 3 months. Secondary outcomes were recurrent pulmonary embolism at 6 months, symptomatic deep vein thrombosis, major bleeding, death at 3 and 6 months, and filter complications.

Results.—In the filter group, the filter was successfully inserted in 193 patients and was retrieved as planned in 153 of the 164 patients in whom retrieval was attempted. By 3 months, recurrent pulmonary embolism had occurred in 6 patients (3.0%; all fatal) in the filter group and in 3 patients (1.5%; 2 fatal) in the control group (relative risk with filter, 2.00 [95% CI, 0.51-7.89]; $P = .50$). Results were similar at 6 months. No difference was observed between the 2 groups regarding the other outcomes. Filter thrombosis occurred in 3 patients.

Conclusions and Relevance.—Among hospitalized patients with severe acute pulmonary embolism, the use of a retrievable inferior vena cava filter plus anticoagulation compared with anticoagulation alone did not reduce the risk of symptomatic recurrent pulmonary embolism at 3 months. These findings do not support the use of this type of filter in patients who can be treated with anticoagulation.

Trial Registration.—clinicaltrials.gov Identifier: NCT00457158.

▶ The previous published PREPIC-1 study showed that placement of a permanent inferior vena cava (IVC) filter in addition to anticoagulation for patients with proximal deep vein thrombosis (DVT) with or without pulmonary embolism (PE) significantly reduced the risk of recurrent PE compared with anticoagulation alone, but that benefit was offset by a greater delayed risk of recurrent DVT and IVC filter thrombosis.[1,2] Although PREPIC-1 focused on permanent filters, based on the delayed risk noted, PREPIC-2 employs a strategy of retrievable filter use plus anticoagulation versus anticoagulation alone. PREPIC-1 showed early benefit favoring filters, but the key finding noted in PREPIC-2 that IVC filter plus anticoagulation compared with anticoagulation alone in patients with symptomatic did not reduce the risk of symptomatic recurrent PE at 3 months was surprising. It is important to note that a single retrievable filter type was used for all patients, not all patients had filters retrieved (filter retrieval attempted in 91.1% and successful in 93.3%), and sample size may have been underpowered with some patients lost to follow-up. Although this is an important randomized trial, the key finding should only be applied within the specific scope of the study question of whether adding a filter to therapeutic anticoagulation in those patients without contraindications to anticoagulation is beneficial. These findings should not be applied to patients with DVT/PE who cannot receive anticoagulation or to the more polarizing question of the role of retrievable IVC filters for prophylaxis.

M. Passman, MD

References

1. Decosus H, Leizorovicz A, Parent F, et al. A clinical trial of vena caval filter in the prevention of pulmonary embolism in patients with proximal deep vein thrombosis. Prevention du Risque d'Embolie Pulmonaire par Interruption Cave Study. *N Engl J Med.* 1998;338:409-415.
2. PREPIC Study Group. Eight year follow-up of patients with permanent vena cava filter in the prevention of pulmonary embolism: the PREPIC (Prevention du Risque d'Embolie Pulmonaire par Interruption Cave) randomized study. *Circulation.* 2005;112:416-422.

Endovascular management of symptomatic gastrointestinal complications associated with retrievable inferior vena cava filters

Genovese EA, Jeyabalan G, Marone LK, et al (Univ of Pittsburgh Med Ctr, PA)

J Vasc Surg Venous Lymphat Disord 3:276-282, 2015

Objective.—With the increase in retrievable inferior vena cava (IVC) filter use, a higher than expected reported rate of pericaval tine penetration is observed. Symptomatic gastrointestinal (GI) complications associated with retrievable IVC filters have been documented; however, their management remains controversial. We describe a series of GI complications of retrievable IVC filters, detailing the spectrum of presenting symptoms and multiple treatment options, including the safety of endovascular retrieval.

Methods.—A retrospective chart review was performed to describe the presentation, diagnosis, and treatment of patients with symptomatic GI complications associated with retrievable IVC filters from 2008 to 2014.

Results.—Nine patients had symptomatic GI complications associated with a retrievable IVC filter (two G2 Recovery [Bard Peripheral Vascular, Tempe, Ariz], seven Celect [Cook Medical, Bloomington, Ind]; six women; age range, 17-81 years). All patients had small bowel perforation on computed tomography scan, four confirmed by esophagogastroduodenoscopy. Concomitant aortic and vertebral penetration occurred in seven and five patients, respectively. Patients presented with various abdominal complaints; one patient presented in acute sepsis. Two patients underwent laparotomy without complications. The remaining seven patients had attempted endovascular retrieval, six of which were successful. One patient's IVC filter was unable to be retrieved, and he was managed medically. Of the six patients who had successful endovascular retrieval, all had resolution of their symptoms with no complications, except for transient sepsis in a single patient who was not receiving periprocedural antibiotics. A follow-up computed tomography scan was performed 48 to 72 hours after endovascular retrieval and ruled out duodenal leak in all patients. Long-term follow-up demonstrated continued resolution of GI symptoms without further episodes of deep venous thrombosis or pulmonary embolism.

Conclusions.—GI complications of retrievable IVC filters are manifested with a wide spectrum of symptoms and frequent concomitant aortic and vertebral penetration. Endovascular retrieval can be safely used as a first-line therapy even in the setting of small bowel and aortic penetration.

▶ The complications associated with inferior vena cava (IVC) filters are relatively infrequent but highly publicized when they occur. Caval penetration by the filter is a relatively common finding and on occasion is implicated in the cause of abdominal pain for certain patients. Although conceptually risky, this case series shows that, for the most part, standard endovascular retrieval can be performed even with radiographic visceral penetration, obviating the need for laparotomy. The authors recommend diligent perioperative antibiotics and postretrieval CT imaging with oral and intravenous contrast. A larger question remains: how many patients with abdominal pain and an IVC filter in place did not have the IVC filter removed as the culprit? Importantly, even with caval penetration by the struts, most retrievable filters are, indeed, retrievable. Tilting of the hook, which permits it to be embedded within the wall of the IVC, remains one of the main reason that filters are unsuccessfully retrieved if attempted. Nevertheless, the interaction of the IVC filter and the caval wall and pericaval structures, and, more importantly, the clinical significance of that interaction, will hopefully be further clarified in the future.

R. J. Feezor, MD, FACS

Inferior vena cava filter retrieval provides no advantage in the average patient

Warner CJ, Richey EA, Tower DE, et al (Dartmouth-Hitchcock Med Ctr, Lebanon, NH; The Dartmouth Inst for Health Policy and Clinical Practice, Lebanon, NH)

J Vasc Surg Venous Lymphat Disord 3:142-146, 2015

Background.—Inferior vena cava (IVC) filter placement is performed to mitigate the risk of pulmonary embolism (PE) when anticoagulation is contraindicated or ineffective. Technical advances now allow catheter-based filter retrieval. Many believe the benefits of retrieval are self-evident, yet retrieval carries an inherent complication risk and cost. The purpose of this study was to quantitatively weigh the risks and benefits of IVC filter retrieval using formal decision analysis.

Methods.—A Markov state-transition model was used to simulate two clinical scenarios: to leave a previously placed IVC filter or to retrieve it. Analysis was performed during the lifetime of the individual, and outcomes were expressed in quality-adjusted life-years (QALYs). The base case is a 60-year-old man with a filter placed within 3 months who no longer requires mechanical thromboprophylaxis. Potential events included PE, filter complications, and death from all other causes during each cycle. Tolls were used to incorporate the disutility of short-term treatment for PE and filter complications. For the base case and sensitivity analyses, we used utilities and probabilities derived from the literature.

Results.—In the base case scenario, leaving the filter in place was preferred to filter retrieval, yielding 22.3 vs 21.9 QALYs. One-way sensitivity analysis demonstrated that filter retrieval may be preferable if the utility of living with a filter is <0.98. For all probabilities of retrieval and PE mortality, leaving the filter in place is preferred.

Conclusions.—Leaving a previously placed IVC filter provides a 0.4 QALY benefit over retrieving the filter for the average patient. This decision is sensitive to the utility of living with the IVC filter.

▶ There is little doubt that inferior vena cava (IVC) filters were previously overused, certainly if the medical profession were truly held to "data-driven" statistics. Now, there is growing pressure ignited by US Food and Drug Administration warnings and fueled by the lay press about the inherent dangers of an indwelling IVC filter. This is a reasonable attempt to provide published data for complications of a filter, including pulmonary embolism, in an effort to guide the question "should a filter be removed." Likely due to the overwhelmingly uncommon occurrences of the negative outcomes, the overarching answer is "leave it" in the average patient. Filters may be overused, but the presence of a filter has a very small chance of causing direct harm. However rational and statistically sound this argument may be, fear is a motivating decision maker: fear of complications for patients and fear of legal ramifications for providers.

R. J. Feezor, MD, FACS

Retrievable inferior vena cava filters can always be removed using "fall-back" techniques

Etkin Y, Glaser JD, Nation DA, et al (Hosp of the Univ of Pennsylvania, Philadelphia; et al)

J Vasc Surg Venous Lymphat Disord 3:364-369, 2015

Objective.—Retrievable inferior vena cava filters (IVCFs) left in place for a prolonged period can lead to complications including filter migration, fracture, and caval thrombosis. "Fall-back" techniques for IVCF retrieval that can be used when standard snaring is unsuccessful have been recently described. The purpose of this study was to analyze how incorporation of these new techniques affected the outcomes of IVCF retrievals at our institution during the past 5 years.

Methods.—Data were collected of all patients undergoing IVCF removal by vascular surgeons at a tertiary academic medical center between 2009 and 2013, including demographics and procedural and filter characteristics. A standard technique of snaring the retrieval hook was attempted first in all cases; if this was unsuccessful, a number of fall-back techniques were employed, including the use of endoscopic graspers, 18F sheaths, and snaring a second wire below the collar of the filter to collapse it into the sheath.

Results.—IVCF retrieval was attempted in 275 patients; 3 were excluded intraoperatively because of thrombus in the filter. Most filters (97%) were Günther Tulips (Cook Medical, Bloomington, Ind); 70% had been placed prophylactically before bariatric surgery. A total of 268 filters (98.5%) were retrieved successfully, 213 (79%) by standard snaring and 55 (21%) with fall-back techniques. In patients undergoing fall-back techniques, technical success was achieved 100% of the time. The median time since insertion was significantly longer in the fall-back group (173 days vs 83 days; $P < .0001$). Four intraoperative complications occurred; fractured wires embolized to the right atrium or pulmonary artery and were successfully removed endovascularly. The majority of the procedures (80%) were performed under sedation in both groups.

Conclusions.—Incorporation of fall-back techniques may allow 100% technically successful and safe removal of retrievable IVCFs and is especially useful in removing filters with prolonged dwell time.

▶ Although retrievable inferior vena cava filters (IVCF) were developed to avoid long-term complications of permanent filters, reported rates continue to vary despite continued efforts to promote IVCF removal. For those patients who undergo possible retrieval, technical success also varies from 82% to 98%, with retrieval limited by prolonged dwell time and tilted or embedded IVCF that prevent success retrieval. This study reviews a large collective IVCF retrieval experience (N = 275), of which 79% were retrieved using standard snare techniques, and 21% required advanced retrieval techniques, thereby significantly increasing successful retrieval. Most retrievals were facilitated using a lasso technique: upsizing the sheath to 18 Fr, directing a wire placed through the apical interstices of the filter, and snaring the wire to allow directing the sheath over the apical hook. Occasional addition techniques of using a double 22 Fr/18 Fr sheath and endobronchial forceps were also used. Overall, this study supports safety of these advanced techniques to increase technical success but operator comfort with these alternative and realizations of associated limitations are required. More importantly, because retrieval success as supported by this and other studies is directly related to IVCF dwell time, further efforts toward earlier retrieval are warranted.

M. Passman, MD

13 Chronic Venous

Progression of varicose veins and chronic venous insufficiency in the general population in the Edinburgh Vein Study

Lee AJ, Robertson LA, Boghossian SM, et al (Univ of Aberdeen, UK; Univ of Edinburgh, UK; et al)

J Vasc Surg Venous Lymphat Disord 3:18-26, 2015

Objective.—The natural history in the general population of chronic venous disease in the legs is not well understood. This has limited our ability to predict which patients will deteriorate and to assign clinical priorities. The aims of this study were to describe the progression of trunk varicose veins and chronic venous insufficiency (CVI) in the general population, to identify important lifestyle and clinical prognostic factors, and to determine the relationship between venous reflux and progression.

Methods.—The Edinburgh Vein Study is a population-based cohort study in which randomly selected adults aged 18 to 64 years had an examination at baseline. This included a questionnaire on lifestyle and clinical factors, standardized assessment and classification of venous disease in the legs, and duplex scan to detect venous reflux in eight segments of each leg. A follow-up examination 13 years later included a reclassification of venous disease to ascertain progression in the development or increase in severity of varicose veins and CVI.

Results.—Among 1566 adults seen at baseline, 880 had a follow-up examination, of whom 334 had trunk varicose veins or CVI at baseline and composed the study sample. The mean (standard deviation) duration of follow-up was 13.4 (0.4) years. Progression was found in 193 (57.8%), equivalent to 4.3% (95% confidence interval [CI], 3.7-4.9) annually. In 270 subjects with only varicose veins at baseline, 86 (31.9%) developed CVI, with the rate increasing consistently with age ($P = .04$). Almost all subjects (98%) with both varicose veins and CVI at baseline deteriorated. Progression of chronic venous disease did not differ by gender or leg, but a family history of varicose veins and history of deep venous thrombosis increased risk (odds ratio [OR], 1.85 [95% CI, 1.14-1.30] and 4.10 [95% CI, 1.07-15.71], respectively). Overweight was associated with increased risk of CVI in those with varicose veins (OR, 1.85; 95% CI, 1.10-3.12). Reflux in the superficial system increased the likelihood of progression, especially in combination with deep reflux (OR, 2.57; 95% CI, 1.55-4.25) and when located in the small saphenous vein (OR, 4.73; 95% CI, 1.37-16.39).

Conclusions.—Nearly half of the general population with chronic venous disease deteriorated during 13 years, and almost one third with varicose veins developed skin changes of CVI, increasing their risk of ulceration. Age, family history of varicose veins, history of deep venous thrombosis, overweight, and superficial reflux, especially in the small saphenous vein and with deep reflux, might influence the risk of progression.

▶ The Edinburgh Vein study is a general population-based longitudinal examination of venous disease that has potential of being akin to the Framingham study on the arterial side. This specific article examines the progression of venous disease and confirms what most practitioners already presume: that in patients with varicose veins or documented insufficiency at baseline, there is a steady progression in severity of disease over time. The overall rate was the equivalent of nearly 5% per year and seemed to be more pronounced with patients who had a history of a deep vein thrombosis or a family history of varicosities. The questions that remain from population studies like these include, as always, selection bias and the potential to alter natural history with preventative measures (daily compression usage). Akin to aspirin usage for stroke prevention, there may be a small effort required to prevent larger more terminal pathology, but given that the progression of chronic venous insufficiency documented here still amounted to relatively mild disease, the impact of minor interventions may be blunted. At the least, efforts such as these bring the prevalence of venous disease to light even more clearly within the medical community.

R. J. Feezor, MD, FACS

A longitudinal single-center cohort study on the prevalence and risk of accessory saphenous vein reflux after radiofrequency segmental thermal ablation of great saphenous veins

Proebstle TM, Möhler T (Univ Med Ctr Mainz, Germany; et al)
J Vasc Surg Venous Lymphat Disord 3:265-269, 2015

Objective.—Endothermal ablation has become a commonly used technology for occlusion of refluxing great saphenous veins (GSVs). However, the risk for primarily untreated accessory saphenous veins (ASVs) to develop reflux during follow-up has not yet been defined. Here, the prevalence and risk of ASV reflux is explored.

Methods.—During a prospective multicenter cohort study on radiofrequency segmental thermal ablation of refluxing GSVs, the presence and reflux status of ASVs were monitored in 93 legs in a single center. Control examinations were performed after 1 week and at 12, 24, 36, and 48 months. Life-table and multiple regression analyses were used to describe frequency and risk factors for presence of reflux in untreated ASVs.

Results.—Of 93 legs, 82 (88%) were available for 4-year follow-up. At baseline, 43 legs (46%) had an anterior ASV detectable by duplex ultrasound, with only two legs (2%) presenting with reflux. During 4 years of follow-up, according to life-table analysis, the proportion of legs with a detectable anterior ASV increased to 71% (n = 65); 32% of all legs and 55% of legs with a detectable anterior ASV exhibited refluxing anterior ASVs. Remarkably, in 35% of all legs with an anterior ASV, this reflux presented as a source of axial reflux, suggesting hemodynamic relevance. Posterior ASVs were detected in only 10 legs during 4-year follow-up, exhibiting reflux in only two cases.

Conclusions.—Whereas posterior ASVs were meaningless, refluxing anterior ASVs occurred in a significant proportion of legs after thermal ablation of GSVs. Whether nonrefluxing anterior ASVs should be treated at the time of GSV ablation needs further examination.

▶ Ablation of truncal veins is an established procedure to treat symptomatic venous insufficiency, and the most often found, and therefore treated, vein is the great saphenous vein (GSV). The incidence of other, potentially more variable venous anatomy and its corresponding pathology is now being investigated. The authors report on a subset of patients in a trial for GSV ablation who have accessory saphenous veins, and the incidence of nearly 46% at baseline is noteworthy, but more notably, only 2% had reflux. Over the duration of follow-up, all after GSV ablation, there is a steady incidence of the development of ASV incompetence. The larger question that is posited in the conclusions is does the ablation of the GSV alter the flow pattern of other leg veins to increase the chance of non-GSV leg vein insufficiency? It is more likely that the underlying pathology that is identified first in the long saphenous vein affected most by hydrostatic pressure is also seen in less physically disadvantaged veins. Certainly, therapy for venous incompetence should be driven by actual symptoms and not chance of progression to symptoms.

R. J. Feezor, MD, FACS

A randomized clinical trial of endovenous laser ablation versus conventional surgery for small saphenous varicose vein

Nandhra S, El-sheikha J, Carradice D, et al (Univ of Hull, UK)

J Vasc Surg 61:741-746, 2015

Background.—This randomized clinical trial compared endovenous laser ablation (EVLA) and surgical ligation with attempted stripping in the treatment of small saphenous vein (SSV) insufficiency. The early results demonstrated that EVLA was more likely to eradicate axial reflux and was also associated with a faster recovery, lower periprocedural pain, and fewer sensory complications. The aim of this 2-year follow-up was to establish whether these benefits remained stable over time and whether these improved technical outcomes were associated with less clinical recurrence.

Methods.—Patients with primary saphenopopliteal junction and SSV reflux were randomized to EVLA or saphenopopliteal junction ligation and attempted stripping/excision. Outcomes assessed at 2 years included the presence of residual or recurrent reflux, clinical recurrence, sensory complications, the need for secondary intervention, and patient-reported quality of life on the Aberdeen Varicose Veins Questionnaire, SF-36, and EuroQol.

Results.—Of 106 patients who were equally randomized and successfully treated according to the protocol, 88 (83%) were successfully assessed at 2 years. The groups were comparable at baseline. At 2 years, EVLA remained superior to surgery in eradicating axial reflux in 36 patients (81.2%) compared with 29 (65.9%) in the surgery group (P =.002). There was no significant difference in clinical recurrence (EVLA: seven of 44 [16%] vs surgery: 10 of 44 [23%]; P =.736), sensory disturbance (EVLA: one [2.4%] vs surgery vs three [6.8%]; P = 1.000) or any quality of life domain.

Conclusions.—The results of treatment of SSV insufficiency with EVLA appear durable up until 2 years. The study does not appear to suggest that the improved abolition of reflux after EVLA compared with surgery is associated with superior outcomes than those seen after surgery by this time point, because equal effect was shown in both groups. The sensory disturbance associated with surgery appears to settle over this time frame. EVLA is therefore superior in the short-term and not inferior by 2 years.

▶ Although most evidence regarding endovenous ablation is directed at treatment of great saphenous vein, insufficiency of the small saphenous vein (SSV) may have different therapeutic implications. As follow-up of a prior randomized study showing endovenous laser ablation of the SSV to more likely have complete abolition of axial reflux, less pain, faster recovery and less sensory complications to conventional surgery (ligation and stripping),[1] this study shows that outcomes remain durable, but that effect equalized. These results are tempered by a sample size limited to detect differences in technical efficacy, not long-term outcomes. However, as the authors note, to do a larger randomized study comparing endovenous techniques with conventional surgery given the success of the former may be difficult because of the lack of equipoise. That said, when combined with the findings from the earlier randomized study, endovenous ablation is still favored over conventional surgery for SSV venous insufficiency.

M. Passman, MD

Reference

1. Samuel N, Carradice D, Wallace T, et al. Randomized clinical trial of endovenous laser ablation versus conventional surgery for small saphenous varicose veins. *Ann Surg*. 2013;257:419-426.

Durability of treatment effect with polidocanol endovenous microfoam on varicose vein symptoms and appearance (VANISH-2)

Todd KL III, VANISH-2 Investigator Group (Southeast Vein and Laser Ctr, Dothan, AL; et al)

J Vasc Surg Venous Lymphat Disord 3:258-264, 2015

Objective.—The objectives of this study were to assess the durability of response to treatment with polidocanol endovenous microfoam (Varithena; Provensis Ltd, a BTG International group company) and to assess the long-term safety of the study patients.

Methods.—This report presents efficacy and safety data from the day after visit 5/week 8 (the primary end point of the study) through the 1-year study visit. As the approved dose concentration is 1%, this analysis focuses on those patients who were randomized to polidocanol endovenous microfoam 1% at study visit 2. Because the objective of the 1-year analysis was to assess the durability of response to treatment with polidocanol endovenous microfoam 1%, the 1-year efficacy analyses based on the efficacy population included all patients who were randomized and received at least one treatment with polidocanol endovenous microfoam 1%. Efficacy end points in the Polidocanol Endovenous Microfoam Versus Vehicle for the Treatment of Saphenofemoral Junction Incompetence (VANISH-2) trial were evaluated at 1 year (n = 221; 96% of those completed the primary end-point measurement at week 8) and included the following: Varicose Vein Symptoms Questionnaire (VVSymQ, Provensis Ltd) score, an assessment of symptoms by patients using electronic daily diaries; Independent Photography Review: Visible Varicose Veins (IPR-V^3) and Patient Self-assessment of Visible Varicose Veins (PA-V^3) scores, the assessment of appearance by an Independent Physician Review panel and by patient self-assessment, respectively; duplex ultrasound response (physiologic response to treatment); Venous Clinical Severity Score (disease severity); and Venous Insufficiency Epidemiological and Economic Study on Quality of Life (VEINES-QOL) score (quality of life).

Results.—Of the 230 patients who completed visit 5/week 8, 56 received polidocanol endovenous microfoam 1% at visit 2/week 0 and were subsequently assessed for efficacy at visit 5/week 8 and visit 10/1 year (one patient of the 57 who completed visit 5/week 8 received a non-polidocanol endovenous microfoam intervention and was not included in the assessment). At 1 year after the first study treatment, patients treated with polidocanol endovenous microfoam demonstrated consistent, durable, and clinically meaningful improvements in symptoms, as measured by reductions in mean VVSymQ score; appearance, as measured by IPR-V^3 (clinician assessment) and PA-V^3 (patient self-assessment) scores; disease severity, as measured by the Venous Clinical Severity Score; and quality of life, as measured by the VEINES-QOL score. At 1 year, there were no new venous thrombus adverse events (VTAEs) and no clinically important sequelae in patients who had a VTAE in the study. In addition, there were no serious adverse events that were determined by the investigator to be related to the study drug. No new safety signals were identified. In patients who previously had a VTAE, none had a recurrence of thrombus or evidence of post-thrombotic syndrome at 1 year.

Conclusions.—Treatment with polidocanol endovenous microfoam 1% led to durable, clinically meaningful, and ongoing improvements at 1 year in varicose vein symptoms and appearance. Serious adverse events were those expected during long-term follow-up of the population of patients studied and were unrelated to treatment.

▶ VANISH-2 evaluated safety and efficacy of polidocanol microfoam 0.5% and 1.0% versus placebo (N = 232) and showed efficacy at 8 weeks, but a higher reported adverse event rate of 60% receiving polidocanol microfoam versus 39% of placebo, most of which were related to retained coagulum, leg pain, and superficial thrombophlebitis and resolved without sequelae.[1] As a follow-up to VANISH-2, this study focuses on long-term outcomes of those patients who received polidocanol endovenous microfoam 1.0% and reached the 1-year end point (N = 57 of 58 randomized). Despite the earlier minor issues noted in VANISH-2, those who received polidocanol microfoam 1.0% had durable and clinically meaningful improvement including patient-reported outcomes at 1 year without any additional adverse events, thereby supporting polidocanol microfoam 1.0% as an additional endovenous therapeutic option. With recent Food and Drug Administration approval of polidocanol microfoam, practitioners have expanded nontumescent endovenous options for treating saphenous reflux.

M. Passman, MD

Reference

1. Todd KL 3rd, Wright D, the VANISH-2 Investigators. The VANISH-2 study: a randomized, blinded, multicenter study to evaluate the efficacy and safety of polidocanol endovenous microfoam 0.5% and 1.0% compared with placebo for the treatment of saphenofemoral junction incompetence. *Phlebology.*. 2014;29: 608-618.

Postoperative hemodynamic changes after endovenous laser ablation and phlebectomy in varicose vein surgery

Park Y, Kim Y-W, Park Y-J, et al (Sungkyunkwan Univ School of Medicine, Seoul, Korea)
J Vasc Surg Venous Lymphat Disord 3:54-57, 2015

Objective.—This study was designed to examine postoperative venous hemodynamic changes at 1 and 6 months after endovenous laser ablation (EVLA) and phlebectomy for primary great saphenous varicose veins.

Methods.—We retrospectively analyzed 116 limbs from 102 patients who were treated with EVLA from 2011 to 2013 at Samsung Medical

Center. Venous hemodynamic changes were evaluated by air plethysmography preoperatively and at 1 month and 6 months postoperatively. The measured hemodynamic changes included venous volume (VV), venous filling index (VFI), residual volume fraction (RVF), and ejection fraction (EF).

Results.—The study included 52 limbs from men (44.8%) and 64 limbs from women (55.2%; male/female ratio, 1:1.23). The mean age of the patients was 54.8 ± 12.3 years. The preoperative median values were VV of 99.1 mL, VFI of 3.6 mL/s, RVF of 39.2%, and EF of 55.5%. The 1-month and 6-month postoperative median values were VV of 77.6 and 75.5 mL, VFI of 1.4 and 1.5 mL/s, RVF of 32.5% and 26.4%, and EF of 60.5% and 66.2%, respectively. The postoperative reduction rates between preoperative and 1-month measurements for VV, VFI, and RVF were 18.6%, 63.9%, and 22.2%, and the increase in EF was 7.9%. ($P < .001$, $P < .001$, $P < .001$, $P = .043$). Comparing 1-month and 6-month measurements, the reduction rates of VV and RVF were 1.9% and 15%, and the increase rates of VFI and EF were 3.2% and 7.6%, respectively. EF was significantly increased at 6 months compared with 1 month after EVLA ($P = .013$), but the other parameters showed no statistically significant differences between 1 month and 6 months after EVLA.

Conclusions.—This study demonstrated that the venous hemodynamic parameters of primary varicose veins improved after performance of EVLA and phlebectomy.

▶ In the surveillance of arterial occlusive pathology, in addition to patient symptoms, the objective measures are centered on the pressure of blood delivered to an extremity, and clinicians use anatomic images as surrogate markers for that intraprocedurally. For venous disease, the capacitance of the venous system and the dynamic nature of pathology as it relates to changes such as postural changes make the study of venous insufficiency more challenging. Concepts such as venous volume and ejection fraction can be measured by air plethysmography (APG), but the application remains limited because of the low availability or willingness to perform APG. The authors performed simultaneous saphenofemoral ligation and laser ablation of incompetent saphenous veins and showed that venous filling predictably decreased and ejection fraction increased. What is curious is that, over time, the reduction in filling diminished, suggesting, although not nearly significant statistically, that there may be negative adaptation over time. As we become more sophisticated in our assessment of venous disease and surveillance after intervention, we may find that treatment of truncal pathology may devolve over time in efficacy as the pathology no doubt effects more than a solitary vein in the lower extremity.

R. J. Feezor, MD, FACS

Randomized trial comparing cyanoacrylate embolization and radiofrequency ablation for incompetent great saphenous veins (VeClose)

Morrison N, Gibson K, McEnroe S, et al (Morrison Vein Inst, Scottsdale, AZ; Lake Washington Vascular, Bellevue; Sentara Vascular Specialists, Virginia Beach, VA; et al)

J Vasc Surg 61:985-994, 2015

Background.—Whereas thermal ablation of incompetent saphenous veins is highly effective, all heat-based ablation techniques require the use of perivenous subfascial tumescent anesthesia, involving multiple needle punctures along the course of the target vein. Preliminary evidence suggests that cyanoacrylate embolization (CAE) may be effective in the treatment of incompetent great saphenous veins (GSVs). We report herein early results of a randomized trial of CAE vs radiofrequency ablation (RFA) for the treatment of symptomatic incompetent GSVs.

Methods.—Two hundred twenty-two subjects with symptomatic GSV incompetence were randomly assigned to receive either CAE (n = 108) with the VenaSeal Sapheon Closure System (Sapheon, Inc, Morrisville, NC) or RFA (n = 114) with the ClosureFast system (Covidien, Mansfield, Mass). After discharge, subjects returned to the clinic on day 3 and again at months 1 and 3. The study's primary end point was closure of the target vein at month 3 as assessed by duplex ultrasound and adjudicated by an independent vascular ultrasound core laboratory. Statistical testing focused on showing noninferiority with a 10% delta conditionally followed by superiority testing. No adjunctive procedures were allowed until after the month 3 visit, and missing month 3 data were imputed by various methods. Secondary end points included patient-reported pain during vein treatment and extent of ecchymosis at day 3. Additional assessments included general and disease-specific quality of life surveys and adverse event rates.

Results.—All subjects received the assigned intervention. By use of the predictive method for imputing missing data, 3-month closure rates were 99% for CAE and 96% for RFA. All primary end point analyses, which used various methods to account for the missing data rate (14%), showed evidence to support the study's noninferiority hypothesis (all $P < .01$); some of these analyses supported a trend toward superiority ($P = .07$ in the predictive model). Pain experienced during the procedure was mild and similar between treatment groups (2.2 and 2.4 for CAE and RFA, respectively, on a 10-point scale; $P = .11$). At day 3, less ecchymosis in the treated region was present after CAE compared with RFA ($P < .01$). Other adverse events occurred at a similar rate between groups and were generally mild and well tolerated.

Conclusions.—CAE was proven to be noninferior to RFA for the treatment of incompetent GSVs at month 3 after the procedure. Both treatment methods showed good safety profiles. CAE does not require tumescent anesthesia and is associated with less postprocedure ecchymosis.

▶ Glue is here. This study illustrates that cyanoacrylate is not inferior to radiofrequency ablation for treatment of incompetent great saphenous veins (GSVs) at 3 months, with added benefit of avoiding tumescent anesthesia and less ecchymosis. Although longer term follow-up is still needed, there certainly seems to be advantages to glue as an option for endovenous ablation. As part of expanding evidence supporting cyanoacrylate and other nontumescent techniques for endovenous ablation, we may be witnessing the beginning of a shift away from endothermal techniques that require tumescent anesthesia. With US Food and Drug Administration approval in 2015, options for use of cyanoacrylate are now commercially available, but with lack of appropriate CPT coding, most insurance carriers still consider these technique investigational, and currently limit its wider dissemination. Whether these techniques will be selectively used or represent a true transformational shift, time will tell.

M. Passman, MD

Superficial venous reflux duration and cessation with two concurrent duplex probes

Lattimer CR, Mendoza E (Ealing Hosp, Middlesexa, UK; the Venenpraxis, Wunstorf, UK; et al)

J Vasc Surg Venous Lymphat Disord 3:154-160, 2015

Background.—Venous reflux is the principal hemodynamic disorder and therapeutic target in patients with superficial venous insufficiency. To date, no studies have identified where or when it stops, anatomically or regionally, along the course of the refluxive conduit. Duplex measurements of reflux are performed invariably with a single probe. Because many anatomic locations are studied, repeated provocation maneuvers are required. However, this fails to appreciate reflux as a circulation. The use of two probes placed concurrently in different regions may address this limitation. The study compared venous reflux duration and cessation, above the knee and below the knee simultaneously, with two duplex probes.

Methods.—Seventeen legs from 17 consecutive patients (12 female, nine left) with great saphenous vein reflux were studied. Their median (range) age was 51 (28-71) years; weight, 76.8 (63.5-189) kg; height, 169 (153-180) cm; and Venous Clinical Severity Score, 5 (1-12). The clinical class of the Clinical, Etiologic, Anatomic, and Pathophysiologic (CEAP) classification was as follows: C2, 6; C3, 4; C4a, 5; and C4b, 2. After 2 minutes of elevation, the leg was assessed for reflux duration with duplex ultrasound. This occurred when the patient stood up during venous filling. One probe was positioned 10 cm below the saphenofemoral junction over the great saphenous vein (point A) and the other over a refluxive saphenous vein or tributary below the knee (point B). Concurrent images were displayed on adjacent monitors and recorded by a single video camera. Reflux duration was from the onset of dependency, indicated by the start of the video, to the termination of the red color (reflux) on video playback. The probes were swapped to negate for differences in machine sensitivity. Each leg was tested three times. Simultaneous was defined when there was <0.1 second difference between the two sites.

Results.—The median (range) vein diameters at points A and B were 6.1 (2.8-9.3) mm and 5.5 (2.5-8.1) mm, respectively, with an intertransducer distance of 41 (23-59) cm. There was no significant difference in reflux duration between point A with 27 (9-150) seconds and point B with 27 (10-149) seconds ($P = .943$ [Wilcoxon]). The correlation was excellent ($r = .986$; $P < .0005$ [Spearman]).

Conclusions.—This is the first study to investigate reflux cessation by introducing a novel two-probe technique. It has demonstrated that reflux may stop simultaneously above and below the knee with use of the elevation to dependency maneuver to provoke reflux. It has shown that either site may be used to measure reflux duration. Furthermore, the two-probe technique confirms the belief that the mechanism of refluxive venous filling is through the descending path of a recirculation circuit.

▶ Compared with the study of the anatomy and corresponding pathology of arterial disease, venous disease remains somewhat elementary, potentially due in part to the intense variability of the anatomy and the lack of precision to date examining the circulation within the venous system. Reflux of truncal veins is well treated with ablative therapies, but to have reflux or retrograde flow within a conduit, there must be entry points and exit points, and in that regard, the refluxing vein is merely part of a larger circuit. The authors use a "elevation to dependency" method of detection, which is well described in the text and yields a much exaggerated duration of reflux (27 seconds here) compared with the more standard provocative maneuvers such as "calf release." Moreover, the cessation of reflux was seen simultaneously in the proximal leg (proximal in the reflux circuit) and the distal leg (distal in the circuit). Augmenting the anatomic knowledge of the refluxing system, and, chiefly, the recognition that the truncal vein is only part of the circuit, may provide opportunities to provide symptomatic relief for patients and yet perhaps preserve conduit for arterial uses. At the least, it provides a more in-depth understanding of the relationship of anatomy and physiology as they relate to overall pathology.

R. J. Feezor, MD, FACS

The effects of environmental and compositional manipulations on the longevity of Tessari-made foam for sclerotherapy

Patel SB, Ostler AE, Dos Santos SJ, et al (Whiteley Clinic, Guildford, Surrey, UK; et al)

J Vasc Surg Venous Lymphat Disord 3:312-318, 2015

Background.—Tessari-made foam sclerotherapy is performed around the world in a variety of clinics differing in methods, equipment, temperatures, and altitudes. We investigated how the following factors affected the foam's longevity: silicone vs nonsilicone syringes, volume of foam made, ratio of gas to sclerosant, use of air vs 50:50 mixture of carbon dioxide and oxygen, temperature, altitude, and 10 consecutive reuses of the syringes.

Methods.—Sclerosant foam was made by the Tessari double-syringe technique. To calculate the longevity, the time was taken for half of the original volume of sclerosant to settle. Half-lives were compared with use of silicone and silicone-free syringes to make the foam. We investigated how the volume (5 mL vs 2 mL) and different ratios affected the foam by observing the half-life of 4:1, 3.5:1, and 3:1 ratios of gas to sclerosant. Air and a 50:50 mixture of carbon dioxide and oxygen were both used as the gas in changing the ratio and volume to see which produced better foam. These experiments were conducted at room (23.9°C) and refrigerator (3°C) temperatures with a constant pressure. The different ratio, volume, and silicone vs nonsilicone syringe experiments were all repeated at 9314, 7460, 4575, and 2326 feet above sea level in addition to the baseline experiment, which took place at 236 feet above sea level. To test how consecutive uses of syringes affected the foam, we made consecutive batches of foam reusing each pair of syringes 10 times; this was repeated five times with silicone syringes and twice with nonsilicone syringes.

Results.—Switching to nonsilicone syringes can increase longevity by 70%. A larger volume of foam and a 3:1 ratio produced longer half-lives at all temperatures and altitudes. The lower (3°C) temperature increased the longevity of foam in all instances, as did the use of air. A high altitude (low pressure) had a detrimental effect on the foam's longevity. Ten consecutive syringe uses had no significant impact on the foam's half-life (silicone syringe mean between first five and last five uses, $P = .95$).

Conclusions.—The optimum conditions for making foam are nonsilicone syringes, larger volumes, a 3:1 air to sclerosant ratio, and low temperatures. Silicone syringes can be reused until friction becomes a burden. Temperature has a bigger effect than altitude on longevity of the foam. Making foam in larger volumes would allow the foam to last longer. To compensate for high altitudes (low pressures), decreasing the temperature will increase the foam's longevity.

Clinical Relevance.—Foam sclerotherapy is performed widely around the world in different environments, at different temperatures, at different altitudes, and with different ratios of sclerosant to gas, using different gases (air or carbon dioxide–oxygen mixtures) and different syringes. The most commonly used technique is the Tessari method of making foam. Foam sclerotherapy relies on the foam's displacing the blood from the target vein, and so longer lasting foam will keep the blood out of the target vein longer, which is likely to have better results, although that needs to be shown. This study explores the variables to see how they affect the longevity of foam.

▶ Foam sclerotherapy is widely used worldwide in the treatment of varicose veins. There are many conditions in which foam is made, different environmental factors (altitude, temperature), and different ratios of air to liquid as well as components of air. The important aspect of foam is its state, in that the longevity of the foam is important, because the mechanism during foam sclerotherapy is the displacement of blood by the foam to cause endothelial injury. Therefore, increasing the half-life of the foam and which critical constituents are responsible for the optimal conditions to make foam will hypothetically provide the best clinical outcome. In this study, the authors' goals were to determine composition and environmental factors that would provide the best foam longevity, defined as the time taken for half of the original volume of sclerosant to settle. The major findings of the study were the following: (1) switching to nonsilicone syringes can increase longevity by 70%. (2) A larger volume of foam and a 3:1 ratio produced longer half-lives at all temperatures and altitudes. (3) Lower temperature increased the longevity of foam in all instances, as did the use of air. (4) High altitude (low pressure) had a detrimental effect on the foam's longevity. (5) Ten consecutive silicone syringe uses had no significant impact on the foam's half-life. Recommendation by the authors were made based on the study findings that included recommending the use of nonsilicone syringes, a 3:1 gas to sclerosant ratio, larger volumes of STS (1 mL) to increase the longevity of foam, and reuse of both nonsilicone and silicone syringes. It is important to note that the Food and Drug Administration has approved foam sclerotherapy in the United States with Varithena (BTG International, West Conshohocken, PA), which is a proprietary make of 1% polidoconal foam with fixed concentrations of oxygen (65%) and carbon dioxide (35%), mixed in a chamber, and which dispenses uniform-sized microfoam bubbles and uses nonsilicone syringes.

J. D. Raffetto, MD, FACS, FSVM

The European multicenter cohort study on cyanoacrylate embolization of refluxing great saphenous veins

Proebstle TM, Alm J, Dimitri S, et al (Univ Med Ctr, Mainz, Germany, Dermatologikum Hamburg, Germany; Countess of Chester Hosp, UK; et al)
J Vasc Surg Venous Lymphat Disord 3:2-7, 2015

Objective.—Cyanoacrylate (CA) embolization of refluxing great saphenous veins (GSVs) has been previously described. The outcomes from a multicenter study are still lacking.

Methods.—A prospective multicenter study was conducted in seven centers in four European countries to abolish GSV reflux by endovenous CA embolization. Neither tumescent anesthesia nor postinterventional compression stockings were used. Varicose tributaries remained untreated until at least 3 months after the index treatment. Clinical examination, quality of life assessment, and duplex ultrasound evaluation were performed at 2 days and after 1, 3, 6, and 12 months.

Results.—In 70 patients, of whom 68 (97.1%) were available for 12-month follow-up, 70 GSVs were treated. Two-day follow-up showed one proximal and one distal partial recanalization. Three additional proximal recanalizations were observed at 3-month (n = 2) and 6-month (n = 1) follow-up. Cumulative 12-month survival free from recanalization was 92.9% (95% confidence interval, 87.0%-99.1%). Mean (standard deviation) Venous Clinical Severity Score improved from 4.3 ± 2.3 at baseline to 1.1 ± 1.3 at 12 months. Aberdeen Varicose Vein Questionnaire score showed an improvement from 16.3 at baseline to 6.7 at 12 months ($P < .0001$). Side effects were generally mild; a phlebitic reaction occurred in eight cases (11.4%) with a median duration of 6.5 days (range, 2-12 days). Pain without a phlebitic reaction was observed in five patients (8.6%) for a median duration of 1 day (range, 0 - 12 days). No serious adverse event occurred. Paresthesia was not observed.

Conclusions.—Endovenous CA embolization of refluxing GSVs is safe and effective without the use of tumescent anesthesia or compression stockings.

▶ Chronic venous disease is a significant disease affecting a large proportion of the population. The great saphenous vein is pathologic in up to 80% to 90% of patients with chronic venous disease. There are a number of treatment options for patient with insufficient great saphenous vein that include pin stripping; thermal ablations; nonthermal ablations, including glues, mechanical, and sclerosant; and foam sclerotherapy. Surgical and less invasive treatment options have been evaluated in a randomized controlled trial and were found to have nearly equally improved clinical outcomes and quality of life.[1] This study is a prospective study evaluating cyanoacrylate in the treatment of great saphenous vein reflux. The potential advantages of cyanoacrylate glue are that it does not require the use of tumescent anesthesia; by chemically bonding vein walls to each other, it obviates the need for postinterventional compression stockings; and it precludes the risk of treatment-related sensory nerve damage. The study follow-up was at 1 year. Seventy patients enrolled in the study, and 68 were evaluable for the 12-month visit. The outcomes were a 93% occlusion rate, improved Venous Clinical Severity Score and EQ-5D and Aberdeen Varicose Vein Questionnaire quality-of-life questionnaires. Early results appear promising from this technique, and long-term follow-up will be necessary to assess for durability and recurrence of disease, including randomized trials comparing other treatment modalities.

J. D. Raffetto, MD, FACS, FSVM

Reference

1. Rasmussen LH, Lawaetz M, Bjoern L, Vennits B, Blemings A, Eklof B. Randomized clinical trial comparing endovenous laser ablation, radiofrequency ablation, foam sclerotherapy and surgical stripping for great saphenous varicose veins. *Br J Surg*. 2011;98:1079-1087.

Tumescent technique without epinephrine for endovenous laser therapy and serum lidocaine concentration

Hudson AJ, Whittaker DR, Szpisjak DF, et al (Uniformed Services Univ of the Health Sciences, Bethesda, MD; Walter Reed Natl Military Med Ctr, Bethesda, MD; et al)

J Vasc Surg Venous Lymphat Disord 3:48-53, 2015

Objective.—Endovenous laser therapy (EVLT) requires tumescent lidocaine anesthesia. Although it is well known that the absorption of local anesthetic varies according to the injection site, little evidence exists establishing the maximum recommended safe dose for extravascular injections such as those used for EVLT. The aim of this study was to evaluate plasma concentration of lidocaine over time after administration of tumescent lidocaine during EVLT procedures in healthy volunteers.

Methods.—Between January 2011 and February 2013, 10 healthy patients scheduled for an EVLT procedure performed in a hospital setting were recruited to participate in an observational study. For each subject, a total of 10 venous samples were obtained for analysis after surgical injection of the tumescent lidocaine solution (0.1% concentration). Samples were collected at baseline (before the surgical procedure start) and then every 30 minutes for the first 2 hours after the initial lidocaine injection. Thereafter, venous samples were obtained every 2 hours, with the last sample drawn 12 hours after the surgeon's initial lidocaine injection. All specimens were drawn from a dedicated intravenous catheter, immediately placed in a heparinized blood collection tube, and centrifuged for 10 minutes at 3000 rpm. Plasma was then removed with a pipette and stored at −70°C until analyzed. Total and free plasma lidocaine concentrations were determined by immunoassay. Plasma lidocaine concentrations were normalized by peak concentration for statistical comparisons.

Results.—Laboratory data were available for nine of the 10 volunteers. The mean total lidocaine dose administered was 6.38 (± 2.2) mg/kg (range, 3.57-10.7 mg/kg). The total lidocaine blood levels ranged from 0.48 (± 0.28) to 1.3 (± 0.49) mcg/mL. The free lidocaine blood levels ranged from nondetectable to 0.76 (± 0.43) mcg/mL. The average total time of injection for the group was 32.8 (± 10.0) minutes (range, 21-49 minutes). Among all dose ranges, both total and free lidocaine peak blood level ratios occurred at times 60 to 120 minutes ($P < .05$). No value considered in the statistical analysis exceeded 5 mcg/mL at any time.

Conclusions.—Tumescent lidocaine without epinephrine for EVLT procedures produces a peak serum concentration at 60 to 120 minutes. The peak plasma concentration as observed with the standard institutional dosing of tumescent lidocaine appeared below the threshold for human toxicity.

▶ Endovenous ablation has all but replaced saphenous vein stripping, and the treatment of venous disease in general has propelled vascular surgeons into new clinical realms. Whereas classical vascular surgery deals with critically ill patients under general anesthesia, with lower priority on patient comfort and cosmesis, patients receiving care for symptomatic venous disease are often ambulatory and reflect more of a purely elective procedure. Infiltration of local anesthetic is a vital part of any thermal ablation procedure. However, because the injections are not intravascular, the serum absorption and risk of toxicity should be quantified. As shown here, there is little risk of systemic toxicity, but certainly clinicians should be keenly aware of the total amount of any pharmacologic agent that is used. These concerns may ultimately be minimized if nonthermal ablative techniques become more popular, as one of the arguments in favor of such includes the avoidance of tumescent anesthesia.

R. J. Feezor, MD, FACS

Embolization techniques for high-flow arteriovenous malformations with a dominant outflow vein

Conway AM, Qato K, Drury J, et al (Lenox Hill Hosp, NY)
J Vasc Surg Venous Lymphat Disord 3:178-183, 2015

Objective.—The aim of this study was to assess the management and outcomes of arteriovenous malformations (AVMs) with a dominant outflow vein (DOV) treated with retrograde venous embolization.

Methods.—A retrospective review was performed from November 2010 to May 2014 on all patients with a high-flow AVM and associated DOV who underwent transvenous embolization of the DOV. Indications, techniques, complications, and outcomes were reviewed.

Results.—Fourteen patients (five male; 36%) underwent transvenous embolization of high-flow AVMs with a DOV. Median age was 41.6 years (15.7-65.8 years). The AVM was located on an extremity in eight patients (57%) and in the pelvis in six patients (43%). The indication for the procedure was pain in 11 patients (79%), swelling in 3 patients (21%), a nonhealing wound in 1 patient (7%), and impotence in 1 patient (7%). The median number of prior procedures to treat the AVM was 2.5 (0-13). Transvenous embolization with coils was performed in 13 patients (93%). The Amplatzer vascular plug and Amplatzer septal occluder (St. Jude Medical, St. Paul, Minn) were used in four patients (29%). Concurrent percutaneous puncture embolization of the AVM nidus was used in seven patients (50%) and transcatheter arterial embolization in eight patients (57%). Technical angiographic success was seen in all patients. Five patients (36%) experienced a complete response to treatment, whereas eight (57%) experienced a partial response. Seven patients (50%) required further procedures for residual symptoms.

Conclusions.—AVMs with a DOV can be successfully treated by a transvenous approach. Percutaneous puncture embolization of the nidus or draining vein and transcatheter arterial embolization may assist in reducing flow.

▶ The treatment of arteriovenous malformations (AVMs) tends to be clustered in certain centers of excellence; relative rarity and complex nature of AVMs preclude hard guidelines from being written. Anatomic descriptors include location and inflow/outflow vessel descriptors. An uncommon configuration is an AVM with a dominant outflow vein, and the authors describe an elegant technique of outflow occlusion and then "proximal" embolization either from an arterial approach, adjacent venous approach, or direct cutaneous approach. The extreme heterogeneity even in subselected case series limits the widespread applicability except for "techniques." However, it is noteworthy that even with presumed expertise and impressive numbers of cases, a "complete clinical response" was achieved in less than half of the cases. This statistic is worthwhile to share with patients when helping them make an informed decision to proceed with intervention.

R. J. Feezor, MD, FACS

Management of perforator vein aneurysms in the lower extremities

Labropoulos N, Comito M, De Zolt P, et al (Stony Brook Univ Med Ctr, NY; MediClinic, Pozzonovo, Italy)

J Vasc Surg Venous Lymphat Disord 3:270-275, 2015

Objective.—Perforator vein aneurysms (PVAs) of the lower extremity have not been defined or reported. This study reports the clinical presentation of patients, the PVA characteristics, and the clinical outcome of their management.

Methods.—Patients with signs and symptoms of chronic venous disease who had a PVA were included. Diagnosis of a PVA was made with duplex ultrasound. Normal perforator veins have a diameter of <3 mm. A PVA was defined as a diameter dilation of >9 mm, and it was always found below the deep fascia. The topography and morphology of the aneurysms were described in detail. All PVAs were treated with subfascial ligation with or without aneurysm excision. All patients were followed up for a minimum of 3 months with clinical examination and duplex ultrasound, and complications were noted.

Results.—There were 21 aneurysms identified in 19 patients. Fourteen (73.7%) patients were female. The mean age at diagnosis was 49 years with a standard deviation of 9. Aneurysm size ranged from 9.8 to

22.2 mm, with a mean diameter of 15.7 mm and a standard deviation of 3.8. Seventeen aneurysms were fusiform, one was saccular, and one was multilobar. The perforators of the great saphenous vein distribution were most frequently involved, whereas only one involved deep vein disease. Few patients had symptoms, such as pressure and pain directly over the affected perforator. There was no association between the location and size of the PVA and the severity of chronic venous disease. Fourteen patients were treated surgically; five patients preferred conservative treatment with elastic compression stockings. Fourteen patients (73.7%) had ligation with (n = 9) or without (n = 5) excision of the aneurysm. All underwent concomitant phlebectomies, and eight of them also had ultrasound-guided foam sclerotherapy. Endovenous thermal ablation of saphenous veins was performed in seven patients, whereas two had ligation and stripping. There were four minor postoperative complications in four patients, all of which resolved within 6 weeks. The median follow-up was 21 months, ranging from 3 to 52 months. There were no recurrences of a PVA. Five patients preferred conservative treatment. The diameter changed from 0 to 13 mm during the follow-up, and the patients' symptoms remained the same or had mild worsening.

Conclusions.—PVAs are rare without causing significant symptoms locally. Diagnosis is made with duplex ultrasound because the affected vein is located below the deep fascia. As only one case in our series of 19 involved the deep veins, we believe that PVAs originate from superficial veins. The condition is relatively benign, and the treatment outcomes are very good with limited complications experienced. However, selective treatment of PVAs may not be needed for most of them as treatment of the superficial veins connecting with the PVA may be sufficient.

► Because of the variability and relative lack of attention paid to venous anatomy, abnormalities such as aneurysms have been poorly described. Other venous aneurysms are felt to be a potential nidus of thrombus, although the incidence is unknown. The authors report on a series of 21 perforator vein aneurysms among a larger group of patients presumably seen for symptoms of venous insufficiency. Most received surgical ligation or excision, although some patients opted for conservative (nonoperative) management. Few, if indeed any, of these patients were symptomatic from these perforator aneurysms. What remains unclear is the true incidence of such aneurysms and the "natural history" if only the more established truncal insufficiency is treated. As more detailed venous ultrasounds are performed for symptoms of venous insufficiency, the incidence of discovering such anatomic anomalies will likely increase.

R. J. Feezor, MD, FACS

The effect of stent placement for May-Thurner syndrome combined with symptomatic superficial venous reflux disease

Yin M, Huang X, Cui C, et al (Shanghai Ninth People's Hosp Affiliated to Shanghai JiaoTong Univ, China)

J Vasc Surg Venous Lymphat Disord 3:168-172, 2015

Objective.—The current study aimed to determine whether it is necessary to correct May-Thurner syndrome (MTS) simultaneously with superficial venous reflux disease (S-VRD) in limbs of combined symptomatic MTS/S-VRD.

Methods.—A retrospective analysis of patients with S-VRD combined with MTS was conducted in a single institution from January 2001 to December 2010. Doppler ultrasound and phlebography were performed in patients with VRD. Computed tomography angiography or transfemoral venography was selectively performed in patients with severe symptoms or findings on phlebography suggestive of MTS. MTS was found in 207 patients. Among these, 121 patients were successfully treated with stent placement combined with endovenous laser ablation (EVLA); the remaining 86 patients, who were treated with EVLA for S-VRD alone, served as a control group. Clinical results, venous reflux, and quality of life were evaluated before and after treatment. Stent patency was followed up with Doppler ultrasound.

Results.—There was no significant difference in age, female to male ratio, clinical symptoms, comorbidities, or percentage with S-VRD between the two groups. A total of 125 stents were placed in 121 patients in the EVLA + stent group. The rate of technical success was 100%. Follow-up periods ranged from 1 to 91 months (mean, 70.4 ± 21.3 months). The 4-year primary patency rate was 93.3%. The incidence of pain, edema, and ulceration was decreased significantly in the stent + EVLA group. However, there was a high rate of S-VRD recurrence in the EVLA-alone group. Quality of life improved significantly in the EVLA + stent group; improvements included relief of pain, edema, and fatigue and increased physical activity. For deep venous reflux, there was no significant improvement after stent placement for MTS.

Conclusions.—Stent placement is an effective and durable treatment of MTS combined with symptomatic S-VRD; it results in a high level of long-term patency and a significant relief of pain, edema, and ulceration. Furthermore, correction of MTS plays an important role in decreasing the recurrence rate of S-VRD after EVLA.

► The combination of saphenous ablation and iliac vein outflow stenting provided more relief from symptoms compared with ablative therapy alone. If one thinks hemodynamically, this is not entirely surprising because the goal of venous insufficiency interventions is to improve efficiency of venous return from the extremity, and leaving a stenosis in the iliac vein will naturally thwart this. The real clinical challenge is selecting the subset of patients with venous insufficiency to evaluate for May-Thurner compression. In the current study, almost 10% of patients with truncal insufficiency also had May-Thurner syndrome by CT scan. Once identified, correcting the anatomic lesions at multiple levels, if present, will provide a greater clinical benefit for patients who have them.

R. J. Feezor, MD, FACS

Treatment of nutcracker syndrome with open and endovascular interventions

Erben Y, Gloviczki P, Kalra M, et al (Mayo Clinic, Rochester, MN)
J Vasc Surg Venous Lymphat Disord 3:389-396, 2015

Objective.—Nutcracker syndrome (NS) is a rare cause of hematuria, flank pain, and renal venous hypertension due to compression of the left renal vein (LRV) between the aorta and the superior mesenteric artery. To evaluate outcomes of open surgery and endovascular interventions, we reviewed our experience.

Methods.—A retrospective review of clinical data of all patients treated at our institution with an intervention for NS between January 1, 1994, and February 28, 2014, was performed. Primary outcomes were morbidity and mortality. Secondary outcomes included late complications, patency, freedom from reintervention, and resolution of symptoms.

Results.—Thirty-seven patients (30 female, seven male) with a mean age of 27 years (range, 14-62 years) were treated. The most frequent symptom was flank pain (97%); the most frequent sign was hematuria (68%). NS was diagnosed with duplex ultrasound scanning with measurement of LRV diameters and flow velocities (87%), with computed tomography or magnetic resonance venography (94%), and with contrast venography with measurement of pressure gradients (93%). Initial treatment was open surgery in 36 patients, endovascular in 1. Distal transposition of the LRV into the inferior vena cava (IVC) was performed in 31 patients. Adjunctive procedures to optimize venous outflow included great saphenous vein cuff in six patients, great saphenous vein patch in four, and both cuff and patch in four. Three patients had patch alone; two had transposition of the left gonadal vein into the IVC. Two patients had anterior reimplantation of retroaortic LRV into the IVC. There were no major early complications, renal failure, or mortality. Three patients underwent early reinterventions within 30 days (stent, two; open revision, one). All LRVs and left gonadal veins were patent at discharge. Follow-up was 36.8 ± 52.6 months (range, 1-216 months). Reinterventions after 30 days were performed in eight patients because of LRV stenosis (n = 7) or LRV occlusion (n = 1). One stent migrated into the IVC and required endovascular removal with repeated stenting. Six patients required stenting. Primary, primary assisted, and secondary patencies at 24 months were 74%, 97%, and 100%, respectively. Freedom from reintervention at 12 and 24 months was 76% and 68%, respectively. Resolution of symptoms occurred in 33 patients (87%).

Conclusions.—Open surgery, mostly LRV transposition, remains a safe and effective treatment of patients with NS. However, one of three patients after open repair required reintervention, most frequently LRV stenting. Open reconstruction should be tailored to the patient's anatomy, and placement of vein cuff or patch may reduce restenosis. Although renal vein stents improved patency, the safety and durability of currently available stents need to be established.

▶ Compression of the left renal vein between the aorta and superior mesenteric artery is increasingly recognized on imaging, but is associated with true renal venous hypertension and/or pelvic venous congestion in a minority of patients. For those with clinically significant nutcracker syndrome, several operative and endovascular interventions have been described. This study focuses on uncommon (n = 37 over 20 years) operative techniques, mostly involving left renal transposition (n = 31) and occasional patch (n = 3) or left gonadal transposition (n = 2) options. There are additional technical descriptions and diagrams of adjunctive patch and cuffs for left renal vein transpositions. As a review of open techniques, this series shows safety and efficacy and sets the bar for comparison of newer endovascular options. Interestingly, approximately 30% had restenosis and needed reintervention, most commonly endovascular stent placement. Although endovascular stenting options were used secondarily in this study, stents are being used with increasing frequency as a primary treatment, although the durability of stent options remains unclear.

M. Passman, MD

14 Miscellaneous

Historical Perspectives

The shirt off his back

Pories WJ (East Carolina Univ, Greenville, NC)
J Vasc Surg 62:1366-1367, 2015

Background.—Surgery doesn't always go as planned, but a case involving Dr. Charles Rob, renowned surgeon and decorated veteran of World War II, shows that challenging situations can lead to innovation.

Case Report.—The patient required repair of an aortic aneurysm but presented an unusual situation. Once the abdomen was opened and the aneurysm was exposed, measuring about 9 cm in diameter, the surgical team saw that the aorta was encased in a sheath of cheese-like inflammation and the lumen was difficult to locate. To address the situation, much of the wall of the mycotic aneurysm was debrided away to reveal clearly defined proximal and distal segments of the aorta that could support a graft. An aortic homograft was ordered from the tissue bank, but the nurse reported back that there were none left. Dr. Rob and the other surgeons were left staring at the empty aortic bed and two large clamps beating in rhythm.

Dr. Rob recalled that he had heard a Dr. Wesolowski report the successful use of cloth grafts to repair aortas in pigs. Then he asked the nurse to get his shirt out of his locker. The shirt was a new type, made totally of nylon, and were popular with travelers because they dried quickly and did not need to be ironed. However, multiple washings caused them to turn a dirty yellow and to develop brown spots in the armpits where the material interacted with deodorant. The shirt in question was well worn and badly discolored. The nurse was instructed to drop it in a steel dish and pour iodine over it. After a short time of soaking the material, Dr. Rob cut a rectangle out of the shirt and sewed it into a tube, then sewed it in place in the patient. He warned those present that it might bleed a bit—but it bled significantly. Once it stopped, the patient had an excellent pulse, his legs were pink and warm, and the surgical site was closed up. Everyone expected that it wouldn't hold, but the patient recovered quickly with no complications.

Follow-up.—Eight years later, one of the surgeons saw the patient again, doing well with good circulation in both legs. The graft was significantly dilated, but it was left in place.

Conclusions.—This report documents what was possibly the first use of a synthetic vascular graft in a human. It is also likely the first time that a surgeon literally gave the patient the shirt off his back (Fig 1).

▶ This wonderful historical tribute from Walter J. Pories is worth the read in its entirety. I personally knew Charles Rob when I was a surgical resident at Walter Reed Army Medical Center in the early 1990s. I had no idea at the time how greatly he influenced the field I would eventually call my own. He was retired as a surgeon but still came to all of our vascular conferences. Always the gentleman and plenty of historical vignettes of his own! I feel privileged to have known him.

My year as the Chief Resident at Strong Memorial Hospital had barely begun in 1961 when I assisted Dr Charles Rob (Fig) in the repair of an aortic aneurysm. Rob was not only one of the two "gods" of vascular surgery, along with [Michael] DeBakey, but he was also decorated for bravery in World War II,

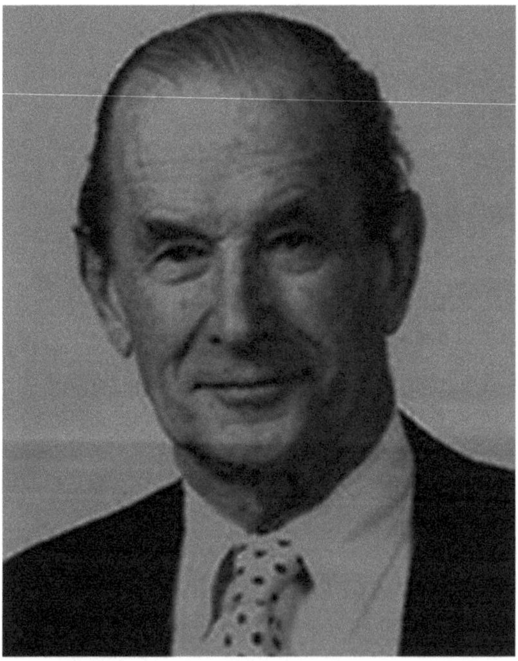

FIGURE 1.—Charles Rob, MD, FACS. (Reprinted from Pories WJ. The shirt off his back. *J Vasc Surg.* 2015;62:1366-1367, with permission from the Society for Vascular Surgery.)

assisted on the resection of the lung of Britain's George VI, and cared for Winston Churchill's ischemic great toe. He was a brilliant surgeon and, on top of that, had a formidable English accent. As far as the house staff was concerned, he could do no wrong.

After we opened the abdomen and exposed the aneurysm, perhaps 9 cm in diameter, and secured proximal and distal control, it became evident that this was an unusual case. The aorta was encased in a sheath of inflammation, and the lumen was difficult to find. Rather than the usual straight incision into the aneurysm and evacuating the grumous contents, we ended up debriding much of the wall of this apparent mycotic aneurysm. Fortunately, after resection of this cheeselike material, there we found clearly defined proximal and distal segments of the aorta that could hold a graft. Accordingly, Rob instructed the nurse to bring an aortic homograft, the only method available for reconstructing the aorta at that time. She returned all too soon from the tissue bank with the news that Dr James DeWeese, the other vascular surgeon in the department, had used the last one.

There was total silence. We all stared at the empty aortic bed and the two large clamps beating in a deadly rhythm. Now what?

Finally, Dr Rob, a man of few words, spoke. "Just a couple of weeks ago, I heard a Doctor Wesolowski report the successful use of cloth grafts to repair aortas in pigs.[1] ... Mary, please get my shirt out of my locker."

By "shirt," he meant one of the new shirts, totally made of nylon, that were sold for travelers because they dried quickly and required no ironing. They also turned a dirty yellow after multiple washings with brown spots in the armpits owing to interaction with deodorants. Rob's shirt was well worn and badly discolored. When the nurse returned to the operating room with an expression of disgust and her arm outstretched to keep it away, Rob quietly told her to drop it into a steel dish and pour iodine over it.

The intern and I stared at each other in disbelief as he let the shirt soak for a very short time and then sat down, cut out a rectangle of cloth and sewed it into a tube. It did not take long and he promptly sewed it in place. Taking the clamps off, he warned us that it "might bleed a bit." Actually, the blood poured out, especially compared with the few leaks seen with the implantation of homografts. Miraculously the bleeding stopped, there was an excellent pulse, the legs were pink and warm, and the professor flipped off his gloves and commanded us to "close up." We did so but were also convinced that we would be called at four in the morning with an impossible situation. What would we tell the family?

To our surprise, he recovered quickly without complications. By chance, I saw the patient again in 1969, 8 years later, when I returned from the Air Force to join the faculty at the University of Rochester. He was doing well with good circulation to both legs. The graft was significantly dilated. We chose to leave it alone and I never saw him or his medical record again.

To my knowledge, this incident was the first use of a synthetic vascular graft in a human, although there may have been earlier applications. I am certain, however, that this case represents the first time when a surgeon literally gave the shirt off his back.

B. W. Starnes, MD

Reference

1. Wesolowski SA, Fries CC, Liebig WJ, Sawyer PN, Deterling RA. The synthetic vascular graft. *Arch Surg*. 1962;84:74-90.

Vascular Infection

In vitro efficacy of antibiotic beads in treating abdominal vascular graft infections

Charlton-Ouw KM, Kubrusly F, Sandhu HK, et al (Univ of Texas Med School at Houston)

J Vasc Surg 62:1048-1053, 2015

Objective.—Abdominal aortic vascular graft infection often involves several different organisms. Antibiotic polymethyl methacrylate (PMMA) beads may be effective in controlling infection after débridement, but bacterial species identification and antibiotic susceptibility are often not available at the time of operation, generating a need for a broad-spectrum drug combination for empirical use. We sought to determine an effective antibiotic in PMMA beads for use in abdominal vascular graft infection.

Methods.—PMMA beads were impregnated with combinations of antibiotics, consisting of daptomycin, tobramycin, and meropenem. Antibiotics were selected on the basis of activity spectrum and heat stability. Beads were placed on separate agar plates with vancomycin-resistant *Enterococcus faecalis, Klebsiella pneumoniae, Staphylococcus epidermidis*, and methicillin-resistant *Staphylococcus aureus*. Antibiotic inhibition was recorded by use of a modified agar-based disk-diffusion method.

Results.—Daptomycin alone was not active against *K. pneumoniae* (average = 0 mm). Tobramycin alone was not active against vancomycin-resistant *E. faecalis, K. pneumoniae*, or methicillin-resistant *S. aureus*. Tobramycin and daptomycin in combination had moderate broad-spectrum activity with 8- to 14-mm mean inhibition halos. Meropenem showed strong activity against all tested organisms with >15-mm mean inhibition halos. The addition of daptomycin to meropenem provided improved coverage of gram-positive organisms. The presence of tobramycin reduced the efficacy of meropenem.

Conclusions.—Antibiotic PMMA beads containing 10% meropenem with 2.5% daptomycin had excellent in vitro activity against typical bacterial species associated with abdominal vascular graft infections. The addition of antibiotic beads may be a useful adjunct in managing such cases. Further studies are required to determine efficacy in clinical practice (Figs 2 and 3, Table 1).

▶ Abdominal vascular graft infections continue to portend a poor prognosis with standard techniques of debridement of infected nonviable tissue and resection and replacement of the graft along with systemic antibiotics the hallmark of treatment. Even with meticulous treatment, the recurrence rate and mortality of these patients continue to be high. The authors of this study sought to determine the optimal bead concentration of antibiotics for commonly encountered abdominal vascular graft infection in vitro. Using polymethylmethacrylate (PMMA) and various concentrations of meropenem, tobramycin, and daptomycin on culture plates (Fig 2), they found that beads containing 10% meropenem and 2.5% daptomycin had the best activity against commonly encountered abdominal pathogens (Table 1).

Although antibiotic beads are used in other specialties such as orthopedic surgery to "sterilize" the operative field this modality has been described in other vascular beds as well. The University of South Florida group described their results with the PMMA beads impregnated with antibiotics for adjunctive treatment of prosthetic lower extremity graft infections. They were able to

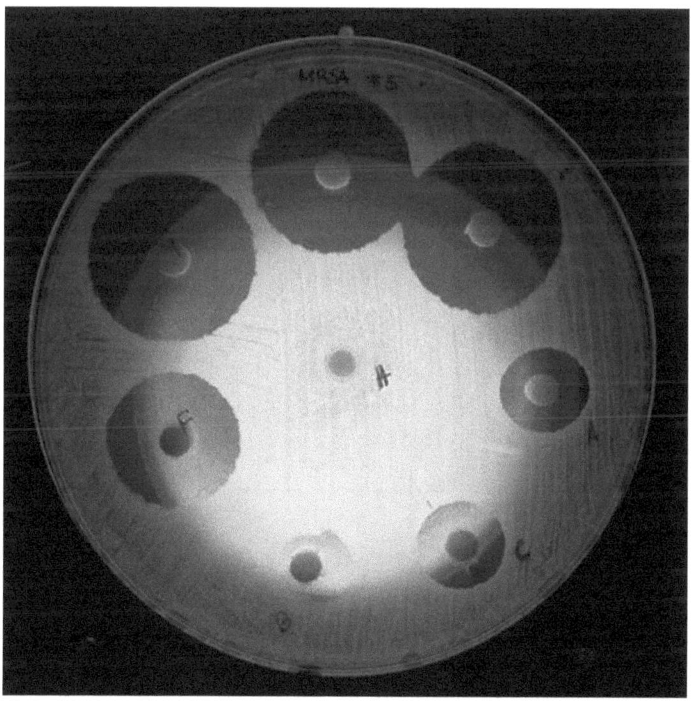

FIGURE 2.—Inhibition halos surround polymethyl methacrylate (PMMA) beads on culture plates after incubation. (Reprinted from Charlton-Ouw KM, Kubrusly F, Sandhu HK, et al. In vitro efficacy of antibiotic beads in treating abdominal vascular graft infections. *J Vasc Surg*. 2015;62:1048-1053, with permission from the Society for Vascular Surgery.)

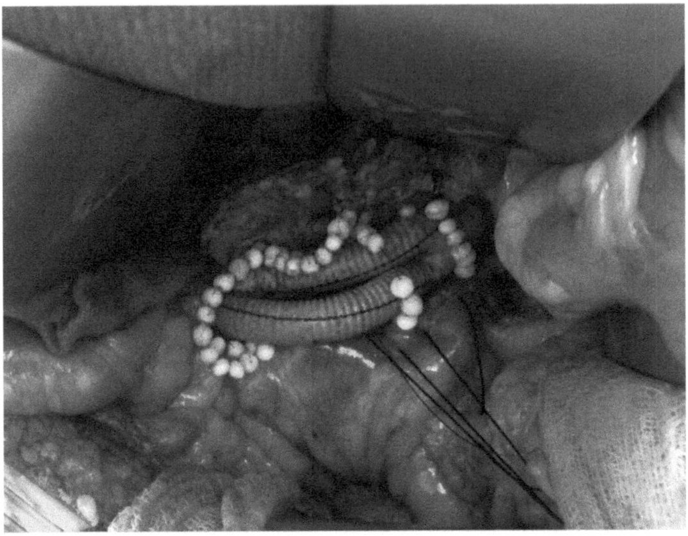

FIGURE 3.—Intraoperative picture of antibiotic-laden polymethyl methacrylate (PMMA) beads around a new aortobi-iliac Dacron graft after resection of previous infected prosthetic vascular graft. (Reprinted from Charlton-Ouw KM, Kubrusly F, Sandhu HK, et al. In vitro efficacy of antibiotic beads in treating abdominal vascular graft infections. *J Vasc Surg*. 2015;62:1048-1053, with permission from the Society for Vascular Surgery.)

TABLE 1.—Average Inhibition Halo Radius (in Millimeters and with Standard Deviation) of Low-Dose, Antibiotic Polymethyl Methacrylate (PMMA) Beads in Bacterial Culture

Antibiotic	*VRE*	Klebsiella *sp*	Staphylococcus Epidermidis	*MRSA*
DA	9.8 ± 1.5	0	10.2 ± 0.4	9.6 ± 0.5
TO	2.0 ± 3.1	10.7 ± 0.8	14.0 ± 1.3	4.7 ± 3.8
DA + TO	8.0 ± 1.1	10.8 ± 0.8	14.3 ± 1.0	9.9 ± 1.1
ME	17.0 ± 0.9	15.3 ± 0.6	21.0 ± 2.5	17.3 ± 1.5
ME + DA	17.2 ± 1.0	16.0 ± 1.3	21.7 ± 2.3	17.7 ± 2.1
ME + TO	13.8 ± 3.4	13.5 ± 2.6	16.7 ± 6.2	13.4 ± 4.2
ME + DA + TO	16.9 ± 2.0	15.0 ± 1.6	21.0 ± 5.2	17.0 ± 2.1
No antibiotic	3.2 ± 3.5	6.9 ± 3.9	8.7 ± 3.1	4.2 ± 6.5

DA, Daptomycin; *ME*, meropenem; *MRSA*, methicillin-resistant *Staphylococcus aureus; TO*, tobramycin; *VRE*, vancomycin-resistant *Enterococcus faecalis*.

Reprinted from Charlton-Ouw KM, Kubrusly F, Sandhu HK, et al. In vitro efficacy of antibiotic beads in treating abdominal vascular graft infections. *J Vasc Surg*. 2015;62:1048-1053, with permission from the Society for Vascular Surgery.

achieve a sterile field based on growth on tissue culture in 87% of graft preservation cases and in situ replacement of the of the infected graft and had a limb salvage rate of 100% with an 11%.[1] The difference in their population was the fact that the patients had groin infections, and the majority were Gram-positive species versus a potential abdominal graft infection, which may have more virulent organisms and does not have the tissue coverage options a groin wound might allow. However, this study does add to our potential armamentarium when dealing with this difficult problem, and perhaps if adding it to debridement, adequate tissue coverage and systemic antibiotics would lead to better results (Fig 3).

N. Singh, MD, FACS

Reference

1. Stone PA, Amstrong PA, Bandyk DF, et al. Use of antibiotic-loaded polymethylmethacrylate beads for the treatment of extracavitary prosthetic vascular graft infections. *J Vasc Surg*. 2006;44:757-761.

Predictors of surgical site infection after hospital discharge in patients undergoing major vascular surgery

Wiseman JT, Fernandes-Taylor S, Barnes ML, et al (Univ of Wisconsin School of Medicine and Public Health, Madison)

J Vasc Surg 62:1023-1031, 2015

Objective.—Surgical site infection (SSI) is one of the most common postoperative complications after vascular reconstruction, producing significant morbidity and hospital readmission. In contrast to SSI that develops while patients are still hospitalized, little is known about the cohort of patients who develop SSI after discharge. In this study, we explore the factors that lead to postdischarge SSI, investigate the differences between risk factors for in-hospital vs postdischarge SSI, and develop a scoring system to identify patients who might benefit from postdischarge monitoring of their wounds.

Methods.—Patients who underwent major vascular surgery from 2005 to 2012 for aneurysm and lower extremity occlusive disease were identified from the American College of Surgeons National Surgical Quality Improvement Program Participant Use Files. Patients were categorized as having no SSI, in-hospital SSI, or SSI after hospital discharge. Predictors of postdischarge SSI were determined by multivariable logistic regression and internally validated by bootstrap resampling. Risk scores were assigned to all significant variables in the model. Summative risk scores were collapsed into quartile-based ordinal categories and defined as low, low/moderate, moderate/high, and high risk. Multivariable logistic regression was used to determine predictors of in-hospital SSI.

Results.—Of the 49,817 patients who underwent major vascular surgery, 4449 (8.9%) were diagnosed with SSI (2.1% in-hospital SSI; 6.9% postdischarge SSI). By multivariable analysis, factors significantly associated with increased odds of postdischarge SSI include female gender, obesity, diabetes, smoking, hypertension, coronary artery disease, critical limb ischemia, chronic obstructive pulmonary disease, dyspnea, neurologic disease, prolonged operative time >4 hours, American Society of Anesthesiology class 4 or 5, lower extremity revascularization or aortoiliac procedure, and groin anastomosis. The model exhibited moderate discrimination (bias-corrected C statistic, 0.691) and excellent internal calibration. The postdischarge SSI rate was 2.1% for low-risk patients, 5.1% for low/moderate-risk patients, 7.8% for moderate/high-risk patients, and 14% for high-risk patients. In a comparative analysis, comorbidities were the primary driver of postdischarge SSI, whereas in-hospital factors (operative time, emergency case status) and complications predicted in-hospital SSI.

Conclusions.—The majority of SSIs after major vascular surgery develop following hospital discharge. We have created a scoring system that can select a cohort of patients at high risk for SSI after discharge. These patients can be targeted for transitional care efforts focused on early detection and treatment with the goal of reducing morbidity and preventing readmission secondary to SSI.

▶ Surgical site infections (SSI) are one of the most common complications after vascular procedures, but SSI after discharge, a period in which the patients are not aggressively monitored, has not been extensively studied. The authors used an analysis of the American College of Surgeons National Surgical Quality Improvement Program (NSQIP) database of all patients undergoing open abdominal aortic aneurysm repair, open aortoiliac repair, and open lower extremity revascularization from 2005 to 2012 to determine rates of postdischarge SSI and risk factors for its development and to create a risk prediction model to better identify at-risk patients. Over this period, 49 817 patients underwent procedures, and 8.9% were diagnosed with SSI (2.1% in hospital and 6.9% after discharge). Risk factors for postdischarge SSI on multivariate analysis were female gender, obesity, diabetes, smoking status, hypertension, coronary artery disease, chronic obstructive pulmonary disease, neurologic disease, American Society of Anesthesiologits class of 4 or 5, groin anastomoses, prolonged operative time, and critical limb ischemia. Those patients at high risk with multiple risk factors had a 14% risk of developing SSI. Interestingly, patient comorbidities were the main risk factors for development of postdischarge SSI, whereas intraoperative factors and hospital complications predicted in-hospital SSI. Although this article has the limitations of any large database study, it suggests that the majority of SSI after vascular procedures occur postdischarge, and a certain subset of patients can be identified and more closely monitored who are at higher risk, thus hopefully preventing readmission and decreasing costs of this complication.

M. R. Smeds, MD, FACS

Lymphedema

A novel method of edema fluid drainage in obstructive lymphedema of limbs by implantation of hydrophobic silicone tubes

Olszewski WL, Zaleska M (Polish Academy of Sciences, Warsaw, Poland; Ministry of Home Affairs, Warsaw, Poland)

J Vasc Surg Venous Lymphat Disord 3:401-408, 2015

Objective.—Lymphedema of limbs is caused by partial or total obstruction of lymphatic collectors as a consequence of skin and deep soft tissue inflammation, trauma of soft tissues and bones, lymphadenectomy, and irradiation in cancer therapy. According to the statistics of the World Health Organization, around 300 million people are affected by pathologic edema of limbs. Effective treatment of such large cohorts has been a challenge for centuries. However, none of the conservative and surgical methods applied so far proved to restore the shape and function of limbs to normal conditions. Actually, physiotherapy is the therapy of choice as a main modality or supplementary to surgical procedures divided into two groups: the bridging drainage and excisional techniques. The microsurgical operations can be performed if some parts of the peripheral collecting lymphatics remain patent and partially drain edematous regions. However, in advanced cases of lymphedema, all main lymphatics are obstructed and tissue fluid accumulates in the interstitial spaces, spontaneously forming "blind channels" or "lakes." The only solution would be to create artificial pathways for edema fluid flow away to the nonobstructed regions where absorption of fluid can take place. The aim of this study was to form artificial pathways for edema fluid flow by subcutaneous implantation of silicone tubes placed along the limb from the lower leg to the lumbar or hypogastric region.

Methods.—In a group of 20 patients with obstructive lymphedema of the lower limbs that developed after lymphadenectomy and irradiation of the pelvis because of uterine cancer with unsuccessful conservative therapy, implantationwas done, followed by external compression as intermittent pneumatic compression and elastic support of tissues. Postoperative circumference measurements, lymphoscintigraphy, and ultrasonography of tissues were carried out during 2 years of follow-up.

Results.—There was a fast decrease of calf circumference since the day of implantation during weeks by a mean 3% with stabilization afterward. Patency of tubes and accumulation of fluid around them were seen on ultrasonography and lymphoscintigraphy in all cases. No tissue cellular reaction to silicone tubes was noted.

Conclusions.—The simplicity of the surgical procedure, decrease of limb edema, and lack of tissue reaction to the implant make the method worth applying in advanced stages of lymphedema with large volumes of accumulated tissue edema fluid.

▶ This article describes a novel approach to treating lymphedema by surgically implanted silicone tubes. The premise is based on the observation that in patients with complete obstruction of all main lymphatics, tissue fluid will accumulate in interstitial spaces forming irregularly shaped lakes that are sometimes interconnected. With three 2-cm-long incisions in the calf, groin, and at the border of the hypogastrium region through, 3 silicone tubes are tunneled in the subcutaneous plane and secured to the fascia thereby facilitating direct drainage from the leg into the hypogastrium region. Sterile medical grade silicone tubes 3 mm outer and 2 mm inner diameter are used and have advantages of hydrophobic properties that prevents ingrowth of connective tissue and facilitates drainage of lymphatic fluid. When combined with further compression-based therapy, there was decrease in calf circumference noted and minimal problems with the silicone tubes. Overall, this is an interesting concept, and based on this preliminary study, it may become a viable treatment option, but only after further properly conducted investigation.

M. Passman, MD

Vascular Pharmacology

Idarucizumab for Dabigatran Reversal

Pollack CV Jr, Reilly PA, Eikelboom J, et al (Pennsylvania Hosp, Philadelphia; Boehringer Ingelheim Pharmaceuticals, Ridgefield, CT; McMaster Univ, Hamilton, Ontario, Canada)

N Engl J Med 373:511-520, 2015

Background.—Specific reversal agents for non–vitamin K antagonist oral anticoagulants are lacking. Idarucizumab, an antibody fragment, was developed to reverse the anticoagulant effects of dabigatran.

Methods.—We undertook this prospective cohort study to determine the safety of 5 g of intravenous idarucizumab and its capacity to reverse the anticoagulant effects of dabigatran in patients who had serious bleeding (group A) or required an urgent procedure (group B). The primary end point was the maximum percentage reversal of the anticoagulant effect of dabigatran within 4 hours after the administration of idarucizumab, on the basis of the determination at a central laboratory of the dilute thrombin time or ecarin clotting time. A key secondary end point was the restoration of hemostasis.

Results.—This interim analysis included 90 patients who received idarucizumab (51 patients in group A and 39 in group B). Among 68 patients with an elevated dilute thrombin time and 81 with an elevated ecarin clotting time at baseline, the median maximum percentage reversal was 100% (95% confidence interval, 100 to 100). Idarucizumab normalized the test results in 88 to 98% of the patients, an effect that was evident within minutes. Concentrations of unbound dabigatran remained below 20 ng per milliliter at 24 hours in 79% of the patients. Among 35 patients in group A who could be assessed, hemostasis, as determined by local investigators, was restored at a median of 11.4 hours. Among 36 patients in group B who underwent a procedure, normal intraoperative hemostasis was reported in 33, and mildly or moderately abnormal hemostasis was reported in 2 patients and 1 patient, respectively. One thrombotic event occurred within 72 hours after idarucizumab administration in a patient in whom anticoagulants had not been reinitiated.

Conclusions.—Idarucizumab completely reversed the anticoagulant effect of dabigatran within minutes. (Funded by Boehringer Ingelheim; RE-VERSE AD ClinicalTrials.gov number, NCT02104947.)

▶ Limitation of bleeding and the absence of reversal agents have dampened enthusiasm for the recent introduction of the new oral anticoagulants thrombin and factor Xa inhibitors. This study shows that idarucizumab completely reversed the anticoagulant effect of dabigatran and offers an important option for patients on dabigatran who need emergent reversal. It should be noted that idarucizumab is specific to dabigatran and should not be used for other agents. This study is also sponsored by Boehringer Ingelheim Pharmaceuticals but is an important steppingstone for reversal options as other pharmaceutical companies develop and evaluate other reversal agents for the other oral anticoagulants. Whether the availability of a reversal agent will eliminate the late-night class-action lawsuit ads, time will tell.

M. Passman, MD

Radiation Safety

Radiation exposure in endovascular repair of abdominal and thoracic aortic aneurysms

Monastiriotis S, Comito M, Labropoulos N (Stony Brook Univ Hosp, NY)
J Vasc Surg 62:753-761, 2015

Background.—Endovascular aortic repair has become increasingly popular the last years for the treatment of abdominal aortic aneurysms (EVAR) and thoracic aortic aneurysms. EVAR is less invasive compared with the classic open approach, related to a decreased immediate postoperative morbidity and mortality. Those beneficial characteristics of EVAR do not come without a cost, since EVAR requires that the patient will be exposed to a significant amount of radiation during preoperative planning, graft placement, and consecutive follow-up. This systematic review examines the periprocedural radiation exposure to patients and staff as well as ways to ameliorate it.

Methods.—A systematic literature search was conducted using the MEDLINE electronic database. All articles reporting radiation exposure to alive humans during EVAR were eligible for review. Only studies publishing numerical data regarding radiation exposure were included in the Results section. Other relevant articles were used for further discussion.

Results.—Twenty-four studies, both prospective and retrospective in nature, were included. These studies revealed that the radiation exposure depends on the specific type of procedure, with more complex procedures carrying greater radiation burden. Variations in the positioning and operating of the fluoroscopic unit may significantly alter radiation dose to both patients and staff. There was an apparent lack of education among vascular specialists and trainees in terms of radiation safety awareness. At follow-up, a significant number of patients needed additional procedures, and all required radiographic imaging, further increasing the radiation exposure to alarming levels.

Conclusions.—Every effort should be made to decrease radiation exposure related to endovascular aortic procedures. Attempts must be directed towards maximizing the operator's awareness, welcoming new imaging technology emitting less radiation, and shifting to follow-up strategies that require minimal or no radiation.

▶ In the current review, the authors collate 24 reports highlighting patient and surgeon radiation exposures during endovascular aneurysm repair (EVAR) procedures. Much effort has been focused on reducing peri-procedural EVAR radiation doses to patients; however, 96% of lifetime radiation exposure is attributed to CT utilization in both the preoperative and postoperative periods. Duplex ultrasound surveillance has been increasingly used to survey EVAR patients to offset lifetime radiation exposure. The reintervention rate for EVAR further increases radiation exposure, which typically requires not only an additional procedure but also more frequent CT examination. As long as the reintervention rate is 10% to 20% for EVAR, lifetime radiation dose will be a concern; endograft technology should be designed to mitigate intermediate and late failures.

Anesthesia providers and operators are subjected to higher radiation exposures compared with circulators and scrub technicians. When comparing over-the-lead apron to under apron radiation monitoring, there is a 95% reduction in exposure, highlighting the effectiveness of barrier techniques. Surgeons' hands receive the highest exposure, followed by head and cornea. Advanced EVAR procedures (fenestrated repairs or complex anatomy) can increase the radiation exposure 5- to 7-fold compared with routine EVAR. It is important to recognize that altering the angle of image acquisition to any position other than direct anterior-posterior increases the thickness of tissue and directly increases the radiation necessary to penetrate the tissue. For these reasons, surgeons should be prudent while using obliquity during procedures. In addition, surgeons should use advanced software programs that allow prepositioned onlay images for advanced procedures; advanced imaging techniques have shown to reduce the overall radiation necessary to complete complex procedures.[1]

Z. M. Arthurs, MD, FACS

Reference

1. Mohapatra A, Greenberg RK, Mastracci TM, Eagleton MJ, Thornsberry B. Radiation exposure to operating room personnel and patients during endovascular procedures. *J Vasc Surg*. 2013;58:702-709.

Radiation exposure to eye lens and operator hands during endovascular procedures in hybrid operating rooms

Attigah N, Oikonomou K, Hinz U, et al (Ruprecht-Karls Univ, Heidelberg, Germany; Paracelsus Med Univ, Nuremberg, Austria)

J Vasc Surg 63:198-203, 2016

Objective.—The purpose of this study was to evaluate the radiation exposure of vascular surgeons' eye lens and fingers during complex endovascular procedures in modern hybrid operating rooms.

Methods.—Prospective, nonrandomized multicenter study design. One hundred seventy-one consecutive patients (138 male; median age, 72.5 years [interquartile range, 65-77 years]) underwent an endovascular procedure in a hybrid operating room between March 2012 and July 2013 in two vascular centers. The dose-area product (DAP), fluoroscopy time, operating time, and amount of contrast dye were registered prospectively. For radiation dose recordings, single-use dosimeters were attached at eye level and to the ring finger of the hand next to the radiation field of the operator for each endovascular procedure. Dose recordings were evaluated by an independent institution. Before the study, precursory investigations were obtained to simulate the radiation dose to eye lens and fingers with an Alderson phantome (RSD, Long Beach, Calif).

Results.—Interventions were classified into six treatment categories: endovascular repair of infrarenal abdominal aneurysm ($n = 65$), thoracic endovascular aortic repair ($n = 32$), branched endovascular aortic repair for thoracoabdominal aneurysms ($n = 17$), fenestrated endovascular aortic repair for complex abdominal aortic aneurysm, ($n = 25$), iliac branched device ($n = 8$), and peripheral interventions ($n = 24$). There was a significant correlation in DAP between both lens ($P < .01$; $r = 0.55$) and finger ($P < .01$; $r = 0.56$) doses. The estimated fluoroscopy time to reach a radiation threshold of 20 mSv/y was 1404.10 minutes (90% confidence limit, 1160, 1650 minutes). According to correlation of the lens dose with the DAP an estimated cumulative DAP of 932,000 mGy/m^2 (90% confidence limit, 822,000, 1,039,000) would be critical for a threshold of 20 mSv/y for the eyes.

Conclusions.—Radiation protection is a serious issue for vascular surgeons because most complex endovascular procedures are delivering measurable radiation to the eyes. With the correlation of the DAP obtained in standard endovascular procedures a critical threshold of 20 mSv/y to the eyes can be predicted and thus an estimate of a potential harmful exposure to the eyes can be obtained.

▶ The current article adds to an increasing number of reports evaluating surgeon radiation exposure. The vascular surgery practice has dramatically changed in the past 10 years. Seventy to eighty percent of vascular procedures now rely on radiation. In addition, the annual number of cases has increased to 300 to 500 per surgeon. The current report is unique in that it specifically addresses exposure to the operator's hands and lens using a direct measurement as opposed to estimations. It is important to note that lead shields were used for this study.

The authors examined multiple endovascular procedures. Peripheral interventions demonstrated the lowest radiation dose, whereas branched and fenestrated endografts demonstrated the highest radiation doses to surgeons. The numbers are astonishing. The maximum recommended radiation does to the lens is 20 mSV/year. In the current study, this maximum dose equates to 22 fenestrated endograft cases, 74 endovascular aneurysm repairs, or 116 lower extremity interventions. It seems that most surgeons likely meet the maximum allowable dose to the lens. Radiation safety is a constant process within each institution; however, it is critical that surgeons drive this process and ensure our own safety as well as our operative team.

Z. M. Arthurs, MD, FACS

Article Index

Chapter 1: Basic Consideration

Chapter 2: Epidemiology

Chapter 3: Vascular Imaging

Chapter 4: Perioperative Considerations

Chapter 5: Abdominal Aorta

Chapter 6: Thoracic Aorta

Chapter 7: Leg Ischemia

Chapter 8: Nonatherosclerotic

Chapter 9: Upper Extremity

Chapter 10: Carotid and Cerebrovascular

Chapter 11: Vascular Trauma

Chapter 12: Venous Thrombosis

Chapter 13: Chronic Venous

Chapter 14: Miscellaneous

Author Index

A

B

C

D

E

F

G

H

J

K

L

M

FSC
www.fsc.org
MIX
Papier | Fördert gute Waldnutzung
FSC® C083411

Kolibri 360 GmbH
Ferdinand-Jühlke-Straße 7
99095 Erfurt, Deutschland
produktsicherheit@kolibri360.de